Study Guide for

Brunner & Suddarth's Textbook of Medical-Surgical Nursing

13th EDITION

Wolters Kluwer | Lippincott Williams & Wilkins
Health

Philadelphia · Baltimore · New York · London
Buenos Aires · Hong Kong · Sydney · Tokyo

Publisher: Lisa McAllister
Executive Editor: Sherry Dickinson
Supervisor, Product Development: Betsy Gentzler
Product Development Editor: Roxanne Halpine Ward
Editorial Assistant: Dan Reilly
Design Coordinator: Joan Wendt
Art Director, Illustration: Jennifer Clements
Production Project Manager: Priscilla Crater
Manufacturing Coordinator: Karin Duffield
Prepress Vendor: Aptara, Inc.

13th edition

9 8 7 6 5 4 3 2 1

Printed in China

ISBN: 978-1-4511-4668-4

Care has been taken to confirm the accuracy of the information presented and to describe generally accepted practices. However, the author(s), editors, and publisher are not responsible for errors or omissions or for any consequences from application of the information in this book and make no warranty, expressed or implied, with respect to the currency, completeness, or accuracy of the contents of the publication. Application of this information in a particular situation remains the professional responsibility of the practitioner; the clinical treatments described and recommended may not be considered absolute and universal recommendations.

The author(s), editors, and publisher have exerted every effort to ensure that drug selection and dosage set forth in this text are in accordance with the current recommendations and practice at the time of publication. However, in view of ongoing research, changes in government regulations, and the constant flow of information relating to drug therapy and drug reactions, the reader is urged to check the package insert for each drug for any change in indications and dosage and for added warnings and precautions. This is particularly important when the recommended agent is a new or infrequently employed drug.

Some drugs and medical devices presented in this publication have Food and Drug Administration (FDA) clearance for limited use in restricted research settings. It is the responsibility of the health care provider to ascertain the FDA status of each drug or device planned for use in his or her clinical practice.

LWW.com

Contributor

Leigh W. Moore, MSN, RN, CNOR, CNE
Associate Professor of Nursing
ADN Program
Southside Virginia Community College
Alberta, Virginia

Reviewers

Carol Anneser, MSN, RN, BC, CNE
Assistant Professor
Department of Nursing
Mercy College of Ohio
Toledo, Ohio

Mary Jo Ardis, MSN
Department Chair, Nursing
Central Carolina Technical College
Sumter, South Carolina

Jo Ann Baker, MSN, FNP-C
Department Chair, Nursing
Delaware Technical Community College
Dover, Delaware

Tena Barnwell, MSN/ED
Assistant Professor
Department of Nursing
North Carolina Central University
Durham, North Carolina

Antoinette Barton-Gooden, MScN, BSc, RN
Lecturer
School of Nursing
The University of the West Indies School
   of Nursing
Mona, Jamaica

Marilyn Boatman, MSN/Ed
Assistant Professor
Department of Nursing
MacMurray College
Jacksonville, Illinois

Arica Branford-Dixon, MSN, JD, RN
Instructor
Department of Nursing
Bluegrass Community and Technical College
Lexington, Kentucky

Patricia Brown-O'Hara, PhD
Assistant Professor
Department of Nursing
Gwynedd-Mercy College
Gwynedd Valley, Pennsylvania

Barbara Brunow, MSN, MEd
Assistant Director/Faculty Member
School of Nursing
Firelands Regional Medical Center
Sandusky, Ohio

Kristine Carey, MSN
Faculty
Department of Nursing
Normandale Community College
Bloomington, Minnesota

Cheryl Cassis, MSN
Professor of Nursing
Belmont College
Clairsville, Ohio

Pamella Chavis, MSN ED(c)
Clinical Assistant Professor
Department of Nursing
North Carolina Agricultural & Technical State
   University
Greensboro North Carolina

Lynette Coffey, MSN
RN,MSN Nurse Educator
Ivy Tech community College
Terre Haute, Indiana

Linda Coleman, MSN
Instructor
School of Nursing
Ivy Tech-Gary campus
Gary, Indiana

Lynette Debellis, MA, RN
Assistant Professor
Department of Nursing
Westchester Community College
Valhalla, New York

Nancy DeMetro, MSN
Assistant Clinical Professor
Department of Nursing
Walsh University
Canton, Ohio

Janice Di Falco, MSN,CNS,CMSRN, FAACVPR
Professor
Department of Nursing
San Jacinto College, Central Campus
Pasadena, Texas

Carrin Dvorak, MSN
Assistant Professor
Department of Nursing
Cuyahoga Community College
Cleveland, Ohio

Donna Gause, MSN, BSN, ADN
Nursing Lecturer, RN, RN-BC
Lander University
Greenwood, South Carolina

Ruth Gladen, MSN/Ed
Associate Professor, RN Program Director
North Dakota State College of Science
Wahpeton, North Dakota

Denise Catherine Hall, MSN
Assistant Professor
Department of Nursing
Albany State University
Albany, Georgia

Darlene Hanson, MS, RN, PhD(c)
Clinical Associate Professor
College of Nursing
University of North Dakota
Grand Forks, North Dakota

Lori Hendrickx, MSN, EdD
Professor
Department of Nursing
South Dakota State University
Brookings, South Dakota

Nancy Hinzman, MSN, DNP
Associate Professor
Department of Nursing
College of Mount St. Joseph
Cincinnati, Ohio

Faith Johnson, MA
Faculty
Department of Nursing
Ridgewater College
Willmar, Minnesota

Judith Johnson, MSN, RN
Associate Professor
Sentara College of Health Sciences
Chesapeake, Virginia

Christine Krause, MSN
First and Second Level Chair
Department of Nursing
Aria Health School of Nursing
Trevose, Pennsylvania

Mary McKay, DNP, ARNP
Assistant Professor
Department of Nursing
University of Miami School of Nursing
   and Health Studies
Coral Gables, Florida

Kassie McKenny, MSN
Associate Professor
Department of Undergraduate Nursing
Clarkson College
Omaha, Nebraska

Janis McMillan, MSN, RN
Nursing Faculty
Coconino Community College
Flagstaff, AZ

Anita Mobrak, MSN
Curriculum Chair and Associate Professor
Department of Nursing
Baptist College of Health Sciences
Memphis, Tennessee

Nancy Noble, MSN, BSN
Associate Professor
Department of Nursing
Marian University
Fond du Lac, Wisconsin

Velma Norwood, MSN
Instructor
Department of Nursing
Delaware Technical Community College
Georgetown, Delaware

Debora Nutt, DNP, MN, BSN, RN
Assistant Professor
College of Nursing
Georgia Regents University
Athens Georgia

Regina O'Drobinak, MSN, APRN, ANP
Chair, Department of Nursing
Ivy Tech Community College
Gary, Indiana

Catherine Page, MSN
Professor, Gerontology Content Expert
Department of Health Science and Nursing
Rio Hondo College
Whittier, California

Valerie Pauoli, MSN, BSN
Nursing Faculty Instructor
Mercy College of Ohio
Toledo, Ohio

Norma Perez, MSN/Ed, RN
Assistant Professor
Department of Nursing
Ivy Tech Community College
Valparaiso, Indiana

Patricia Pfeiffer, MSN, MSA
Division Chair, Allied Health & Public Services
Wayne Community College
Goldsboro, North Carolina

Linda Phelps, DNP
Instructor
Department of Nursing
Ivy Tech Community College
Indianapolis, Indiana

Barbara Pinchera, DNP
Associate Professor
Department of Nursing
Curry College
Milton, Massachusetts

Cynthia Pitter, MScN
Lecturer
School of Nursing
The University of the West Indies
Mona, Jamaica

Loretta Quigley, MS, RN
Academic Dean
Saint Joseph's College of Nursing
Syracuse, New York

Barbara Rauscher, MSN, RN
Professor of Nursing
Lenoir-Rhyne University
Hickory, North Carolina

Pat Recek, MSN
Assistant Dean Health Sciences
Department of Vocational Nursing
Austin Community College
Austin, Texas

Susan Rouse, PhD
Associate Professor
Department of Nursing
Indiana University Northwest
Gary, Indiana

Shamel Sands, MSN/Ed
Lecturer
College of Nursing
The College of The Bahamas
New Providence, Bahamas

Jeanne Saunders, EdD
Professor
Department of Nursing
Daytona State College
Daytona Beach, Florida

Brian Schroeder, MSN, RN
Professor of Nursing
Santa Ana College
Santa, Ana, California

Susan Seiboldt, MS, Nursing Administration
Assistant Professor
College of Nursing
Carl Sandburg College
Victoria, Illinois

Diana Stanfort, MSN
Clinical Assistant Professor
Department of Nursing
Indiana University
Richmond, Indiana

Jennifer Sugg, MSN
Instructor
Department of Nursing
Wayne Community College
Goldsboro, North Carolina

Patricia Taylor, MSN Ed, RN
Instructor
Kapiolani Community College
Department of Nursing
Honolulu, Hawaii

Valerie Taylor-Haslip, PhD
Associate Professor
Department of Health Sciences/Nursing
LaGuardia Community College
Island City, New York

Winni Tucker, MSN, CNE
Professor
School of Nursing
Daytona State College
DeLand, Florida

Daryle Wane, PhD ARNP, FNP-BC
Professor
Department of Nursing-Health Occupations
Pasco-Hernando College
New Port Richey, Florida

Terri Wenzig, MSN/ED
Faculty
Department of Nursing
Chemeketa Community College
Salem, OR

Amy Williams, MSN, RN
Faculty
Department of Nursing
Bossier Parish Community College
Bossier City, Louisiana

Cheryl Winter, MSN, FNP
Associate Professor of Nursing,
Bluefield State College
Beaver, West Virginia

Victoria Young, MSN, RN
Assistant Professor
Department of Nursing
Louisiana State University
Alexandria, Louisiana

Katrice Ziefle, MA, Nursing Education
Nursing Faculty
Minneapolis Community and Technical College
Minneapolis, Minnesota

Preface

This Study Guide was developed by Leigh W. Moore, MSN, RN, CNOR, CNE, to accompany *Brunner and Suddarth's Textbook of Medical-Surgical Nursing, Thirteenth Edition*, by Janice L. Hinkle and Kerry H. Cheever. The Study Guide is designed to help you review and apply important concepts from the textbook to prepare for exams as well as for your nursing career. The following types of exercises are provided in each chapter of the Study Guide.

ASSESSING YOUR UNDERSTANDING

The first section of each Study Guide chapter reviews the basic information of the textbook chapter and helps you to remember key concepts, vocabulary, and principles.

- **Fill in the Blanks:** Fill-in-the-blank exercises test important chapter information, encouraging you to recall key points.
- **Short Answers:** Short-answer questions cover facts, concepts, procedures, and principles of the chapter. These questions ask you to recall information as well as demonstrate your comprehension of the information.
- **Matching:** Matching questions test your knowledge of the definition of key terms.
- **Labeling:** Labeling exercises are used where you need to remember certain visual representations of the concepts presented in the textbook.
- **Sequencing:** Sequencing exercises ask you to remember particular sequences or orders, such as in normal or abnormal physiologic processes.

APPLYING YOUR KNOWLEDGE

The second section of each Study Guide chapter consists of case study–based exercises that ask you to begin to apply the knowledge you gained from the textbook chapter and reinforced in the first section of the Study Guide chapter. A case study scenario based on the chapter's content is presented, followed by related short-answer questions. The questions could cover topics such as lab values, next steps in nursing care, and anticipated diagnoses.

PRACTICING FOR NCLEX

The third and final section of the Study Guide helps you practice NCLEX-style questions while further applying the knowledge you have gained and reinforced through reading the textbook chapter and completing the first two sections of the Study Guide chapter. Including both multiple-choice and alternate-item formats, the questions are scenario based, asking you to reflect, consider, and apply what you know and to choose the best answer out of those offered.

ANSWERS

The answers for all of the exercises and questions in the Study Guide are provided at the back of the book, so you can assess your own learning as you complete each chapter.

We hope that you will find this Study Guide to be helpful and enjoyable, and we wish you every success in your studies and future profession.

The Publisher

Contents

UNIT **1**

BASIC CONCEPTS IN NURSING   1

CHAPTER **1**

Health Care Delivery and Evidence-Based
Nursing Practice   3

CHAPTER **2**

Community-Based Nursing Practice   9

CHAPTER **3**

Critical Thinking, Ethical Decision Making,
and the Nursing Process   13

CHAPTER **4**

Health Education and Health Promotion   19

CHAPTER **5**

Adult Health and Nutritional
Assessment   23

UNIT **2**

**BIOPHYSICAL AND PSYCHOSOCIAL
CONCEPTS IN NURSING PRACTICE   29**

CHAPTER **6**

Individual and Family Homeostasis, Stress,
and Adaptation   31

CHAPTER **7**

Overview of Transcultural Nursing   37

CHAPTER **8**

Overview of Genetics and Genomics in
Nursing   41

CHAPTER **9**

Chronic Illness and Disability   45

CHAPTER **10**

Principles and Practices of
Rehabilitation   49

CHAPTER **11**

Health Care of the Older Adult   53

UNIT **3**

**CONCEPTS AND CHALLENGES IN PATIENT
MANAGEMENT   57**

CHAPTER **12**

Pain Management   59

CHAPTER **13**

Fluid and Electrolytes: Balance and
Disturbance   65

CHAPTER **14**

Shock and Multiple Organ Dysfunction
Syndrome   73

CHAPTER **15**

Oncology: Nursing Management in
Cancer Care   79

CHAPTER **16**

End-of-Life Care   85

UNIT 4

PERIOPERATIVE CONCEPTS AND NURSING MANAGEMENT   89

CHAPTER 17

Preoperative Nursing Management   91

CHAPTER 18

Intraoperative Nursing Management   97

CHAPTER 19

Postoperative Nursing Management   103

UNIT 5

GAS EXCHANGE AND RESPIRATORY FUNCTION   109

CHAPTER 20

Assessment of Respiratory Function   111

CHAPTER 21

Respiratory Care Modalities   117

CHAPTER 22

Management of Patients With Upper Respiratory Tract Disorders   123

CHAPTER 23

Management of Patients With Chest and Lower Respiratory Tract Disorders   129

CHAPTER 24

Management of Patients With Chronic Pulmonary Disease   135

UNIT 6

CARDIOVASCULAR AND CIRCULATORY FUNCTION   139

CHAPTER 25

Assessment of Cardiovascular Function   141

CHAPTER 26

Management of Patients With Dysrhythmias and Conduction Problems   147

CHAPTER 27

Management of Patients With Coronary Vascular Disorders   155

CHAPTER 28

Management of Patients With Structural, Infectious, and Inflammatory Cardiac Disorders   161

CHAPTER 29

Management of Patients With Complications From Heart Disease   165

CHAPTER 30

Assessment and Management of Patients With Vascular Disorders and Problems of Peripheral Circulation   169

CHAPTER 31

Assessment and Management of Patients With Hypertension   173

UNIT 7

HEMATOLOGIC FUNCTION   177

CHAPTER 32

Assessment of Hematologic Function and Treatment Modalities   179

CHAPTER 33

Management of Patients With Nonmalignant Hematologic Disorders   185

CHAPTER 34

Management of Patients With Hematologic Neoplasms   191

UNIT 8

IMMUNOLOGIC FUNCTION   197

CHAPTER 35

Assessment of Immune Function   199

CHAPTER 36

Management of Patients With
Immunodeficiency Disorders   205

CHAPTER 37

Management of Patients With HIV Infection
and AIDS   209

CHAPTER 38

Assessment and Management of Patients
With Allergic Disorders   215

CHAPTER 39

Assessment and Management of Patients
With Rheumatic Disorders   219

UNIT 9

MUSCULOSKELETAL FUNCTION   225

CHAPTER 40

Assessment of Musculoskeletal
Function   227

CHAPTER 41

Musculoskeletal Care Modalities   231

CHAPTER 42

Management of Patients With
Musculoskeletal Disorders   237

CHAPTER 43

Management of Patients With
Musculoskeletal Trauma   243

UNIT 10

DIGESTIVE AND GASTROINTESTINAL
FUNCTION   249

CHAPTER 44

Assessment of Digestive and
Gastrointestinal Function   251

CHAPTER 45

Digestive and Gastrointestinal Treatment
Modalities   255

CHAPTER 46

Management of Patients With Oral
and Esophageal Disorders   259

CHAPTER 47

Management of Patients With Gastric
and Duodenal Disorders   265

CHAPTER 48

Management of Patients With Intestinal
and Rectal Disorders   269

UNIT 11

METABOLIC AND ENDOCRINE
FUNCTION   275

CHAPTER 49

Assessment and Management of Patients
With Hepatic Disorders   277

CHAPTER 50

Assessment and Management of Patients
With Biliary Disorders   283

CHAPTER 51

Assessment and Management of Patients
With Diabetes   287

CHAPTER 52

Assessment and Management of Patients
With Endocrine Disorders   293

UNIT 12

KIDNEY AND URINARY FUNCTION   299

CHAPTER 53

Assessment of Kidney and Urinary
Function   301

CHAPTER 54

Management of Patients With Kidney
Disorders   305

CHAPTER 55

Management of Patients With Urinary
Disorders   309

UNIT 13

REPRODUCTIVE FUNCTION   313

CHAPTER 56

Assessment and Management of Female Physiologic Processes   315

CHAPTER 57

Management of Patients With Female Reproductive Disorders   319

CHAPTER 58

Assessment and Management of Patients With Breast Disorders   325

CHAPTER 59

Assessment and Management of Problems Related to Male Reproductive Processes   329

UNIT 14

INTEGUMENTARY FUNCTION   333

CHAPTER 60

Assessment of Integumentary Function   335

CHAPTER 61

Management of Patients With Dermatologic Problems   339

CHAPTER 62

Management of Patients With Burn Injury   345

UNIT 15

SENSORY FUNCTION   351

CHAPTER 63

Assessment and Management of Patients With Eye and Vision Disorders   353

CHAPTER 64

Assessment and Management of Patients With Hearing and Balance Disorders   357

UNIT 16

NEUROLOGIC FUNCTION   363

CHAPTER 65

Assessment of Neurologic Function   365

CHAPTER 66

Management of Patients With Neurologic Dysfunction   369

CHAPTER 67

Management of Patients With Cerebrovascular Disorders   373

CHAPTER 68

Management of Patients With Neurologic Trauma   377

CHAPTER 69

Management of Patients With Neurologic Infections, Autoimmune Disorders, and Neuropathies   381

CHAPTER 70

Management of Patients With Oncologic or Degenerative Neurologic Disorders   387

UNIT 17

ACUTE COMMUNITY-BASED CHALLENGES   393

CHAPTER 71

Management of Patients With Infectious Diseases   395

CHAPTER 72

Emergency Nursing   399

CHAPTER 73

Terrorism, Mass Casualty, and Disaster Nursing   405

Answers   409

Basic Concepts in Nursing

Health Care Delivery and Evidence-Based Nursing Practice

1. Define nursing, health, and wellness.
2. Describe factors causing significant changes in the health care delivery system and their impact on health care and the nursing profession.
3. Describe care planning tools and nursing roles that are useful in coordinating patient care.
4. Discuss behavioral competencies and characteristics of professional nursing practice.
5. Compare and contrast the advanced practice registered nurse roles most relevant to medical–surgical nursing practice.
6. Describe models that foster interdisciplinary collaborative practice and promote safety and quality outcomes in the practice of health care.

SECTION I: ASSESSING YOUR UNDERSTANDING

Activity A *Fill in the blanks.*

1. With the shift from acute to chronic illnesses, practitioners today are facing four major health care concerns: _____, _____, _____, and _____.

2. Four comorbidities associated with the major health concern of obesity are: _____, _____, _____, and _____.

3. In addition to clinical pathways, there are four other evidence-based practice (EBP) tools a nurse can use. They are: _____, _____, _____, and _____.

4. Four categories of advanced practice nurses (APNs) are: _____, _____, _____, and _____.

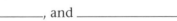 **Activity B** *Briefly answer the following.*

1. List four phenomena frequently identified by the American Nurses Association (ANA) in 2003 as the focus of nursing care and research. An example is provided.

    Pain and discomfort (Example)

    _____, _____, _____, and _____.

2. List six significant changes (socioeconomic, political, scientific, and technological) that have evolved over the last hundred years that have influenced where nurses practice.

    _____, _____, _____, _____, _____, _____.

3. Choose four health and illness problems and write a human response to each that would require nursing intervention. An example is provided.

Health and Illness Problems	Human Response Requiring Nursing Intervention
Fractured right arm (Example)	Self-care limitations (Example)
1. _____	_____
2. _____	_____
3. _____	_____
4. _____	_____

4. According to Hood and Leddy (2010), wellness involves proactively working toward physical, psychological, and spiritual well-being. Four major concepts supporting wellness are:

_____, _____,

_____, and _____.

5. List Maslow's hierarchy of needs, and give an example for each need. The first need is provided as an example.

Need	Example
Physiologic (Example)	Food and water (Example)
_____	_____
_____	_____
_____	_____
_____	_____
_____	_____
_____	_____

6. Health promotion efforts today target negative lifestyle behaviors. List six examples.

_____ _____

_____ _____

_____ _____

7. How can the nurse promote effective nurse–patient relationships and positive outcomes regarding culture?

_____

_____

8. Define the term *evidence-based practice* (EBP).

_____

_____

9. Define the term *clinical pathway* as it relates to the concept of managed care.

_____

_____

10. Explain when care mapping may be more beneficial than clinical pathways for managing care.

_____

_____

11. List five common features of managed care:

_____

_____

12. List the purpose and goals of case management.

_____

_____

13. What is the primary difference between community-based nursing and community-oriented/public health nursing?

_____

_____

Activity C *Complete the following flow charts.*

1. Continuous quality improvement (CQI) mandates the standardization of processes that are implemented and improved on a continuous basis. Complete the blank lines on the flow chart for the process of radial pulse assessment.

Radial Pulse Assessment

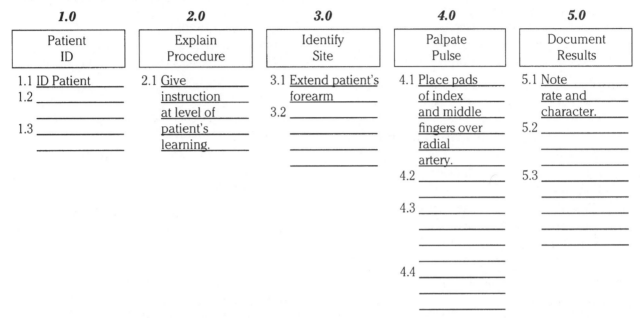

1.0	2.0	3.0	4.0	5.0
Patient ID	Explain Procedure	Identify Site	Palpate Pulse	Document Results

1.1 <u>ID Patient</u>
1.2 _____
_____
1.3 _____
_____

2.1 <u>Give</u>
<u>instruction</u>
<u>at level of</u>
<u>patient's</u>
<u>learning.</u>

3.1 <u>Extend patient's</u>
<u>forearm</u>
3.2 _____
_____
_____
_____

4.1 <u>Place pads</u>
<u>of index</u>
<u>and middle</u>
<u>fingers over</u>
<u>radial</u>
<u>artery.</u>
4.2 _____
_____
4.3 _____
_____
_____
_____
4.4 _____
_____
_____

5.1 <u>Note</u>
<u>rate and</u>
<u>character.</u>
5.2 _____
_____
_____
5.3 _____
_____
_____
_____

2. The Joint Commission mandated in 1992 that health care organizations move toward implementation of CQI. A cause-and-effect diagram can illustrate potential causes of a process so that the cause can be examined and corrected and patient care improved. Complete the following diagram.

CQI Cause and Effect Diagram: Delayed Medication

Possible Causes

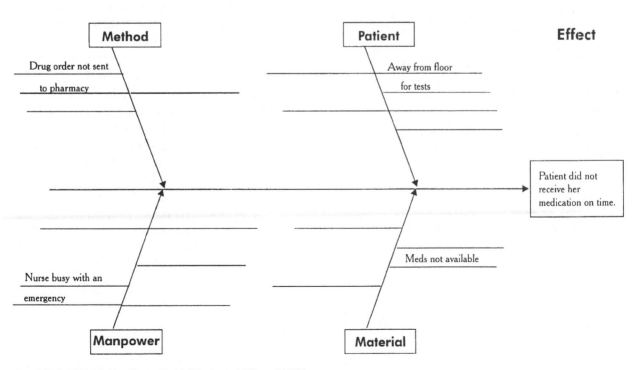

Study Guide for Brunner & Suddarth's Textbook of Medical-Surgical Nursing, 13th Edition.

SECTION II: APPLYING YOUR KNOWLEDGE

Activity D *Consider the scenario and answer the questions.*

The nurse working in the Intensive Care Unit (ICU) at a local community hospital determines a need to improve the care of patients with ventilator-associated pneumonia (VAP).

1. What steps can the nurse take to present the need for a change in care practice to her peers?

   a. Determine best practices from valid research studies.

   b. Inform the nurses that they need to further their education.

   c. Tell the nurse manager that she needs to implement the changes.

   d. Have the physician write orders for all patients at risk for VAP.

2. How can the ICU improve the care of the patients with VAP?

   a. Have respiratory therapy take care of all of the ventilator patients.

   b. Incorporate evidence-based findings into patient care.

   c. Have one of the nurses specialize in the care of patients that are on ventilators.

   d. Adopt another facility's standards of care.

3. The nurse is aware that the Institute for Healthcare Improvement (IHI) Ventilator Bundle has determined interventions that can improve patient outcomes. What interventions can the unit adopt to improve this care for the patients on ventilators? (Select all that apply.)

   a. Provide oral care with chlorhexidine.

   b. Place the patient in the prone position.

   c. Keep the head of the bed elevated at all times.

   d. Keep the patient sedated.

   e. Turn the patient every 4 hours.

SECTION III: PRACTICING FOR NCLEX

Activity E *Answer the following questions.*

1. The registered nurse has a responsibility to practice nursing according to the Social Policy Statement (2003) of the American Nurses Association (ANA). What definition by the ANA best describes the role of registered nurses?

   a. To diagnose and treat medical conditions

   b. To prescribe medications in order to treat a variety of medical conditions

   c. To prevent illness and maintain health

   d. To diagnose and treat the human responses to health and illness

2. What underlying focus in any definition of nursing is the registered nurse's responsibility in practice?

   a. Appraise and enhance an individual's health-seeking perspective.

   b. Coordinate a patient's total health management with all disciplines.

   c. Diagnose acute pathology.

   d. Treat acute clinical reactions to chronic illness.

3. A patient who adheres to the dietary laws of Judaism is in traction and confined to bed. The patient needs assistance with the evening meal of chicken, rice, beans, a roll, and a carton of milk. Which nursing approach is most representative of promoting wellness?

   a. Remove items from the overbed table to make room for the dinner tray.

   b. Push the overbed table toward the bed so that it will be within the patient's reach when the dinner tray arrives.

   c. Ask a family member to assist the patient with the tray and the overbed table, then straighten the area in an attempt to provide a pleasant atmosphere for eating.

   d. Ask whether the patient would like to make any substitutions in the foods and fluids received.

4. Using the concept of the wellness–illness continuum, what would the nurse include in the development of a nursing care plan for a chronically ill patient?

a. Educate the patient about every possible complication associated with the specific illness.

b. Encourage positive health characteristics within the limits of the specific illness.

c. Limit all activities because of the progressive deterioration associated with all chronic illnesses.

d. Recommend activity beyond the scope of tolerance to prevent early deterioration.

5. How should the registered nurse be responsive to the changing health care needs of society?

a. Focus care on the traditional disease-oriented approach to patient care, because hospitalized patients today are more acutely ill than they were 10 years ago.

b. Learn how to delegate discharge planning to ancillary personnel so that registered nurses can spend their time managing the "high-tech" equipment needed for patient care.

c. Place increasing emphasis on wellness, health promotion, and self-care, because the majority of Americans today suffer from chronic debilitative illness.

d. Stress the curative aspects of illness, especially the acute, infectious disease processes.

6. Continuous quality improvement (CQI) was mandated in health care organizations in 1992. What does the nurse understand is the primary purpose of CQI?

a. Identify measures to ensure minimal expectations of care.

b. Assess the impact of financial decisions on patient care delivery.

c. Examine processes that affect patient care and the need for improvement.

d. Review medication errors for individual patients.

7. Which statement by the nurse shows an understanding of the focus of the quality assurance programs developed in the 1980s?

a. "The quality assurance programs focus on individual incidents or errors and minimal expectations."

b. "The quality assurance programs focus on decreasing the cost of health care for the consumer."

c. "The quality assurance programs focus on processes used to provide care and improving those processes."

d. "The quality assurance programs focus on coordinating care for patients."

8. What is the primary focus of the nurse advocacy role in managing a clinical pathway?

a. Continuity of care

b. Cost-containment practices

c. Effective utilization of services

d. A patient's progress toward desired outcomes

9. The nurse is practicing in a community-based setting. What outcomes may be achieved by the nurse's community interventions? (Select all that apply.)

a. Promote wellness.

b. Reduce the spread of disease.

c. Improve the health status of the community.

d. Prevent hospital-acquired illness.

e. Promote the financial health of the community.

10. The nurse is providing care for a patient in the hospital scheduled for discharge in the morning. The patient will require further services after discharge since recovery is not complete. What can the nurse do to ensure quality care delivery for this patient?

a. Inform the family members that someone will have to stay with the patient after discharge.

b. Inform the physician that the patient is not ready to go home yet.

c. Contact the case manager for coordination of care prior to discharge of the patient.

d. Call social services to check on the patient after discharge.

CHAPTER 2

Community-Based Nursing Practice

Learning Objectives

1. Discuss the multiple roles and various settings in which nurses practice in the community.
2. Compare the differences and similarities between community- and hospital-based nursing.
3. Describe the discharge planning process.
4. Explain methods for identifying community resources and making referrals.
5. Discuss how to prepare for a home health care visit and how to conduct the visit.

SECTION I: ASSESSING YOUR UNDERSTANDING

Activity A *Fill in the blanks.*

1. _____ is a philosophy of care in which the care is provided as patients and their families move among various service providers outside of hospitals.

2. Community-based care is generally focused on _____ or their _____.

3. _____, _____, and _____ are three chronic conditions increasing in prevalence and causing an increased need for community health services.

4. The four primary concepts supporting community-based nursing care are _____, _____, _____, and _____.

5. Hospice nursing has become a specialty area of nursing practice in which nurses provide _____ care in patients' homes and within hospice centers.

6. When a nurse makes a home health visit, the agency should know the nurse's _____ and the _____ the visits.

7. Federal legislation, especially the _____, has been enacted to ensure safe and healthy work environments.

Activity B *Briefly answer the following.*

1. List four factors that have affected the shift of health care delivery from inpatient to outpatient settings:

   _____, _____, _____, and _____.

2. List specific skills a nurse will need to function in community-based care.

   _____

   _____

3. Community-based nursing practice focuses on three primary goals: _____, _____, and _____.

4. List several examples of "skilled" nursing services provided by home care.

   _____

   _____

5. The first step in preparing for a home visit is for the nurse to:

_____

_____

6. Explain the purpose of the initial home visit.

_____

_____

7. List the range of nursing responsibilities within ambulatory health care settings.

_____

_____

8. The homeless have high rates of health care problems. List six health care problems frequently experienced by homeless people.

_____   _____

_____   _____

_____   _____

9. Differentiate between primary, secondary, and tertiary levels of preventive care, and provide a clinical case example for each level.

_____

_____

_____

10. What is a major financial incentive for discharging a patient from the acute care facility prior to full recovery?

_____

_____

11. What is "tele-health," and what are its implications for nursing care?

_____

_____

SECTION II: APPLYING YOUR KNOWLEDGE

Activity C *Consider the scenario and assess the patient's need for a home visit.*

CASE STUDY: Assessing the Need for a Home Visit

Mrs. Flynn is an 85-year-old woman who suffered a stroke on December 28. She was admitted to the emergency department and suffered another stroke on December 30. The left occipital area and the cerebellum were affected, resulting in the loss of 50% of vision (right half of each eye) and loss of balance. After 2 weeks in the hospital and 10 days in a rehabilitation treatment center, Mrs. Flynn will be discharged to her one-floor home, where she lives alone. Her son and daughter both live an hour away. She is capable of walking with a walker. Before the stroke, Mrs. Flynn was independent, an active member of several citizens groups, and participated in water walking at the YMCA three times a week. Her driver's license was revoked. Using Chart 2-3, Assessing the Home Environment, in the text, complete the outline to assess Mrs. Flynn's need for a home visit. Create your own answers to several of the questions so that you can complete the assessment.

Current Health Status

1. How well is the patient progressing?
2. How serious are the present signs and symptoms?
3. Has the patient shown signs of progressing as expected, or does it seem that recovery will be delayed?

_____

_____

Home Environment

1. Are worrisome safety factors apparent?
2. Are family or friends available to provide care, or is the patient alone?

_____

_____

Level of Self-Care Ability

1. Is the patient capable of self-care?
2. What is the patient's level of independence?
3. Is the patient ambulatory or bedridden?
4. Does the patient have sufficient energy or is she frail and easily fatigued?

_____

_____

Level of Nursing Care Needed

1. What level of nursing care does the patient require?
2. Does the care require basic skills or more complex interventions?

_____

_____

Prognosis

1. What is the expectation for recovery in this particular instance?
2. What are the chances that complications may develop if nursing care is not provided?

_____

_____

Educational Needs

1. How well has the patient or family grasped the teaching points made?
2. Is there a need for further follow-up and retraining?
3. What level of proficiency does the patient or family show in carrying out the necessary care?

_____

_____

Mental Status

1. How alert is the patient?
2. Are there signs of confusion or thinking difficulties?

_____

_____

Level of Adherence

1. Is the patient following the instructions provided?
2. Does the patient seem capable of following the instructions?
3. Are the family members helpful, or are they unwilling or unable to assist in caring for the patient as expected?

_____

_____

SECTION III: PRACTICING FOR NCLEX

Activity D *Answer the following questions.*

1. The nurse is providing a community education program about sexually transmitted infections for a group of 13- to 16-year-olds at the local YMCA. What type of prevention is the nurse targeting?
   a. Primary prevention
   b. Secondary prevention
   c. Tertiary prevention
   d. Community prevention

2. When would be the best time to begin discharge planning for a patient who will require assistance in the home after leaving the acute care facility?
   a. As the patient is preparing to be picked up from the hospital by family members
   b. At the time of the patient's admission to the hospital
   c. When the patient recovers from the acute phase of the illness
   d. After the patient is discharged from the hospital

3. The nurse is making an initial home visit to assess a patient for home health services. Which patients most frequently require home health services?
   a. Children with chronic, debilitating disorders
   b. Newborns who are sent home with apnea monitors
   c. The frail and elderly who need skilled care
   d. Young adults on prolonged intravenous therapy

4. The home health nurse and the parish nurse have separate roles in health care. What is the common factor that all community-based nurses share?
   a. They all take care of patients in a community setting.
   b. They all take care of patients after they are discharged from the hospital.
   c. They all take care of the patients in their home setting.
   d. They focus on community needs as well as the needs of individual patients.

5. What should the school nurse working in the elementary school setting be aware is one of the most frequent health care problems to affect this population?
   a. Eating disorders
   b. Emotional problems
   c. Infections
   d. Drug abuse

6. The nurse is caring for a patient who is to be discharged from the acute care facility to a rehabilitation unit after having a stroke. What type of prevention is this considered to be?
   a. Primary
   b. Secondary
   c. Tertiary
   d. Rehabilitation

Critical Thinking, Ethical Decision Making, and the Nursing Process

Learning Objectives

1. Define the characteristics of critical thinking, critical thinkers, and the critical thinking process.
2. Define *ethics* and *nursing ethics*.
3. Identify several ethical dilemmas common to the medical-surgical area of nursing practice.
4. Specify strategies that can aid nurses in ethical decision making.
5. Describe the components of the nursing process.
6. Develop a plan of nursing care for a patient using strategies of critical thinking.

SECTION I: ASSESSING YOUR UNDERSTANDING

Activity A *Fill in the blanks.*

1. Five of the most common ethical issues that nurses face today include: _____, _____, _____, _____, and _____.

2. _____ and _____ are two types of "advance directives" that specify a patient's wishes before hospitalization.

3. The term *metacognition* refers to the critical thinking skill of _____.

Activity B *Briefly answer the following.*

1. There are three consistent themes threaded through all definitions of critical thinking. These themes are:

   _____

   _____

   _____

2. List 10 characteristics of critical thinkers as identified by Alfaro-LeFevre (2009).

   _____ _____

   _____ _____

   _____ _____

   _____ _____

   _____ _____

3. List six skills that are needed for nurses to be critical thinkers.

   _____ _____

   _____ _____

   _____ _____

4. Explain this statement: How a nurse perceives a situation and employs critical thinking skills depends on the "lens" through which she or he sees the situation.

_____

_____

5. Compare and contrast the meaning of the following terms: *moral dilemma, moral problem, moral uncertainty,* and *moral distress.*

_____

_____

_____

6. Write the definition of nursing as proposed in Nursing's Social Policy Statement (2010, p. 9.)

_____

_____

_____

7. Explain the concept of a "durable power of attorney."

_____

_____

8. Suggest an opening statement that a nurse can use during the interview process.

_____

9. Discuss how formulation of a nursing diagnosis and identification of collaborative problems differs from making a medical diagnosis.

_____

_____

_____

_____

10. Discuss the significance of establishing expected outcomes during the evaluation phase of the nursing process.

_____

_____

_____

Activity C *Read each statement below. Put "N" in front of every nursing diagnosis and "C" in front of every collaborative problem.*

____ **1.** Anxiety related to impending surgery

____ **2.** Constipation related to altered nutrition

____ **3.** Potential complication: paralytic ileus secondary to postoperative inactivity

____ **4.** Potential complication: sacral decubiti secondary to bed rest

____ **5.** Risk for impaired skin integrity related to prolonged bed rest

____ **6.** Ineffective breastfeeding related to fear of discomfort

____ **7.** Potential complication: hypoglycemia related to inadequate food intake

____ **8.** Potential complication: phlebitis related to intravenous therapy

____ **9.** Risk for posttraumatic syndrome related to an accident

____ **10.** Potential complication: oral lesions related to chemotherapy

Activity D

PART I: Critical Thinking

Match the critical-thinking strategy in Column II with the nursing process skill listed in Column I.

Column I

____ **1.** Categorize information

____ **2.** Design a plan of care

____ **3.** Determine assessment processes

____ **4.** Evaluate outcomes

____ **5.** Implement a standard plan

____ **6.** Make a nursing diagnosis

____ **7.** Manage collaborative problems

Column II

a. Assert a practice role

b. Formulate a relationship

c. Generate a hypothesis

d. Provide an explanation

e. Recognize a pattern

f. Search for information

g. Set priorities

PART II: Ethical Principles

Match the definitions of ethical principles listed in Column II with their associated terms listed in Column I.

Column I

___ **1.** Autonomy

___ **2.** Beneficence

___ **3.** Justice

___ **4.** Nonmaleficence

___ **5.** Paternalism

___ **6.** Veracity

Column II

a. Limiting one's autonomy based on the welfare of another

b. Similar cases should be treated the same

c. The commitment to not deceive

d. Freedom of choice

e. The duty to do good and not inflict harm

f. The expectation that harm will not be done

SECTION II: APPLYING YOUR KNOWLEDGE

Activity E *Consider the scenario and fill in the blanks below.*

CASE STUDY: Ethical Analysis

You are a registered nurse and a board member of American Red Cross Disaster Relief Services. When a smallpox epidemic erupted among thousands in Washington, DC, as a result of terrorist activity, the board was asked by the Office of Homeland Security to allocate limited resources. The board decided that those with the greatest chance of survival and those working for the government would be treated. Those individuals with preexisting or terminal conditions would not be treated. The decision resulted in multiple deaths while preserving the lives of those most likely to survive. The framework for decision making followed the utilitarian approach.

Assessment

1. People involved in the decision:

a. _____

b. _____

c. _____

2. Those affected by the decision:

a. _____

b. _____

c. _____

3. List two possible conflicts between ethical principles and professional obligations.

a. _____

b. _____

Planning

1. Medical facts:

a. _____

b. _____

2. Influencing information:

a. _____

b. _____

3. Ethical/moral issues:

a. _____

b. _____

4. Competing claims:

a. _____

b. _____

5. Treatment options:

a. _____

b. _____

Implementation

Compare the Utilitarian and the Deontological approaches.

Utilitarian	Deontological or Formalist
1. Basis of ethical principles:	
a. _____	a. _____
b. _____	b. _____
2. Predict consequences of actions:	
a. _____	a. _____
b. _____	b. _____

3. Assign a positive or negative value to each consequence:

   a. _____   a. _____

   b. _____   b. _____

4. Choose the consequence, decision, or action that predicts the highest positive value:

   a. _____   a. _____

   b. _____   b. _____

Evaluation

1. The best, morally correct action is to:

   _____

2. This decision is based on the ethical reasoning that:

   _____

3. The decision can be defended based on the following arguments:

   a. _____

   b. _____

   c. _____

SECTION III: PRACTICING FOR NCLEX

Activity F *Answer the following questions.*

1. A patient with chronic obstructive pulmonary disease has asked an adult child to make medical decisions in the event the patient will not be able to make them. What type of advance directive should the patient sign?

   a. Ethical committee form
   b. Financial power of attorney
   c. Do not resuscitate order
   d. Durable power of attorney for health care

2. The nurse working in the operating room is scheduled to circulate for an elective abortion. The nurse tells the supervisor that it will not be possible to assist with this case due to religious beliefs. What problem is the nurse experiencing with this surgical case?

   a. Nonmaleficence
   b. Trust issues
   c. An ethical dilemma
   d. Veracity

3. The patient has become confused and attempts to climb out of bed. What interventions can the nurse provide prior to using restraints?

   a. Call the physician to prescribe sedation for the patient.
   b. Ask a family member to sit with the patient.
   c. Place the patient in a chair at the nurses' station with a sheet tied around the waist.
   d. Place all four side rails of the bed in the upright position.

4. When an ethical decision is made based on the reasoning of the "greatest good for the greatest number," what theory is the nurse following?

   a. Deontological theory
   b. Formalist theory
   c. Moral-justification theory
   d. Utilitarian theory

5. The nurse prepares to administer medication to the patient. The patient states, "I would prefer not to take that medication until I speak with my physician." The nurse honors the patient's desire to make decisions, following which common ethical principle?

   a. Autonomy
   b. Beneficence
   c. Fidelity
   d. Paternalism

6. The nurse moves a confused, disruptive patient to a private room at the end of the hall so that other patients can rest, even though the confused patient becomes more agitated. The nurse's intervention is consistent with what moral theory?

   a. "Consequentialism," by which good consequences for the greatest number are maximized
   b. "Duty of obligation," by which an action, regardless of its results, is justified if the decision making was based on moral principles
   c. "Paternalism," in which the action limits the patient's autonomy
   d. "Veracity," in which the nurse has an obligation to tell the truth

7. A hospital board of directors decides to close a pediatric burn treatment center (BTC) that annually admits 50 patients and to open a treatment center for terminally ill AIDS patients (with an expected annual admission of 200). This decision means that the nearest BTC for children is now 300 miles away. What example of ethical reasoning is this decision consistent with?

   a. A formalist approach

   b. Obligation or duty

   c. "The means justifies the end"

   d. Utilitarianism

8. A terminally ill patient asks the nurse, "Am I dying?" How will the nurse's response be influenced by moral obligation? (Select all that apply.)

   a. Communicate the patient's wishes to the family.

   b. Consult with the physician.

   c. Provide correct information to the patient.

   d. Tell the patient: "You will be fine."

   e. Have the physician disclose the information the patient requires.

9. A patient with a "Do Not Resuscitate" (DNR) order requires large doses of a narcotic for pain that rates a 10 on a 0–10 scale. After the patient requests pain medication, the nurse assesses a respiratory rate of 12 breaths per minute. What intervention by the nurse would be considered ethical?

   a. Ask the patient to wait 20 minutes and reassess.

   b. Give half of the prescribed dose.

   c. Give the pain medication without fear of respiratory depression.

   d. Withhold the pain medication and contact the physician.

10. What does the nurse determine is a moral problem rather than a moral dilemma?

    a. Family members tell the physician that they do not want their father informed of his terminal diagnosis.

    b. A 32-year-old father of three with advanced cancer of the lungs asks that everything be done to prolong his life, even though his chemotherapy treatments are no longer effective.

    c. A confused 80-year-old needs restraints for protection from injury, even though the restraints increase agitation.

    d. A young patient with AIDS has asked not to receive tube feedings to prolong life because of intense pain.

11. Assessment, the first of five steps in the nursing process, begins with initial patient contact. What activities by the nurse are included in this component of the nursing process? (Select all that apply.)

    a. Interviewing and obtaining a nursing history

    b. Observing for altered symptomatology

    c. Collecting and analyzing data

    d. Evaluation of the patient's response to a medication

    e. Developing outcome criteria

12. The nurse is developing a plan of care for a patient. What is the end result of data analysis during the assessment process?

    a. Actualization of the plan of care

    b. Determination of the patient's responses to care

    c. Collection and analysis of data

    d. Identification of actual or potential health problems

13. What therapeutic communication technique validates what the nurse believes to be the main idea of an interaction?

    a. Acknowledgment

    b. Focusing

    c. Restating

    d. Summarizing

14. What statement does the nurse determine is a medical diagnosis rather than a nursing diagnosis?

   a. Fever of unknown origin

   b. Fluid volume excess

   c. Risk for falls

   d. Sleep-pattern disturbances

15. Which priority intervention illustrates planned nursing care prioritized according to Maslow's hierarchy of needs?

   a. Administer pain medication to an orthopedic patient 30 minutes before transportation to physical therapy for crutch-walking exercises.

   b. Discourage a terminally ill patient from participating in a plan of care, to minimize fears about death.

   c. Help a patient walk to the shower while the breakfast tray waits on the overbed table, because the shower area is vacant at this time.

   d. Interrupt a family's visit with a depressed patient to assess blood pressure measurement, because it is time to take the scheduled vital signs.

16. A patient that has had a stroke is not able to eat without maximum assistance and has a nursing diagnosis of "Imbalanced nutrition, less than body requirements, related to inability to feed self." What would be an immediate nursing outcome for the patient to achieve?

   a. Acquire competence in managing cookware designed for handicapped people.

   b. Assume independent responsibility for meeting self-nutrition needs.

   c. Learn about food products that require minimal preparation yet meet individual needs for a balanced diet.

   d. Master the use of special eating utensils to feed self.

17. The registered nurse (RN) is responsible for delegating patient care responsibilities to licensed practical nurses (LPNs) as well as ancillary personnel. What would be the most appropriate task to delegate to a nursing assistant?

   a. Assessing the degree of lower leg edema in a patient on bed rest

   b. Obtaining vital signs for a patient that has been hospitalized for 3 days

   c. Measuring the circumference of a patient's calf for edema

   d. Recording the size and appearance of a decubitus ulcer

Health Education and Health Promotion

1. Describe the purposes and significance of health education.
2. Describe the concept of adherence to a therapeutic regimen.
3. Identify variables that affect learning readiness and adult learning abilities.
4. Describe the relationship of the teaching–learning process to the nursing process.
5. Develop an individualized teaching plan for a patient.
6. Define health promotion and discuss major health promotion models.
7. Describe the components of health promotion: self-responsibility, nutritional awareness, stress reduction and management, and physical fitness.
8. Specify the variables that affect health promotion activities for adolescents, young and middle-aged adults, and older adults.
9. Describe the role of the nurse in health promotion.

SECTION I: ASSESSING YOUR UNDERSTANDING

Activity A *Briefly answer the following.*

1. List three significant factors for a nurse to consider when planning patient education:

   _____

   _____

   _____

2. Explain why health education is so essential for those with a chronic illness:

   _____

   _____

3. List five common examples of specific activities that promote and maintain health:

   _____   _____

   _____   _____

   _____

4. Define the term *adherence* as it relates to a person's therapeutic regimen:

   _____

5. Name four classifications of variables (factors) that influence a person's ability to adhere to a program of care:

   _____   _____

   _____   _____

6. There is a positive correlation between patient motivation and adherence to a teaching plan. Name three significant variables affecting motivation and learning:

   _____   _____

   _____

7. List the six stages of personal change that an individual experiences as he or she moves toward a healthy behavior:

_____ _____

_____ _____

_____ _____

8. Describe the nature of the teaching–learning process:

_____

_____

9. List at least six variables that make adherence to a therapeutic regimen difficult for the elderly:

_____ _____

_____ _____

_____ _____

10. Increased age affects cognition by decreasing:

_____, _____,

and _____.

11. Discuss how learner readiness affects a learner and the learning situation:

_____

_____

_____

12. Identify six teaching techniques that nurses frequently use:

_____ _____

_____ _____

_____ _____

13. Identify two overall goals from the Healthy People 2020 report:

_____

_____

14. Health promotion activities are grounded in four active processes:

_____ _____

_____ _____

15. Explain at least five ways that exercise can promote health.

_____ _____

_____ _____

_____

Activity B *Rewrite each statement correctly. Underline the key concepts.*

1. Health education is a dependent function of nursing practice that requires physician approval.

_____

_____

2. The largest groups of people in need of health education today are children and those with infectious diseases.

_____

_____

3. Patients are encouraged to evidence compliance with their therapeutic regimen.

_____

_____

4. Evaluation, the final step in the teaching process, should be summative (done at the end of the teaching process).

_____

_____

5. Elderly persons rarely experience significant improvement from health promotion activities.

_____

_____

6. About 50% of elderly persons have one or more chronic illnesses.

_____

_____

SECTION II: APPLYING YOUR KNOWLEDGE

Activity C *Consider the scenario and answer the questions.*

The nurse is admitting a patient into the intensive care unit with acute congestive heart failure. The patient was discharged 8 days ago with the same diagnosis. The patient had been instructed prior to discharge to follow up with the primary care physician within 1 week, follow a low-sodium/1.5 L fluid restriction diet, and begin taking two new medications. When performing the assessment of the patient, the nurse found that the patient had not followed the discharge instructions and had been eating and drinking without restriction. The medications had not been started, and the patient had not seen the primary care physician.

1. What variables can determine the patient's adherence to the therapeutic regimen?

_____

_____

_____

2. How can the nurse increase the success of the patient's adherence to the therapeutic regimen after discharge?

_____

_____

SECTION III: PRACTICING FOR NCLEX

Activity D *Answer the following questions.*

1. Which patient is most in need of health education by the nurse?
   a. A 28-year-old female with abdominal pain
   b. A 62-year-old male with chronic kidney injury
   c. A 42-year-old male with acute pericarditis
   d. A 72-year-old female with a respiratory infection

2. What is the priority responsibility for the nurse providing patient teaching? (Select all that apply.)
   a. Determining individual needs for teaching
   b. Motivating each person to learn
   c. Giving a test at the end of a teaching session
   d. Waiting until the patient expresses a desire to learn
   e. Presenting information at the level of the learner

3. The nurse is preparing to educate a patient about the home care of an abdominal wound. What patient behaviors does the nurse notice that demonstrate readiness to learn? (Select all that apply.)
   a. The patient shows the motivation to learn.
   b. The patient has accepted the therapeutic regimen.
   c. The patient is unable to look at the wound.
   d. The patient tells the nurse the family member will take care of it.
   e. The patient requests a contact number if there are questions.

4. Which action by the nurse can negatively affect the patient's ability to learn?
   a. Feedback in the form of constructive encouragement when a person has been unsuccessful in the learning process
   b. Negative criticism when the patient is unsuccessful so that inappropriate behavior patterns will not be learned
   c. The creation of a positive atmosphere in which the patient is encouraged to express anxiety
   d. The establishment of realistic learning goals based on individual needs

5. Since normal aging results in changes in cognition, how should the nurse teach an elderly patient to administer insulin?
   a. Repeat the information frequently for reinforcement.
   b. Present all the information at one time so that the patient is not confused by pieces of information.
   c. Speed up the demonstration because the patient will tire easily.
   d. The elderly patient is not capable of learning self-administration and someone else should be instructed.

6. The home health nurse reviews a medication administration calendar with an elderly patient. In order to consider sensory changes that occur with aging, how should the nurse proceed?

   a. Print directions in large, bold type, preferably using black ink.

   b. Highlight or shade important dates and times with contrasting colors.

   c. Use several different colors to emphasize special dates.

   d. Type out the information on the computer.

7. What nursing action involves modifying a teaching program if a learner is not experientially ready?

   a. Changing the wording in a teaching pamphlet so that a patient with a fourth-grade reading level can understand it

   b. Contacting family members to assist in goal development to help stimulate motivation

   c. Postponing a teaching session with a patient until pain has subsided

   d. Notifying the physician that the patient will not yet be eligible for discharge

8. The nurse identifies a patient's inability to pour a liquid medication into a measuring spoon. This is an example of what part of the nursing process?

   a. Assessment

   b. Planning

   c. Implementation

   d. Evaluation

9. The nurse develops a program of increased ambulation for a patient with an orthopedic disorder. This is an example of what component of the nursing process?

   a. Assessment

   b. Planning

   c. Implementation

   d. Evaluation

10. The nurse develops outcome criteria for a patient with chronic obstructive pulmonary disease. Which outcome criteria are appropriate for this patient?

    a. The patient will have the ability to climb a flight of stairs without experiencing difficulty in breathing.

    b. The patient will not experience an alteration in skin integrity.

    c. The patient will perform passive range-of-motion exercises once daily.

    d. The nurse will obtain a pulse oximetry reading twice a day.

11. Which health promotion model does the nurse identify is the reason some people choose actions to foster health and others refuse to participate?

    a. Health Belief Model

    b. Resource Model of Preventive Health

    c. Achieving Health for All Model

    d. Social Learning Theory Model

12. What does the nurse understand is the single most important factor in determining health status and longevity?

    a. Adherence to a plan

    b. Good nutrition

    c. Motivation to change

    d. Stress reduction

CHAPTER 5

Adult Health and Nutritional Assessment

Learning Objectives

1. Identify ethical considerations necessary for protecting a person's rights related to data collected in the health history and physical assessment.
2. Describe the components of a holistic health history.
3. Explore the concept of spirituality and the assessment of spiritual needs of patients.
4. Apply culturally sensitive interviewing skills and techniques to conduct a successful health history, physical examination, and nutritional assessment.
5. Identify genetic aspects nurses should incorporate into the health history and physical assessment.
6. Identify modifications needed to obtain a health history and conduct a physical assessment for a person with a disability.
7. Describe the techniques of inspection, palpation, percussion, and auscultation to perform a basic physical assessment.
8. Discuss the techniques of measurement of body mass index, biochemical assessment, clinical examination, and assessment of food intake to assess a person's nutritional status.
9. Describe factors that may contribute to altered nutritional status in high-risk groups such as adolescents and older adults.

SECTION I: ASSESSING YOUR UNDERSTANDING

Activity A *Fill in the blanks.*

1. The role of the nurse in assessment includes two primary responsibilities: _____ and _____.

2. When questioning a patient about lifestyle and health-related behaviors, the nurse should ask about: _____, _____, _____, _____, and _____.

3. The *three leading causes of death* in the United States that are related in part to poor nutrition are _____, _____, and _____.

4. Adolescent girls are particularly at risk for nutritional deficits in minerals, such as _____, _____, and _____.

Activity B *Briefly answer the following.*

1. Describe five basic guidelines that a nurse should use while conducting a health assessment:

_____ _____

_____ _____

_____

2. Explain how mutual trust and confidence between the interviewer and the patient facilitate the communication process:

_____

_____

3. Define the term *chief complaint:*

_____

_____

4. A number of diseases of first- or second-order relatives are significant when a nurse takes a patient's family history. List six diseases that are considered significant:

_____   _____

_____   _____

_____   _____

5. A nurse uses the Department of Agriculture's MyPlate (Fig. 5-6 in the textbook) to evaluate a patient's dietary information. About what food groups should the nurse obtain information?

_____

_____

6. Explain the concept of *negative nitrogen balance:*

_____

_____

7. List six questions that a nurse could incorporate into a genetic health assessment:

_____

_____

_____

_____

_____

_____

Activity C

PART I

Identify which type of assessment was most likely used to obtain the data. Write the word on the line provided.

Column I

_____ **a.** Asymmetry of movement is associated with a central nervous system disorder.

_____ **b.** Clubbing of the fingers is a diagnostic symptom of chronic pulmonary disorders.

_____ **c.** Tenderness is present in the area of the thyroid isthmus.

_____ **d.** Tactile fremitus is diagnostic of lung consolidation.

_____ **e.** Tympanic or drum-like sounds are produced by pneumothorax.

_____ **f.** The first heart sound is created by the simultaneous closure of the mitral and tricuspid valves.

_____ **g.** A friction rub is present with pericarditis.

_____ **h.** Nodules present with gout lie adjacent to the joint capsule.

Column II

Inspection

Palpation

Percussion

Auscultation

PART II

Match the body area listed in Column II with the descriptive sign of poor nutrition listed in Column I.

Column I

____ **1.** Atrophic papillae

____ **2.** Brittle, dull, depigmented

____ **3.** Cheilosis

____ **4.** Flaccid, underdeveloped

____ **5.** Fluorosis

____ **6.** Xerophthalmia

Column II

a. Abdomen

b. Eyes

c. Hair

d. Lips

e. Muscles

f. Skeleton

g. Teeth

h. Tongue

SECTION II: APPLYING YOUR KNOWLEDGE

Activity D *Consider the scenario and answer the questions.*

CASE STUDY: Calculating a Healthy Diet

Mrs. Allred is a 40-year-old Hispanic woman, 5 ft 5 in tall, with three children younger than 5 years of age. She weighs 175 lb. She had no known history of any physical illness before experiencing fatigue and irritability that she believed was the result of her parenting responsibilities. Mrs. Allred does not exercise regularly, eats snack foods while watching television with her children, and is too tired to prepare balanced meals for her family. She orders fast food or pizza for dinner at least three times a week.

PART I: Estimate Ideal Body Weight

1. Calculate Mrs. Allred's frame size based on a wrist circumference of 16 cm.

   a. Small frame

   b. Medium frame

   c. Large frame

2. Mrs. Allred's ideal body weight (IBW) is _____ lb. Therefore, she needs to _____ (gain/lose) approximately _____ lb.

3. Her body mass index (BMI) is _____, which is considered (ideal, overweight, obese) _____.

PART II: Calculate a Balanced Diet

Calculate a balanced diet for Mrs. Allred's ideal body weight, as determined in Part I.

1. Convert IBW in pounds to kilograms. _____.

2. Determine basal energy needs (1 kcal/kg/hr): _____ calories.

3. Increase activity by 40% (moderate activity): _____ calories.

4. Divide calories into carbohydrates (50%) _____, fats (30%) _____, and proteins (20%) _____.

5. Estimate grams for each: carbohydrates _____, fats _____, and proteins _____.

PART III: Design a Healthy Diet

Refer to the U.S. Department of Agriculture's MyPlate (Fig. 5-6) to design a healthy diet for Mrs. Allred.

1. Mrs. Allred should eat about _____ servings of fruit daily.

2. What daily minimum of whole grains should she eat? _____

3. Mrs. Allred should be advised to eat about _____ of vegetables daily.

4. What is the daily recommended amount of protein for her? _____

5. What is the daily recommended amount of dairy products she should eat? _____

SECTION III: PRACTICING FOR NCLEX

Activity E *Answer the following questions.*

1. When obtaining a health history from a patient, what should be the nurse's primary focus? (Select all that apply.)

   a. The primary method of payment

   b. A comprehensive body systems review

   c. What the patient ate prior to coming to the clinic

   d. Current and past medical problems

   e. Family history

2. What does the patient have the right to know about the data collected by the nurse? (Select all that apply.)
   a. How the information will be used
   b. Why the information is being obtained
   c. What type of document is being used
   d. Whether the information will be held in confidence
   e. When the facility will be using electronic order entry

3. The nurse is assessing the patient's pain. Which question asked by the nurse is considered an open-ended question?
   a. "Are you having pain?"
   b. "Is the pain sharp and piercing?"
   c. "Point to where it hurts."
   d. "Describe the pain."

4. What priority factor regarding the patient may help the physician arrive at a diagnosis?
   a. Family history
   b. History of the present illness
   c. Past health history
   d. Results of the systems review

5. Which question by the nurse may be used to obtain educational or occupational information?
   a. "Are you a blue-collar worker?"
   b. "Do you have difficulty meeting your financial commitments?"
   c. "Is your income more than $20,000 per year?"
   d. "What college did you attend?"

6. Which statement made by the nurse would be a nontherapeutic response when the patient says, "I will not take pain medication when I am in pain"?
   a. "Is there another way you have learned to lessen pain when you experience it?"
   b. "Let a nurse know when you are in pain so you can be helped to decrease stimuli that may exaggerate your pain experience."
   c. "Refusing medication can only hurt you by increasing your awareness of the pain experience."
   d. "You have the right to make that decision. How can the nurses help you cope with your pain?"

7. Which question asked by the nurse will provide information about a patient's lifestyle? (Select all that apply.)
   a. "Have you always lived in this geographic area?"
   b. "Do you have any food preferences?"
   c. "How many hours of sleep do you require each day?"
   d. "What type of exercise do you prefer?"
   e. "What are the names of your children?"

8. When obtaining a health history from an older adult patient, what should the nurse remember to do? (Select all that apply.)
   a. Ask questions slowly, directly, and in a voice loud enough to be heard by those who are hearing impaired.
   b. Clarify the frequency, severity, and history of signs and symptoms of the present illness.
   c. Conduct the interview in a calm, unrushed manner using eye-to-eye contact.
   d. Have a family member in the room when asking questions to make sure the patient's answers are accurate.
   e. Frequently touch the patient so that you may bring his or her attention back to the interview.

9. The nurse assesses the patient's posture, stature, and body movements. What part of the physical examination process is this?
   a. Auscultation
   b. Inspection
   c. Palpation
   d. Percussion

10. When the nurse is percussing for measurement of the patient's liver span, what type of response should be heard?
    a. Dull sound
    b. Flat sound
    c. Resonant sound
    d. Tympanic sound

11. The nurse notes hyperresonance over inflated lung tissue when performing a physical assessment on a patient with emphysema. What process does the nurse use for this assessment?

    a. Auscultation

    b. Inspection

    c. Palpation

    d. Percussion

12. The nurse detects a heart murmur when performing a physical assessment on a patient. What process does the nurse use for this assessment?

    a. Auscultation

    b. Inspection

    c. Palpation

    d. Percussion

13. The nurse is discussing lifestyle changes and weight reduction with a female patient who has excess abdominal fat. What waist circumference should the patient maintain in order to remain healthy?

    a. 30 to 34 inches

    b. 35 inches

    c. 36 to 38 inches

    d. 39 to 41 inches

14. The nurse observes a serum albumin level of 2.50 g/dL in an older adult patient who lives at home alone. What does this level indicate?

    a. A severe protein deficiency

    b. Low levels of serum protein

    c. An acceptable amount of protein

    d. An extremely high measurement of protein

15. What primary nutritional nursing consideration should be included in the physical assessment of an older adult patient?

    a. Altered metabolism and nutrient use secondary to an acute or chronic illness

    b. Decreased appetite related to loneliness

    c. Limited financial resources

    d. The patient's ability to shop for and prepare food

Biophysical and Psychosocial Concepts in Nursing Practice

Individual and Family Homeostasis, Stress, and Adaptation

Learning Objectives

1. Relate the principles of internal constancy, homeostasis, stress, and adaptation to the concept of steady state.
2. Identify the significance of the body's compensatory mechanisms in promoting adaptation and maintaining the steady state.
3. Compare physical, physiologic, and psychosocial stressors.
4. Describe the general adaptation syndrome as a theory of adaptation to biologic stress.
5. Compare the sympathetic-adrenal-medullary and hypothalamic-pituitary responses to stress.
6. Identify ways in which maladaptive responses to stress can increase the risk of illness and cause disease.
7. Describe the relationship of the process of negative feedback to the maintenance of the steady state.
8. Compare the adaptive processes of hypertrophy, atrophy, hyperplasia, dysplasia, and metaplasia.
9. Describe the inflammatory and reparative processes.
10. Assess the health patterns of a person and families; determine their effects on maintenance of the steady state.
11. Identify individual, family, and group measures that are useful in reducing stress.

SECTION I: ASSESSING YOUR UNDERSTANDING

Activity A *Fill in the blanks.*

1. Stress is a change in the environment that is perceived as _____, _____, or _____.

2. Maladaptive compensatory mechanisms result in disease processes in which cells may be _____, _____, or _____.

3. The neural and hormonal activities that respond to stress and maintain homeostasis are located in the _____.

4. Cell injury results when stressors interfere with the body's optimal balance by altering cellular ability to _____, _____, and _____.

5. Research has shown that the single most important factor influencing an individual's health is _____.

6. Four concepts that are key to understanding a steady state of dynamic balance are _____, _____, _____, and _____.

7. Five bodily functions that are regulated by negative feedback mechanisms include the following: _____, _____, _____, _____, and _____.

8. The five cardinal signs of inflammation are:
_____, _____, _____,
_____, and _____.

Activity B *Briefly answer the following.*

1. Define a *maladaptive* response to a stressor:

_____

_____

2. Explain why *hyperpnea,* after intense exercise, is considered an adaptive response to a physiologic stressor:

_____

_____

3. Give several examples of acute, *time-limited* stressors and chronic, *enduring* stressors:

_____

_____

4. Psychosocial stressors are classified as day-to-day occurrences (daily hassles), major events that affect large groups, and those infrequently occurring situations that directly affect a person. List two examples from your personal experiences that could be included under each classification.

   a. Day-to-day occurrences:

   _____

   _____

   b. Major events that affect large groups of people:

   _____

   _____

   c. Infrequently occurring major stressors:

   _____

   _____

5. Discuss the correlation between stress, illness, and critical life events:

_____

_____

6. Discuss how internal cognitive processes and external resources are used by an individual to manage stress:

_____

_____

7. Define stress according to Hans Selye's Theory of Adaptation (1976):

_____

_____

8. According to Hans Selye's Theory of Adaptation (1976), there are about 12 diseases of maladaptation. List six:

_____   _____

_____   _____

_____   _____

9. List four possible nursing diagnoses for individuals suffering from stress:

_____   _____

_____   _____

10. How does a person with positive self-esteem, energy, and health typically respond to stressors in a positive way?

_____

_____

11. What is the difference between physical, physiologic, and psychosocial stressors?

_____

_____

Activity C *Match the primary category of stressors listed in Column II with its associated stressors listed in Column I.*

Column I

____ **1.** Anxieties

____ **2.** Genetic disorders

____ **3.** Hypoxia

____ **4.** Infectious agents

____ **5.** Life changes

____ **6.** Nutritional imbalance

____ **7.** Social relationships

____ **8.** Trauma

Column II

a. Physiologic

b. Psychosocial

SECTION II: APPLYING YOUR KNOWLEDGE

Activity D *Consider the scenario and answer the questions.*

David, a 52-year-old corporate attorney, comes to the clinic and informs the nurse that he has been suffering from chest pain, an inability to sleep at night, and anxiety. He states, "I am working 70 or more hours a week and there is no time to enjoy life." David has a physical examination with an electrocardiogram and laboratory studies that rule out any physical cause for the symptoms.

1. The nurse attempts to educate David about relaxation techniques. What is the goal of relaxation techniques?

   _____

   _____

2. What type of commonly used relaxation techniques can the nurse educate David about?

   _____

   _____

3. What does the nurse understand are four similar factors in all relaxation techniques?

   _____

   _____

SECTION III: PRACTICING FOR NCLEX

Activity E *Answer the following questions.*

1. A patient has been paralyzed from the chest down for 7 years and is diagnosed with pneumonia. The nurse realizes that the patient will need additional support to cope with the infection for what reason?

   a. Coping measures become less effective with advancing age.

   b. The patient's available coping resources are already being used to manage the problems of immobility.

   c. An acute infectious process requires more adaptive mechanisms than a chronic stressor does.

   d. This additional physical stressor places unmanageable demands on the patient's internal and external resources.

2. A patient is admitted to the medical unit with periodic episodes of shortness of breath, tightness in the throat, and crying. What should the nurse do to evaluate the impact of physiologic and psychological components on the patient's illness?

   a. Perform a thorough physical examination and include subjective patient statements as well as objective laboratory data.

   b. Focus primary attention on the respiratory system, because this is the patient's chief complaint.

   c. Determine that the patient is not in acute distress, then perform a complete physical examination, including data about the patient's lifestyle and social relationships.

   d. Attempt to discover the reasons behind the patient's anxieties, because stress can cause breathing difficulties.

3. The nurse is interviewing a patient with shortness of breath. The patient reveals that she is in the process of getting a divorce. What does this information alert the nurse to do?

   a. Try to determine whether there is a psychological basis for the patient's physical symptoms.

   b. Restrict family members from visiting, because their presence may aggravate the patient's symptoms.

   c. Teach the patient specific breathing exercises that can be used to manage symptoms.

   d. Request that the physician recommend counseling services.

4. A patient is admitted to the emergency department for observation after a minor automobile accident. On the basis of an understanding of the sympathetic nervous system's response to stress, what would the nurse expect to find during assessment? (Select all that apply.)

   a. Cold, clammy skin

   b. Decreased heart rate

   c. Rapid respirations

   d. Skeletal muscle tension

   e. Seizure activity

5. A patient is experiencing lower leg pain associated with lactic acid accumulation. When does the nurse expect the pain to decrease?

   a. When aerobic metabolism is reinstated

   b. When anaerobic metabolism becomes the major pathway for energy release

   c. When muscle use and subsequent glucose catabolism increase

   d. When vasoconstriction diminishes blood flow, thereby slowing the removal of waste products

6. A patient has a diagnosis of hypertrophy of the heart muscle, which correlates with cellular adaptation to injury. What findings does the nurse expect to occur? (Select all that apply.)

   a. Compromised cardiac output

   b. Muscle mass changes evident on radiologic examination

   c. Cellular alteration compensatory to some stimulus

   d. Decreased cell size, leading to more effective ventricular contractions

   e. Increased cardiac output

7. A pregnant patient is having changes in her breast and asks the nurse if this should be cause for concern. What does the nurse understand is the cellular adaptation to stress in the pregnant woman?

   a. Dysplasia

   b. Hyperplasia

   c. Hypertrophy

   d. Metaplasia

8. A patient has a hemoglobin level of 7 g/dL. What should the nurse be alert to assess for?

   a. Hyperemia

   b. Hypertension

   c. Hypoglycemia

   d. Hypoxia

9. A patient with diabetes is admitted to the hospital with a blood sugar level of 320 mg/dL. Why should the nurse monitor fluid intake and output for this patient?

   a. Decreased blood osmolarity causes fluid to shift into the interstitial spaces, resulting in polydipsia.

   b. Polydipsia occurs when glucose catabolism is accelerated, thereby increasing the body's need for fluids.

   c. Polyuria results from osmotic diuresis, which is compensatory to hyperglycemia.

   d. The blood's hypotonicity will result in tissue fluid retention and weight gain.

10. The nurse is caring for a patient with a fever. Care for this patient should be based on what body responses? (Select all that apply.)

   a. Diaphoresis, which is a compensatory mechanism that cools the body

   b. Vasodilation of surface blood vessels, which prevents excessive heat loss

   c. Increased heart rate, which helps to meet increased metabolic demands

   d. Increased nutrient catabolism, which influences the body's caloric needs

   e. Decrease in cellular metabolism, which decreases metabolic demand

11. The patient wants to be prescribed an anti-infective drug for the flu. The nurse understands that anti-infective medications would not be useful against which biologic agents?

   a. Bacteria

   b. Fungi

   c. Mycoplasmas

   d. Viruses

12. The nurse is talking with a patient who is considering becoming pregnant and is concerned about genetic disorders. Which genetic disorders does the nurse inform the patient arise from inherited traits? (Select all that apply.)

   a. Hemophilia

   b. Meningitis

   c. Phenylketonuria

   d. Sickle cell anemia

   e. Encephalitis

13. A nurse is caring for a patient with a localized response to bee stings. What symptoms does the nurse know to look for? (Select all that apply.)

    a. Hyperemia due to increased blood flow

    b. Cool skin around the site of the sting

    c. Blanching due to compensatory vasoconstriction

    d. Pain due to pressure on the nerve endings

    e. Swelling due to increased vascular permeability

14. The nurse is caring for a patient with an infected surgical incision. Which signs demonstrating systemic response does the nurse observe? (Select all that apply.)

    a. A febrile state caused by the release of pyrogens

    b. Anorexia, malaise, and weakness

    c. Leukopenia owing to increased white blood cell production

    d. Loss of appetite and complaints of aching

    e. Subnormal body temperature caused by vasoconstriction

15. The nurse is performing an assessment to determine the patient's social support systems. Which question is important for the nurse to ask?

    a. Does the patient believe that he or she belongs to a group that is mutually dependent and communicative?

    b. Does the patient have adequate insurance coverage to take care of health costs?

    c. What does the patient do for a living?

    d. Does the patient have any significant past medical problems?

16. A patient with a strong history of breast malignancy in her family is scheduled for a breast biopsy in the morning. What would be the most appropriate nursing action when caring for this patient the evening before surgery?

    a. Administer a soothing back massage to promote relaxation and decrease stress.

    b. Make sure she eats all of her evening meal, because she will be NPO after midnight.

    c. Minimize the emotional impact of surgery by encouraging her to socialize with other patients.

    d. Sit with her and provide an opportunity for her to talk about her concerns.

Overview of Transcultural Nursing

Learning Objectives

1. Identify key components of cultural assessment.
2. Apply transcultural nursing principles, concepts, and theories when providing nursing care to individuals, families, groups, and communities.
3. Develop strategies for planning, providing, and evaluating culturally competent nursing care for patients from diverse backgrounds.
4. Critically analyze the influence of culture on nursing care decisions and actions for patients.
5. Discuss the impact of diversity and health care disparities on health care delivery.

SECTION I: ASSESSING YOUR UNDERSTANDING

Activity A *Fill in the blanks.*

1. The founder of transcultural nursing is

   _____.

2. Three elements frequently used to identify diversity are _____, _____, and _____.

3. The two underlying goals of transcultural nursing are to provide _____ and _____ care.

4. The three major paradigms used to explain the causes of disease and illness are _____, _____, and _____.

5. The most common non-English language spoken in the United States is _____.

6. The theory of transcultural nursing supports providing care that _____, _____, and _____.

Activity B *Briefly answer the following.*

1. Name four basic characteristics of all ethnic cultures.

   _____   _____

   _____   _____

2. Define the term *culturally competent nursing care.*

   _____

   _____

   _____

3. List four examples of American subcultures based on ethnicity.

   _____   _____

   _____   _____

4. Give at least five examples of other groupings that can be used to identify subcultures.

   _____

   _____

5. Explain the concept of *culturally competent or congruent nursing care.*

_____

_____

_____

6. List four strategies that individuals tend to use when communication has broken down.

_____   _____

_____   _____

7. Name five religious groups that routinely incorporate fasting into their religious practices.

_____   _____

_____   _____

_____

8. Explain the concept of yin/yang.

_____

_____

_____

Activity C *Match the classification of a complementary or alternative therapy listed in Column II with a specific type of holistic care listed in Column I. Answers can be used more than once.*

Column I

____ **1.** Hypnosis

____ **2.** Reiki

____ **3.** Acupuncture

____ **4.** Chiropractic

____ **5.** Dietary plans

____ **6.** Ayurveda

____ **7.** Therapeutic touch

____ **8.** Homeopathic medicine

____ **9.** Dance and music

____ **10.** Qi gong

Column II

a. Alternative medical systems

b. Biologically based systems

c. Energy therapies

d. Manipulative methods

e. Mind–body interventions

SECTION II: APPLYING YOUR KNOWLEDGE

Activity D *Consider the scenario and answer the questions.*

A 72-year-old Egyptian woman who speaks no English and is a devout Muslim is visiting her son in the United States for 2 months. While she is going down the steps of her son's home, her foot misses the top step and she falls down nine steps and fractures her left femur. She has an open reduction and internal fixation of her left hip and is admitted to the surgical unit.

1. What activities could the nurse use to overcome language barriers when interacting with this patient?

_____

_____

_____

2. The patient receives a lunch tray that she pushes away. The nurse observes the food on the tray and determines why the patient refuses to eat it. What food item may be offensive to this patient?

_____

SECTION III: PRACTICING FOR NCLEX

Activity E *Answer the following questions.*

1. The nurse is assigned to care for a patient with a cultural background that is different than the nurse's. Prior to delivering care, what is important for the nurse to do?

a. The nurse should explore his/her own cultural beliefs.

b. Request to be reassigned to a patient with a culture the nurse is familiar with.

c. Be determined to provide care the same way to every patient, regardless of cultural background.

d. Determine what type of dietary restrictions the patient will have.

2. The nurse is assigned to prepare a patient who speaks only Spanish for a surgical procedure. Prior to the patient signing the permit, what should the nurse do?

a. Allow the patient's family member to interpret the surgical permit.

b. Obtain an impartial interpreter to explain the permit with the nurse.

c. After pointing to the place for the patient to sign, tell him or her to make an X.

d. Ask the family to provide an interpreter.

3. The nurse is providing education to the patient about wound care and the patient changes the subject to talk about the weather. What does the nurse understand may be the cause of the abrupt change of subject?

a. The patient is bored with the conversation.

b. The patient has a hearing deficit.

c. The patient may not understand what is being explained by the nurse.

d. The patient already knows how to do the wound care.

4. The nurse is speaking to a patient who is Native American. During the conversation, the patient maintains downcast eyes. What does the nurse understand is the most likely reason for this behavior?

a. The patient feels that the nurse holds a lesser position of authority.

b. It is a sign of appropriate deferential behavior.

c. The patient is fearful of the nurse.

d. The patient is not interested in what the nurse is saying.

5. What cultural group does the nurse understand may be late for a scheduled appointment at the clinic because of a wide frame of reference?

a. Hispanic

b. Arabian

c. Native American

d. Asian

6. The nurse should anticipate making an appointment with a female physician in the medical practice for a female patient of which culture?

a. Arabian

b. Asian

c. Japanese

d. Latin American

7. When performing a physical assessment, the nurse should be aware that in which culture would it be impolite to touch the patient's head?

a. Arabian

b. Hispanic

c. Jewish

d. Asian

8. The nurse is admitting an Asian-American patient to the medical-surgical floor. When calling the dietary department, the nurse tells the dietitian that all Asians eat rice. What attitude is the nurse displaying?

a. Ethnocentrism

b. Cultural sensitivity

c. Cultural humility

d. Stereotyping

9. A patient tells the nurse that she will be researching an alternative method of treatment for her disease. What is the best response by the nurse?

a. "You should comply with what the physician tells you is the best treatment."

b. "Those types of treatments are not reliable and can be harmful to you."

c. "If you use an alternative method of treatment, you cannot use traditional medicine as a treatment."

d. "You are within your right to search for other methods of treatment. Just be sure to inform your physician what treatments you are using."

10. A patient who is Asian practices the yin/yang theory of harmony and illness. What paradigm of health and illness is this practice rooted in?

a. Biomedical

b. Holistic

c. Religious

d. Scientific

CHAPTER 8

Overview of Genetics and Genomics in Nursing

Learning Objectives

1. Describe the role of the nurse in integrating genetic and genomic in nursing care.
2. Identify the common patterns of inheritance of genetic disorders.
3. Conduct a genetic- and genomic-based assessment.
4. Apply the principles, concepts, and theories of genetics and genomics to individuals, families, groups, and communities.
5. Identify ethical issues in nursing related to genetics and genomics.

SECTION I: ASSESSING YOUR UNDERSTANDING

Activity A *Fill in the blanks.*

1. A person's individual genetic makeup (composed of 30,000–40,000 genes) is called a _____; the person's set of characteristics of physical appearance and other traits is called a _____.

2. Genes are working subunits of DNA. Genes are arranged in linear order within _____. Twenty-two pairs of chromosomes, also called _____, are the same in males and females. The 23rd pair, the _____, is composed of two _____ for the female and _____ for the male. At conception, the sex of a child is determined because each parent gives _____.

3. With autosomal dominant inheritance, a woman with the *BRCA1* hereditary breast cancer gene has a lifetime risk of _____% of acquiring breast cancer and a _____% chance of passing the gene to each child.

4. _____ is a common chromosomal condition that occurs with greater frequency in pregnancies of women who are 35 years of age or older.

5. The frequency of chromosomal abnormalities in newborns is _____; this accounts for _____% of all spontaneous first-trimester pregnancy losses.

6. _____, which can be identified with parasympathetic testing, is the most common adult-onset condition in the Caucasian population.

7. _____ is the study of all the genes in the human genome and their interactions.

8. Chromosomes are located within the nucleus of a cell. The human body has _____ chromosomes.

9. Gene mutations have significant implications for health and illness. _____ is a mutation in protein structure that alters the configuration of hemoglobin.

10. _____ is a multifactorial genetic condition that tends to cluster in families.

11. Three examples of adult-onset conditions believed to be the result of multifactorial genetic mutations include _____, _____, and _____.

Activity B *Briefly answer the following.*

1. Define the term *genomic medicine.*

    _____

    _____

    _____

2. What are the essential nursing competencies for genetics and genomics?

    _____

    _____

3. Cite five examples of multifactorial-inherited conditions.

    _____   _____

    _____   _____

    _____

4. Define the term *pharmacogenetics.*

    _____

    _____

5. List five nursing activities in genetics-related nursing practice.

    _____   _____

    _____   _____

    _____

Activity C

PART I: Terminology

Match the genetic term listed in Column II with its specific definition listed in Column I.

Column I

____ 1. The number of chromosomes normally present in humans (N = 46)

____ 2. The presence of one extra chromosome (e.g., Down syndrome)

____ 3. The genes and variations that a person inherits from his or her parents

____ 4. A single chromosome from any of the 22 pairs not involved in sex determination (XX or XY)

____ 5. A person's entire physiologic and biologic makeup as determined by genotype and environment

____ 6. Primary genetic material (DNA)

____ 7. A heterozygous person who carries two different alleles of a gene pair

____ 8. The microscopic cell nucleus that contains genetic information

Column II

a. Autosome

b. Carrier

c. Chromosome

d. Deoxyribonucleic acid

e. Diploid

f. Genotype

g. Phenotype

h. Trisomy

PART II: Adult-Onset Disorders

Match the age of adult onset in Column II with the specific disorder listed in Column I.

Column I	Column II
____ **1.** Spinocerebellar ataxia, type 2	**a.** Mean age of 30 years
____ **2.** Huntington's disease	**b.** 30 to 40 years
____ **3.** Early-onset familial Alzheimer's disease	**c.** 35 to 44 years
____ **4.** Hereditary hemochromatosis	**d.** 40 to 60 years
____ **5.** Spinocerebellar ataxia, type 3	**e.** 60 to 65 years
____ **6.** Polycystic kidney disease	**f.** 50 to 70 years
____ **7.** Familial hypercholesterolemia	
____ **8.** Amyotrophic lateral sclerosis (ALS)	

SECTION II: APPLYING YOUR KNOWLEDGE

Activity D *Consider the scenario and answer the questions.*

Maggie and Josh are planning to have another child. Maggie has had four spontaneous pregnancy losses, and they have a 3-year-old son with Down syndrome.

1. Maggie has a "balanced" chromosomal rearrangement. What can this mean for future pregnancies?

_____

_____

2. Prior to Maggie becoming pregnant, what should the nurse suggest to the couple?

_____

3. Why would fluorescent in situ hybridization (FISH) be performed?

_____

SECTION III: PRACTICING FOR NCLEX

Activity E *Answer the following questions.*

1. A pregnant patient has had an amniocentesis. She has been told that the fetus has a condition in which cellular division results in an extra chromosome. What condition may affect the fetus?

a. Down syndrome

b. Sickle cell anemia

c. Tay-Sachs disease

d. Turner syndrome

2. A patient understands that her diagnosis of ovarian cancer syndrome is an autosomal-dominant inherited condition. What is the chance that her daughter will inherit the gene mutation for this disease?

a. 10%

b. 25%

c. 50%

d. 80%

3. A patient has an autosomal recessive inherited condition. For what type of disorder does the nurse anticipate the patient will be treated?

a. Cystic fibrosis

b. Hereditary breast cancer

c. Huntington disease

d. Familial hypercholesterolemia

4. A 32-year-old patient has just been told that she has the *BRCA1* hereditary breast cancer gene mutation. What is her risk of developing cancer by the age of 65 years?

a. 25%

b. 50%

c. 80%

d. 100%

5. A couple considering starting a family is told that they are both carriers for thalassemia. What does the nurse tell them is the risk that their child will inherit the gene?

a. 25%

b. 50%

c. 75%

d. 100%

6. A couple is considering starting a family but is concerned about the risk of Tay-Sachs disease. What cultural group does the nurse understand is most at risk for the disease?

   a. Ashkenazi Jewish

   b. Italian Americans

   c. Native Americans

   d. African Americans

7. What target cultural population is a priority for the nurse to educate about prevention of hypertension?

   a. Italian Americans

   b. Native Americans

   c. African Americans

   d. Hispanics

8. Parents request that a test be done to determine if the fetus has Down syndrome. What type of test does the nurse anticipate the physician will order?

   a. Presymptomatic testing

   b. Prenatal screening

   c. Predisposition testing

   d. A family pedigree

9. The daughter of a patient with Huntington disease has requested that she be tested for the disease even though she has no symptoms at this time. What type of test does the nurse anticipate the physician will order?

   a. Presymptomatic testing

   b. Prenatal testing

   c. Predisposition testing

   d. A family pedigree

10. In order to develop an awareness of genetics and genomic concepts, what is essential that the nurse do first?

    a. Examine his or her own beliefs and values.

    b. Make judgments based on the type of patients being treated.

    c. Do an Internet search on genetics.

    d. Ask the physician what he or she thinks.

CHAPTER 9

Chronic Illness and Disability

Learning Objectives

1. Define "chronic conditions."
2. Identify factors related to the increasing incidence of chronic conditions.
3. Describe characteristics of chronic conditions and implications for people with chronic conditions and for their families.
4. Describe advantages and disadvantages of various models of disability.
5. Describe implications of disability for nursing practice.

SECTION I: ASSESSING YOUR UNDERSTANDING

Activity A *Fill in the blanks.*

1. The four causes of major chronic illnesses that are preventable by lifestyle changes are _____, _____, _____, and _____.

2. In 2009, approximately _____ people in the United States had one or more chronic illnesses.

3. The three most frequently occurring chronic diseases that result from four preventable causes are _____, _____, and _____.

4. The three categories used to classify disabilities are _____, _____, and _____.

Activity B *Briefly answer the following.*

1. Three characteristics common to all forms of chronic illness are:

   _____

   _____

   _____

2. Identify six challenges commonly associated with chronic conditions.

   _____   _____

   _____   _____

   _____   _____

3. List six common medical and nursing management problems related to chronic conditions.

   _____   _____

   _____   _____

   _____   _____

4. Define the concept of the Trajectory Model as it relates to chronic illness.

   _____

   _____

5. What is the difference between the terms *disability* and *impairment* according to the definitions approved by the World Health Organization's (2001) classification system?

_____

_____

6. What psychological and emotional reactions to chronic illness and its consequences (e.g., lifestyle changes, financial resources) affect adjustment?

_____

_____

7. What is the difference between the Rehabilitation Act of 1973 and the Disabilities Act of 1990, and how they have helped protect disabled people from discrimination?

_____

_____

Activity C *The following statements list some characteristics of chronic illness. For each statement, write an explanation of how nursing care can improve the patient's and family's response to management and adaptation.*

1. Managing chronic illness involves more than managing medical problems.

_____

_____

2. Chronic conditions are associated with different phases over a course of time.

_____

_____

3. Managing chronic conditions requires persistent adherence to a therapeutic regimen.

_____

_____

4. Chronic illness affects the whole family.

_____

_____

SECTION II: APPLYING YOUR KNOWLEDGE

Activity D *Consider the scenario and answer the questions.*

The focus of care for patients with chronic illness is determined by their phase of illness. Each of the nine phases can be correlated to a step in the nursing process. For each of the following steps, discuss the role of nursing intervention. Julie, a 32-year-old mother of one, works full-time as a teacher and has just been diagnosed with rheumatoid arthritis. She is in the trajectory onset/stable phase of chronic illness. She is seen by a rheumatologist and will be placed on immunosuppressant medication to control the autoimmune response.

Step 1: Using assessment, identify the specific problems and the trajectory phase.

_____

_____

_____

Step 2: Establish and prioritize goals.

_____

_____

_____

Step 3: Define a plan of action to achieve desired outcomes.

_____

_____

_____

Step 4: Implement the plan and interventions.

_____

_____

_____

Step 5: Follow-up and evaluate outcomes.

_____

_____

_____

SECTION III: PRACTICING FOR NCLEX

Activity E *Answer the following questions.*

1. The nurse is caring for a patient who had a stroke and has right-sided hemiparesis. The patient is receiving physical therapy that will continue when discharged through home health care services. After what minimum period of time could this patient's medical condition be termed *chronic*?
   a. 8 weeks
   b. 3 months
   c. 16 weeks
   d. 6 months

2. Which chronic illness directly related to an unhealthy lifestyle does the nurse understand is increasing rapidly?
   a. Diabetes mellitus
   b. Breast cancer
   c. Emphysema
   d. Colorectal cancer

3. Which aspect of a healthy lifestyle can the nurse encourage a patient to improve that can significantly enhance quality of life with a chronic condition?
   a. Diet
   b. Exercise
   c. Hydration
   d. Rest

4. A patient who is at risk for developing a chronic condition because of genetic factors is said to be in which phase of the Trajectory Model?
   a. Pretrajectory
   b. Trajectory
   c. Unstable
   d. Acute

5. Chronic illness can be monitored using the Trajectory Model. In what phase can the nurse's nursing diagnosis help in care planning?
   a. Pretrajectory
   b. Trajectory
   c. Crisis
   d. Downward course

6. Which phase of the Trajectory Model does the nurse recognize is present when the patient is in remission, after an exacerbation of illness?
   a. Acute
   b. Crisis
   c. Comeback
   d. Downward course

7. The nurse recognizes which disorder as a developmental disability in a patient?
   a. Cerebral palsy
   b. Spinal cord injury
   c. Stroke
   d. Osteoarthritis

8. Which disability model is most appropriate for the nurse to use as a guide for planning care?
   a. Biopsychosocial Model
   b. Interface Model
   c. Medical and Rehabilitation Model
   d. Social Model

9. When providing education to the patient with a chronic illness, what is a priority intervention for the nurse to perform?
   a. Educate all patients the same.
   b. Provide written information only so that patients will have a reference.
   c. Adapt teaching strategies and materials to the individual patient.
   d. If the patient is hearing impaired, teach a family member instead.

10. A patient has had a traumatic amputation of the left leg above the knee following an industrial accident. What type of disability does this patient have?
    a. Chronic disability
    b. Impaired disability
    c. Developmental disability
    d. Acquired disability

CHAPTER 10

Principles and Practices of Rehabilitation

Learning Objectives

1. Describe the goals of rehabilitation.
2. Discuss the interdisciplinary approach to rehabilitation.
3. Describe components of a comprehensive assessment of functional capacity.
4. Use the nursing process as a framework for care of patients with self-care deficits, impaired physical mobility, impaired skin integrity, and altered patterns of elimination.
5. Describe the significance of continuity of care and community reentry from the health care facility to the home or extended care facility for patients who need rehabilitative assistance and services.

SECTION I: ASSESSING YOUR UNDERSTANDING

Activity A *Fill in the blanks.*

1. The initial sign of pressure is _____, which is caused by _____; unrelieved pressure results in _____ and _____.

2. Two areas that are the most susceptible to the effects of shear and therefore pressure ulcer formation are the _____ and the _____.

3. Four microorganisms that contribute to infection in pressure ulcers are: _____, _____, _____, and _____.

4. Serum albumin levels less than _____ increase the risk of pressure ulcers. Therefore, a protein intake of _____ is recommended to promote ulcer healing.

5. Two assessment scales that nurses can use to quantify a patient's risk for pressure ulcer formation are the _____ and _____ scales.

6. Two common musculoskeletal complications for patients who are in bed for prolonged periods are: _____ and _____.

7. Four factors that contribute to foot drop are _____, _____, _____, and _____.

8. To maintain use, a joint should be moved through its range of motion at least _____ times per day.

9. A life-threatening complication of a stage IV pressure ulcer is _____.

10. Alkaline-producing beverages such as

_____, _____,

_____, _____,

and _____ promote bacterial growth in the urine and should be avoided for patients who suffer from incontinence.

Activity B *Briefly answer the following.*

1. Name the three goals of rehabilitation.

_____

_____

2. List eight specialty rehabilitation programs accredited by the Commission for the Accreditation of Rehabilitation Facilities (CARF).

_____   _____

_____   _____

_____   _____

_____   _____

3. List five major goals for rehabilitation that are associated with the nursing diagnosis of self-care deficit in activities of daily living (ADL): bathing/hygiene, dressing/grooming, feeding, and toileting..

_____   _____

_____   _____

_____

4. Five nursing diagnoses for patients with impaired physical mobility could be

_____, _____,

_____, _____,

and _____.

Four major rehabilitative goals are

_____, _____,

_____, and _____.

5. List four collaborative problems for a patient with impaired physical mobility.

_____   _____

_____   _____

6. Name three complications commonly associated with prolonged or impaired physical immobility.

_____   _____

_____

7. List five types of therapeutic exercises and describe the nursing activity required to support the exercise.

Therapeutic Exercise   Nursing Activity

_____   _____

_____   _____

_____   _____

_____   _____

_____   _____

8. List 6 of 10 risk factors for pressure ulcer formation.

_____   _____

_____   _____

_____   _____

9. List 6 of a possible 12 areas susceptible to pressure ulcer formation.

_____   _____

_____   _____

_____   _____

10. Eschar covering an ulcer should be removed surgically for what reason?

_____

Activity C *Match the explanations of range-of-motion techniques listed in Column II with their associated terms in Column I.*

Column I

____ **1.** Adduction

____ **2.** Dorsiflexion

____ **3.** Extension

____ **4.** Inversion

____ **5.** Pronation

____ **6.** Abduction

Column II

a. Bending of the foot toward the leg

b. Increasing the angle of a joint

c. Movement away from the midline of the body

d. Movement that turns the sole of the foot inward

e. Movement toward the midline of the body

f. Rotating the forearm so that the palm is down

SECTION II: APPLYING YOUR KNOWLEDGE

Activity D *Consider the scenario and answer the questions.*

CASE STUDY: Assisted Ambulation: Crutches

Rita, a 17-year-old high school student, is in a full leg cast because of a compound fracture of the left femur. Rita is to be discharged from the hospital in several days.

1. What exercise can the nurse recommend to strengthen Rita's upper extremity muscles?

2. Rita is 5 ft 5 inches tall. When the nurse measures Rita's crutches, what should they measure?

3. Before teaching a crutch gait, the nurse directs Rita to assume the tripod position. In this basic crutch stance, the crutches are placed in front and to the side of Rita's toes. What should the approximate distance be?

4. Rita is not allowed to bear weight on her casted leg. What gait should the nurse educate her to use?

SECTION III: PRACTICING FOR NCLEX

Activity E *Answer the following questions.*

1. When is the optimal time for the nurse to begin the rehabilitation process for a patient with a cervical spine injury?
   a. After the patient feels comfortable in the clinical setting
   b. After the physician has prescribed rehabilitative goals
   c. When an exercise program has been initiated
   d. With initial patient contact

2. The nurse has developed an evidence-based plan of care for a patient requiring rehabilitation after a total hip replacement. Ultimately, who should approve the plan of care?
   a. The physician
   b. The patient
   c. The physical therapist
   d. The nurse

3. A patient in rehabilitation has become dependent on family members' assistance with self-care. What can the nurse do to encourage the patient to become independent? (Select all that apply.)
   a. Motivate the patient to learn and accept responsibilities for self-care.
   b. Help the patient identify safe limits of independent activity.
   c. Educate the patient in how to perform self-care activities.
   d. Inform the patient that the family will continue to provide care if she won't try.
   e. Have the patient placed in a long-term care facility until able to perform self-care activities.

4. A patient who has a disability is attempting to gain employment via vocational rehabilitation. What should the nurse closely monitor in the patient with a disability attempting to seek employment?
   a. Substance abuse
   b. Cognitive ability
   c. Orientation level
   d. Self-care ability

5. The nurse is using a measurement tool to determine a patient's level of independence in activities of daily living, such as continence, toileting, transfers, and ambulation. What would be the appropriate tool for the nurse to use?
   a. Barthel Index
   b. Patient evaluation conference system
   c. The Pulses Profile
   d. The Braden Scale

6. What position should be avoided when positioning a patient in bed in order to decrease the incidence of musculoskeletal complications?

   a. Prone
   b. Semi-Fowler's
   c. Side-lying
   d. Dorsal

7. The nurse is assisting a patient in assuming a side-lying position. What intervention would be best for the nurse to provide?

   a. Align the lower extremities in a neutral position.
   b. Extend the legs with a firm support under the popliteal area.
   c. Place the uppermost hip slightly forward in a position of slight abduction.
   d. Position the trunk so that hip flexion is minimized.

8. The nurse is fitting a patient for crutches that are required for an ankle injury. What quick method can the nurse use to measure so that the crutches will be of appropriate height?

   a. Use the patient's height and add 6 inches.
   b. Use the patient's height and add 12 inches.
   c. Use the patient's height and subtract 8 inches.
   d. Use the patient's height and subtract 16 inches.

9. How can the nurse prevent continuous moisture on the skin of a patient who is at risk for developing skin breakdown?

   a. Apply powder.
   b. Place an indwelling catheter in the patient.
   c. Administer vitamin B_{12} to the patient.
   d. Practice meticulous hygiene measures.

10. The nurse assesses initial skin redness in a patient who is at risk for skin breakdown. How should the nurse document this finding?

    a. Anoxia
    b. Eschar
    c. Hyperemia
    d. Ischemia

11. The nurse is assessing a patient at risk for the development of a pressure ulcer. What laboratory test will assist the nurse in determining this risk?

    a. Serum albumin
    b. Serum glucose
    c. Prothrombin time
    d. Sedimentation rate

12. What diet can the nurse recommend to a patient with hypoproteinemia that spares protein?

    a. A diet high in carbohydrates
    b. A diet high in fats
    c. A diet high in minerals
    d. A diet high in vitamins

13. The nurse is initiating a bladder-training schedule for a patient. What intervention can be provided for optimal success? (Select all that apply.)

    a. Encourage the patient to wait 30 minutes after drinking a measured amount of fluid before attempting to void.
    b. Give up to 3,000 mL of fluid daily.
    c. Teach bladder massage to increase intra-abdominal pressure.
    d. Require the patient to restrict fluid intake during the day to decrease voiding.
    e. Administer a diuretic every morning.

14. The nurse is developing a bowel training program for a patient. What education can the nurse provide for the patient that will increase the chance of success of the bowel program? (Select all that apply.)

    a. Set a daily defecation time that is within 15 minutes of the same time every day.
    b. Have an adequate intake of fiber-containing foods.
    c. Have a fluid intake between 2 and 4 L/day.
    d. Take a retention enema daily.
    e. Take a laxative daily.

Health Care of the Older Adult

Learning Objectives

1. Describe the demographic trends and the physiologic aspects of aging in older adults in the United States.
2. Describe the significance of preventive health care and health promotion for the older adult.
3. Compare and contrast the common physical and mental health problems of aging and their effects on the functioning of older people and their families.
4. Identify the role of the nurse in meeting the health care needs, including medication therapy, of the older patient.
5. Examine the concerns of older people and their families in the home and community, in the acute care setting, and in the long-term care facility.
6. Discuss the potential economic effect on health care of the large aging population in the United States.

SECTION I: ASSESSING YOUR UNDERSTANDING

Activity A *Fill in the blanks.*

1. Bone changes associated with aging frequently result from a loss of _____.

2. The primary cause of age-related vision loss in the elderly is _____.

3. With aging, there is a gradual decline in _____ and _____; _____ skills tend to remain intact.

4. _____ is the most common affective or mood disorder of old age.

5. _____ are the leading cause of injury in the elderly.

6. _____, the primary source of federal funding, provides nursing home care for the elderly poor.

Activity B *Briefly answer the following.*

1. Define the term *geriatric syndromes*.

_____

_____

2. Age-related changes reduce the efficiency of the cardiovascular system. These changes include _____, _____, _____, and _____, which result in _____.

3. Name two age-related alterations in metabolism.

_____

_____

4. List the five most common infections in the elderly: _____, _____, _____, _____, and _____.

5. Describe the concept of *continuing care retirement communities.*

_____

_____

_____

6. What nursing interventions can be used to help older adults with learning and memory?

_____

_____

7. Determine what nursing interventions can be used to help patients manage their medications and improve compliance.

_____

_____

_____

8. What are the differences between delirium and dementia with regard to clinical manifestations?

_____

_____

_____

9. What is the purpose of the Older Americans Act, and what services does it provide to the elderly?

_____

_____

_____

10. What is the difference between Medicare and Medicaid?

_____

_____

11. What is the purpose of a living will and a durable power of attorney, and what are their limitations?

_____

_____

12. Describe the Patient Self-Determination Act (PSDA).

_____

_____

_____

SECTION II: APPLYING YOUR KNOWLEDGE

Activity C *Consider the scenarios and answer the questions.*

CASE STUDY: Loneliness

Suzanne is an 80-year-old retired schoolteacher. She was recently widowed and lives alone. She is financially secure but socially isolated, because she has outlived most of her friends. Her children are self-sufficient and are very busy with their own lives.

1. What psychological threats may Suzanne experience?

_____

_____

2. Suzanne is concerned about the dryness of her skin. What suggestions can the nurse make for care of her skin?

_____

_____

3. Suzanne notices that food does not taste the same as before. What does she need to be aware that this sensory change is probably related to?

_____

_____

4. An analysis of Suzanne's diet shows that it does not contain adequate protein. For a body weight of 134 lb, what should her daily protein intake be?

_____

_____

5. Most accidents among older people involve falls within the home. What preventive measures can the nurse advise Suzanne to take?

_____

_____

CASE STUDY: Alzheimer's Disease

Thomas, a 75-year-old retired bricklayer, lives at home with Anne, his 65-year-old wife, who is healthy and active. Lately Anne has noticed that Thomas is negative, hostile, and suspicious of her. He gets lost in his own home, and his conversations have been accompanied by forgetfulness. Recently, Thomas's physician has indicated a probable diagnosis of Alzheimer's disease.

1. What can the nurse suggest to help Anne deal with Thomas's behavior?

_____

_____

2. What is an important point for the nurse to communicate to Anne?

_____

_____

3. What can the nurse make patient caregivers aware of?

_____

_____

4. The physician explains that there is no cure for the disease and no way to slow its progression, which intensifies symptoms. What complications should the family be aware of that are the cause of death in patients with Alzheimer's?

_____

_____

CASE STUDY: Dehydration

Vera, an 89-year-old widow, was transferred from a nursing home to a hospital with a diagnosis of dehydration. Vera needs to be in bed because of her generalized weakness. She is occasionally confused and disoriented.

1. What interventions should the nurse provide to ensure adequate temperature regulation?

_____

_____

2. Vera has been incontinent of urine since admission. What nursing intervention would be important for the nurse to provide?

_____

_____

3. The nurse suggests that Vera sit in a rocking chair for 20 minutes, four times a day. Why does the nurse suggest this for her?

_____

_____

SECTION III: PRACTICING FOR NCLEX

Activity D *Answer the following questions.*

1. The nurse is working in a long-term care facility. When assessing her patients, what body system dysfunction should the nurse look for as the leading cause of morbidity and mortality in the older adult population?
   a. Cardiovascular
   b. Genitourinary
   c. Gastrointestinal
   d. Respiratory

2. When performing a respiratory assessment on an older adult patient, what changes associated with aging does the nurse expect to find? (Select all that apply.)
   a. Increased residual volume
   b. Decreased residual volume
   c. Loss of elastic tissue surrounding the alveoli
   d. Reduced vital capacity
   e. Decreased pulmonary resistance

3. The nurse is assessing the genitourinary status of an older adult female patient who is experiencing stress incontinence. What finding is a common gerontologic finding for this population?
   a. Bladder capacity decreases with advanced age.
   b. All patients develop urinary tract infections.
   c. Renal filtration rate increases.
   d. Urine is more dilute in the older population.

4. The nurse is assisting an older adult patient with dietary planning. The nurse emphasizes the importance of adequate intake of fruits, vegetables, and fish. What should the patient's daily carbohydrate intake be?
   a. 20% to 25%
   b. 40% to 45%
   c. 55% to 60%
   d. 70% to 75%

5. The patient asks the nurse why she seems to have bone changes since she has gotten older. What is the best response by the nurse?

   a. "Bone changes from aging result from a loss of calcium."

   b. "Bone changes from aging result from a loss of magnesium."

   c. "Bone changes from aging result from a loss of vitamin A."

   d. "Bone changes from aging result from a loss of vitamin C."

6. When administering medications to an older adult patient, which medication does the nurse understand may remain in the body longer due to increased body fat?

   a. Anticoagulants

   b. Barbiturates

   c. Digitalis glycosides

   d. Diuretics

7. An older adult female patient informs the nurse that she is sexually active but has a problem with vaginal dryness. What can the nurse tell the patient that may help relieve this problem?

   a. Use vaginal douche daily.

   b. Use Monistat vaginal cream to treat the fungal infection she probably has.

   c. Use a water-based lubricant with sexual intercourse.

   d. Find other methods of sexual expression.

8. An older adult female patient tells the nurse, "I have lost an inch of height and have a hump on my back. What can I do about this?" What is the best response by the nurse?

   a. "In order to prevent further bone loss, eat a diet high in calcium and low in phosphorus."

   b. "In order to prevent further bone loss, eat a diet high in magnesium and high in phosphorus."

   c. "You can reverse the bone loss with surgical intervention."

   d. "Supplement your diet with a multivitamin."

9. An older adult male patient tells the nurse that he wakes several times a night to pass his urine but never feels as though he fully empties his bladder. What suggestion can the nurse make to help control this in the evening?

   a. Drink several glasses of fluid prior to going to bed in the evening to dilute the urine.

   b. He probably has developed a urinary tract infection and requires an antibiotic.

   c. Limit drinking a lot of fluid in the evening, especially caffeinated beverages.

   d. Wear a condom catheter at night so that he will not have to get up so much.

10. The nurse brings the older adult patient a dinner tray and observes the patient placing excess amounts of salt on the food. What suggestions for flavoring can the nurse provide to decrease the amount of salt the patient is placing on her food? (Select all that apply.)

    a. Drink water before the meal.

    b. Use low-sodium herbs and spices.

    c. Use an alcohol-based mouthwash prior to eating.

    d. Use pepper instead of salt.

    e. Use lemon instead of salt to flavor food.

Concepts and Challenges in Patient Management

CHAPTER 12

Pain Management

Learning Objectives

1. Identify the fundamental concepts of pain.
2. Distinguish between the types of pain.
3. Describe the four processes of nociception.
4. Explain underlying mechanisms of neuropathic pain.
5. Identify methods to perform a pain assessment.
6. List the first-line analgesic agents from the three groups of analgesic agents.
7. Identify the effects of select analgesic agents on older adults.
8. Identify practical nonpharmacologic methods that can be used in the clinical setting in patients with pain.
9. Use the nursing process as a framework for the care of patients with pain.

SECTION I: ASSESSING YOUR UNDERSTANDING

Activity A *Fill in the blanks.*

1. Pain can be defined according to its _____, _____, and _____.

2. _____, _____, and _____ are the three basic categories of pain.

3. A person's reported intensity of pain is determined by an individual's _____ (the smallest stimulus where pain is felt) and _____ (the maximum amount of pain a person can tolerate).

4. Although the criterion is arbitrary, acute pain can be classified as chronic when it has persisted for _____.

5. After administration of an epidural opioid, the nurse needs to assess for _____, which may occur up to _____ hours but usually peaks between _____ hours.

6. A chemical substance thought to inhibit the transmission of pain is _____.

Activity B *Briefly answer the following.*

1. Pain can be categorized by its etiology. List four of eight pain syndromes.

   _____

   _____

2. Name one pathophysiologic response to chronic pain.

   _____

3. List five algogenic substances that are released into the tissues and affect the sensitivity of nociceptors: _____, _____, _____, _____, and _____.

4. List seven factors that directly influence an individual's response to pain: _____, _____, _____, _____, _____, _____, and _____.

5. Identify seven factors that a nurse needs to consider for complete pain assessment:

   _____, _____,

   _____, _____,

   _____, _____,

   and _____.

6. List eight common physiologic responses to pain: _____, _____, _____, _____, _____, _____, _____, and _____.

7. Define the term *balanced analgesia.*

_____

_____

8. Define the term *placebo effect.*

_____

_____

9. List four nonpharmacologic interventions for pain management: _____, _____, _____, and _____.

10. Distinguish among acute, chronic (persistent, nonmalignant), and cancer-related pain and cite an example of each.

_____

_____

11. What pain management strategies may be used for those at the end of their life?

_____

_____

12. Compare and contrast the precautions and contraindications for the following opioids.

	Precautions	Contraindications
Morphine		
Codeine		
Oxycodone		
Demerol		
Darvon		
Vicodin		

13. What are the nursing responsibilities for management of patient-controlled analgesia?

_____

_____

14. How does the technique of *distraction* work to relieve acute and chronic pain?

_____

_____

Activity C *Match the term listed in Column II with its definition in Column I.*

Column I

____ **1.** Pain receptors sensitive to noxious stimuli.

____ **2.** Nonsteroidal agents that decrease inflammation.

____ **3.** The only commercially available transdermal opioid medication.

____ **4.** Significantly increases a person's response to pain.

____ **5.** Chemicals known to inhibit the transmission or perception of pain.

____ **6.** This substance, released in response to painful stimuli, causes vasodilation.

____ **7.** An inactive substance given in place of pain medication.

____ **8.** Medication administered directly into the subarachnoid space and cerebrospinal fluid.

____ **9.** Transcutaneous stimulation of nonpain receptors in the same area of an injury.

____ **10.** Term used to describe a pain's rhythm.

Column II

a. Fentanyl
b. Endorphins
c. Placebo
d. Waning
e. TENS
f. Nociceptors
g. Histamine
h. Anxiety
i. Epidural
j. NSAIDS

SECTION II: APPLYING YOUR KNOWLEDGE

Activity D *Consider the scenario and answer the questions.*

CASE STUDY: Pain Experience

Courtney is a young, healthy adult who slipped off the stairs going down to the basement and struck her forehead on the cement flooring. Courtney did not lose consciousness but did sustain a mild concussion and a hematoma that was 5 cm in width and protruded outward about 6 cm. She experienced immediate acute pain at the site of injury plus a pounding headache.

1. After an immediate assessment of the localized pain, based on the patient's description, what does the nurse predict about the pain?

   _____

2. During the assessment process, the nurse attempts to determine Courtney's physiologic and behavioral responses to her pain experience. The nurse is aware that a patient can be in pain yet appear to be "pain free." What is a behavioral response indicative of acute pain?

   _____

3. The nurse uses distraction to help Courtney cope with her pain experience. What suggested activities can help her cope?

   _____

   _____

4. After treatment, Courtney is discharged to home while still in pain. What should the nurse do?

   _____

   _____

SECTION III: PRACTICING FOR NCLEX

Activity E *Answer the following questions.*

1. A patient slipped and fell on the floor in the hospital room, which caused a back injury, and the patient now complains of pain. How can the nurse determine that the pain is characteristic of acute pain?
   a. It does not respond well to treatment.
   b. It is associated with a specific injury.
   c. It serves no useful purpose.
   d. It responds well to placebos.

2. The nurse is caring for a patient who has been hospitalized on several occasions for lower abdominal pain related to Crohn's disease. How may this chronic pain be described?
   a. Attributable to a specific cause
   b. Prolonged in duration
   c. Rapidly occurring and subsiding with treatment
   d. Separate from any central or peripheral pathology

3. A patient comes into the clinic frequently with complaints of pain. What would the nurse recognize as chronic benign pain in a patient?
   a. A migraine headache
   b. An exacerbation of rheumatoid arthritis
   c. Low back pain
   d. Sickle cell crisis

4. When the nurse is performing an assessment and finds no physical cause for a patient's pain, what should the nurse do when the patient continues to complain of pain?
   a. Believe a patient when he or she states that pain is present.
   b. Doubt that pain exists when no physical origin can be identified.
   c. Realize that patients frequently imagine and state that they have pain without actually feeling painful sensations.
   d. Assume that the patient may be a drug seeker and should be given other methods for pain control.

5. When a nurse asks a patient to describe the quality of the pain, what type of descriptive term does the nurse expect the patient to use?

   a. Burning

   b. Chronic

   c. Intermittent

   d. Severe

6. The nurse is assessing a patient complaining of severe pain. What physiologic indicator does the nurse recognize as significant of acute pain?

   a. Diaphoresis

   b. Bradycardia

   c. Hypotension

   d. Decreased respiratory rate

7. The nurse is assessing an older adult patient just admitted to the hospital. Why is it important that the nurse carefully assess pain in the older adult patient?

   a. Older people are expected to experience chronic pain.

   b. Older people have a decreased pain threshold.

   c. Older people experience reduced sensory perception.

   d. Older people have increased sensory perception.

8. The nurse is administering an analgesic to an older adult patient. Why is it important for the nurse to assess the patient carefully?

   a. Older people metabolize drugs more rapidly.

   b. Older people have increased hepatic, renal, and gastrointestinal function.

   c. Older people are more sensitive to drugs.

   d. Older people have lower ratios of body fat and muscle mass.

9. The nurse administers an opioid analgesic to a patient. What serious side effect should the nurse carefully monitor for?

   a. Renal toxicity

   b. Respiratory depression

   c. Seizure activity

   d. Hypertension

10. The nurse informs the patient that a preventive approach for pain relief will be used, involving nonsteroidal anti-inflammatory drugs. What will this mean for the patient?

    a. The pain medication will be administered before the pain becomes severe.

    b. The pain medication will be administered before the pain is experienced.

    c. The pain medication will be administered when the pain is at its peak.

    d. The pain medication will be administered when the level of pain tolerance has been exceeded.

11. The nurse's major area of assessment for a patient receiving patient-controlled analgesia is assessment of what system?

    a. Cardiovascular

    b. Integumentary

    c. Neurologic

    d. Respiratory

12. What does the nurse understand is the advantage of using intraspinal infusion to deliver analgesics? (Select all that apply.)

    a. It is easily accessible by the nurse.

    b. Higher doses may be administered.

    c. Side effects of systemic analgesia are reduced.

    d. Effects on pulse, respirations, and blood pressure are reduced.

    e. The need for injections decreases in frequency.

13. The nurse observes the anesthesiologist administer a single-dose, extended-release drug in an epidural catheter for a patient undergoing a major surgical procedure. What drug does she understand is being administered?

    a. Codeine

    b. Demerol

    c. Dilaudid

    d. Depodur

14. The nurse is assisting the anesthesiologist with the insertion of an epidural catheter and the administration of an epidural opioid for pain control. What adverse effect of epidural opioids should the nurse monitor for?

   a. Asystole

   b. Hypertension

   c. Bradypnea

   d. Tachycardia

15. Prior to starting a peripheral intravenous line on a patient, what intervention can the nurse provide to decrease the pain from the needle puncture?

   a. Give an oral opioid analgesic 30 minutes before the procedure.

   b. Apply diclofenac gel over the site 1 hour before the procedure.

   c. Apply eutectic mixture of local anesthetic cream 30 minutes prior to the procedure.

   d. Inject lidocaine 2% with epinephrine locally around the potential procedure site.

16. What medication can the nurse administer to the patient intravenously for the control of pain and fever?

   a. Lortab

   b. Percocet

   c. Dilaudid

   d. Ofirmev

17. The physician has ordered a mu opioid analgesic for a patient with pain. What drug does the nurse anticipate administering?

   a. Nubain

   b. Stadol

   c. Buprenex

   d. Fentanyl

18. The patient develops respiratory depression after the nurse administers fentanyl for pain. What medication can the nurse anticipate administering to counteract the effects of the fentanyl?

   a. Nubain

   b. Morphine

   c. Narcan

   d. Lidocaine

19. The nurse applies a transdermal patch of fentanyl for a patient with pain due to cancer of the pancreas. The patient puts the call light on 1 hour later and tells the nurse that it has not helped. What is the best response by the nurse?

   a. "It will take approximately 12 to 18 hours for the medication to begin to work, so I will give you something else now to relieve the pain."

   b. "It should have begun working 30 minutes ago. I will call the doctor and let him know you need something stronger."

   c. "You have probably developed a tolerance to the medication."

   d. "It will take about 24 hours for the medication to work. I can't give you anything else or you will overdose."

CHAPTER 13

Fluid and Electrolytes: Balance and Disturbance

1. Differentiate between osmosis, diffusion, filtration, and active transport.
2. Describe the role of the kidneys, lungs, and endocrine glands in regulating the body's fluid composition and volume.
3. Identify the effects of aging on fluid and electrolyte regulation.
4. Plan effective care of patients with the following imbalances: fluid volume deficit and fluid volume excess, sodium deficit (hyponatremia) and sodium excess (hypernatremia), and potassium deficit (hypokalemia) and potassium excess (hyperkalemia).
5. Describe the cause, clinical manifestations, management, and nursing interventions for the following imbalances: calcium deficit (hypocalcemia) and calcium excess (hypercalcemia), magnesium deficit (hypomagnesemia) and magnesium excess (hypermagnesemia), phosphorus deficit (hypophosphatemia) and phosphorus excess (hyperphosphatemia), and chloride deficit (hypochloremia) and chloride excess (hyperchloremia).
6. Explain the roles of the lungs, kidneys, and chemical buffers in maintaining acid–base balance.
7. Compare metabolic acidosis and alkalosis with regard to causes, clinical manifestations, diagnosis, and management.

8. Compare respiratory acidosis and alkalosis with regard to causes, clinical manifestations, diagnosis, and management.
9. Interpret arterial blood gas measurements.
10. Identify a safe and effective procedure of venipuncture.
11. Describe measures used for preventing complications of intravenous therapy.

SECTION I: ASSESSING YOUR UNDERSTANDING

Activity A *Fill in the blanks.*

1. About _____% of total body fluid is in the intracellular space; the major positively charged ion in intracellular fluid is _____. The extracellular space is divided into three compartments: _____, _____, and _____; the major positively charged ion in extracellular fluid is _____. About _____% of the _____ L of total blood volume is _____.

2. The primary concentration of phosphorus (85%) is located in the _____, with about 15% located in _____.

3. The normal blood pH is _____.

4. The upper and lower blood pH levels that are incompatible with life are _____ and _____.

5. The average daily urinary output in an adult is _____ L.

6. Cardiac effects of hyperkalemia are usually present when the serum potassium level reaches _____ mEq/L.

7. A normal oxygen saturation value for arterial blood is _____.

8. Sodium, the most abundant electrolyte in extracellular fluid, is primarily responsible for maintaining fluid _____, which _____.

9. Sodium is regulated by _____, _____, and the _____ system.

10. Sodium establishes the electrochemical state necessary for _____ and the _____.

11. The most common buffer system in the body is the _____.

12. The most characteristic manifestations of hypocalcemia and hypomagnesemia is _____.

Activity B *Briefly answer the following.*

PART 1

1. Define the term *osmotic pressure*.

   _____

   _____

2. Distinguish between the terms *urine specific gravity, blood urea nitrogen,* and *creatinine*.

   _____

   _____

3. Distinguish between the terms *baroreceptors* and *osmoreceptors*.

   _____

   _____

4. How are calcium levels regulated?

   _____

   _____

5. Name the primary complication of hyperphosphatemia which occurs when the calcium–magnesium product exceeds 70 mg/dL.

   _____

   _____

6. Write the mathematical formula that a nurse would use to approximate the value of serum osmolality.

   _____

7. Explain why the administration of a 3% to 5% sodium chloride solution requires intense monitoring.

   _____

   _____

8. List four of six symptoms associated with air embolism, a complication of intravenous therapy.

   _____

   _____

PART II

1. Indicate which of the following factors contribute to *hyponatremia* by writing "Low" in the space provided, and indicate which contribute to *hypernatremia* by writing "High" in the space provided.

   a. _____ vomiting

   b. _____ diarrhea

   c. _____ watery diarrhea

   d. _____ inability to quench thirst

   e. _____ burns over a large surface area

   f. _____ diuretics

   g. _____ heat stroke

   h. _____ adrenal insufficiency

   i. _____ syndrome of inappropriate antidiuretic hormone

   j. _____ status post-therapeutic abortion

   k. _____ diabetes insipidus with water restriction

   l. _____ excessive parenteral administration of dextrose and water solution

2. Indicate which of the following factors contribute to *hypokalemia* by writing "Low" in the space provided, and indicate which contribute to *hyperkalemia* by writing "High" in the space provided.

   a. _____ alkalosis

   b. _____ tourniquet too tight when collecting a blood sample

   c. _____ vomiting

   d. _____ gastric suction

   e. _____ leukocytosis

   f. _____ anorexia nervosa

   g. _____ hyperaldosteronism

   h. _____ furosemide (Lasix) administration

   i. _____ steroid administration

   j. _____ kidney failure

   k. _____ penicillin administration

   l. _____ adrenal steroid deficiency

3. Indicate which of the following factors contribute to *hypocalcemia* by writing "Low" in the space provided, and indicate which contribute to *hypercalcemia* by writing "High" in the space provided.

   a. _____ hyperparathyroidism

   b. _____ massive administration of citrated blood

   c. _____ malignant tumors

   d. _____ immobilization because of multiple fractures

   e. _____ pancreatitis

   f. _____ thiazide diuretics

   g. _____ kidney failure

   h. _____ aminoglycoside administration

4. Indicate which of the following factors contribute to *hypomagnesemia* by writing "Low" in the space provided, and indicate which contribute to *hypermagnesemia* by writing "High" in the space provided.

   a. _____ alcohol abuse

   b. _____ kidney failure

   c. _____ diarrhea

   d. _____ gentamicin administration

   e. _____ untreated ketoacidosis

5. Indicate which of the following factors contribute to *hypophosphatemia* by writing "Low" in the space provided, and indicate which contribute to *hyperphosphatemia* by writing "High" in the space provided.

   a. _____ hyperparathyroidism

   b. _____ kidney failure

   c. _____ major thermal burns

   d. _____ alcohol withdrawal

   e. _____ neoplastic disease chemotherapy

6. For each of the following factors, indicate the probable cause by writing "M-ACID" for metabolic acidosis, "M-ALKA" for metabolic alkalosis, "R-ACID" for respiratory acidosis, or "R-ALKA" for respiratory alkalosis.

   a. _____ sedative overdose

   b. _____ lactic acidosis

   c. _____ ketoacidosis

   d. _____ severe pneumonia

   e. _____ hypoxemia

   f. _____ acute pulmonary edema

   g. _____ diarrhea

   h. _____ vomiting

   i. _____ hypokalemia

   j. _____ gram-negative bacterial infection

Activity C *Correlate the associations between body fluid compartments. Match the fluid space in Column II with an associated factor in Column I.*

Column I	Column II
____ 1. Third space fluid shift	a. Intracellular space
____ 2. The smallest compartment of the extracellular fluid space	b. Extracellular fluid compartment
____ 3. Space where plasma is contained	c. Intravascular space
____ 4. Comprises the intravascular, interstitial, and transcellular fluid	d. Transcellular space
____ 5. Comprises about 60% of body fluid	e. Interstitial space
____ 6. Comprises fluid surrounding cell	f. Intravascular fluid volume deficit

SECTION II: APPLYING YOUR KNOWLEDGE

Activity D *Consider the scenarios and answer the questions.*

CASE STUDY: Extracellular Fluid Volume Deficit

Harriet, 30 years old, has been admitted to the burn treatment center with full-thickness burns over 30% of her upper body. Her diagnosis is consistent with extracellular fluid volume deficit (FVD).

1. What symptom would indicate to the nurse that the patient may be experiencing an FVD?

2. What should the nursing plan of care for Harriet include that would indicate to the nurse that there may be an FVD?

3. What interventions provided by the nurse would be appropriate for this patient?

CASE STUDY: Congestive Heart Failure

George, 88 years old, is suffering from congestive heart failure. He was admitted to the hospital with a diagnosis of extracellular fluid volume excess. He was frightened, slightly confused, and dyspneic on exertion.

1. What symptoms does the nurse expect to find when performing the assessment on this patient?

2. What manifestation of extracellular fluid volume excess does the nurse anticipate finding?

3. When developing a plan of care for the patient, what interventions should the nurse be sure to include?

CASE STUDY: Diabetes

Isaac, 63 years old, was admitted to the hospital with a diagnosis of diabetes. On his admission, the nurse observed rapid respirations, confusion, and signs of dehydration.

1. Isaac's arterial blood gas values are pH, 7.27; HCO_3, 20 mEq/L; PaO_2, 33 mm Hg. The nurse understands that the patient is compensating at this time. What do the blood gas results indicate for this patient?

2. What does the nurse recognize are the manifestations associated with an alteration in acid–base balance?

3. In terms of cellular buffering response, what should the nurse expect the major electrolyte disturbance to be?

4. What prescribed intravenous medication does the nurse anticipate administering to correct the acid–base imbalance?

CASE STUDY: Intravenous Therapy

Jill, an 84-year-old woman, was admitted to the hospital for treatment for dehydration. The physician immediately ordered intravenous therapy, 1,000 mL of D5 W, q8h.

1. The nurse understands that, when administering intravenous (IV) fluids to this patient, monitoring for complications is included in the plan of care. What systemic complications should the nurse monitor for in the patient?

2. After several attempts to obtain a peripheral IV site, the nurse requests that a central vein be accessed by the physician. Which vein does the nurse anticipate the physician will cannulate?

3. The nurse is determining the flow rate of the IV fluids. What would be the correct way for her to calculate the flow rate?

SECTION III: PRACTICING FOR NCLEX

Activity E *Answer the following questions.*

1. The nurse should assess the patient for signs of lethargy, increasing intracranial pressure, and seizures when the serum sodium reaches what level?

   a. 115 mEq/L

   b. 130 mEq/L

   c. 145 mEq/L

   d. 160 mEq/L

2. In a patient with excess fluid volume, hyponatremia is treated by restricting fluids to how many milliliters in 24 hours?

   a. 400

   b. 600

   c. 800

   d. 1,200

3. A patient who is semiconscious presents with restlessness and weakness. The nurse assesses a dry, swollen tongue and a body temperature of 99.3°F. The urine specific gravity is 1.020. What is the most likely serum sodium value for this patient?

   a. 110 mEq/L

   b. 140 mEq/L

   c. 155 mEq/L

   d. 165 mEq/L

4. A patient's serum sodium concentration is within the normal range. What should the nurse estimate the serum osmolality to be?

   a. <136 mOsm/kg

   b. 275–300 mOsm/kg

   c. >408 mOsm/kg

   d. 350–544 mOsm/kg

5. With which condition should the nurse expect that a decrease in serum osmolality will occur?

   a. Diabetes insipidus

   b. Hyperglycemia

   c. Kidney failure

   d. Uremia

6. The nurse notes that a patient's urine osmolality is 980 mOsm/kg. What should the nurse assess as a possible cause of this finding?

   a. Acidosis

   b. Fluid volume excess

   c. Diabetes insipidus

   d. Hyponatremia

7. What does the nurse recognize as one of the indicators of the patient's renal function?

   a. Blood urea nitrogen

   b. Serum creatinine

   c. Specific gravity

   d. Urine osmolality

8. A patient has been involved in a traumatic accident and is hemorrhaging from multiple sites. The nurse expects that the compensatory mechanisms associated with hypovolemia would cause what clinical manifestations? (Select all that apply.)

   a. Hypertension

   b. Oliguria

   c. Tachycardia

   d. Bradycardia

   e. Tachypnea

9. What laboratory findings does the nurse determine are consistent with hypovolemia in a female patient? (Select all that apply.)

   a. Hematocrit level of >47%

   b. BUN: serum creatinine ratio of >12.1

   c. Urine specific gravity of 1.027

   d. Urine osmolality of >450 mOsm/kg

   e. Urine positive for blood

10. A patient with mild fluid volume excess is prescribed a diuretic that blocks sodium reabsorption in the distal tubule. Which diuretic does the nurse anticipate administering to this patient?

    a. Bumex

    b. Demadex

    c. HydroDiuril

    d. Lasix

11. The nurse is caring for a patient with a diagnosis of hyponatremia. What nursing intervention is appropriate to include in the plan of care for this patient? (Select all that apply.)
    a. Assessing for symptoms of nausea and malaise
    b. Encouraging the intake of low-sodium liquids
    c. Monitoring neurologic status
    d. Restricting tap water intake
    e. Encouraging the use of salt substitute instead of salt

12. A patient with abnormal sodium losses is receiving a regular diet. How can the nurse supplement the patient's diet to provide 1,600 mg of sodium daily?
    a. One beef cube and 8 oz of tomato juice
    b. Four beef cubes and 8 oz of tomato juice
    c. One beef cube and 16 oz of tomato juice
    d. One beef cube and 12 oz of tomato juice

13. The nurse is caring for a patient with hypernatremia. What complication of hypernatremia should the nurse continuously monitor for?
    a. Red blood cell crenation
    b. Red blood cell hydrolysis
    c. Cerebral edema
    d. Renal failure

14. The physician has prescribed a hypotonic IV solution for a patient. Which IV solution should the nurse administer?
    a. 0.45% sodium chloride
    b. 0.90% sodium chloride
    c. 5% dextrose in water
    d. 5% dextrose in normal saline solution

15. A patient is admitted with severe vomiting for 24 hours as well as weakness and "feeling exhausted." The nurse observes flat T waves and ST-segment depression on the electrocardiogram. Which potassium level does the nurse observe when the laboratory studies are complete?
    a. 4.0 mEq/L
    b. 8.0 mEq/L
    c. 2.0 mEq/L
    d. 2.6 mEq/L

16. What foods can the nurse recommend for the patient with hypokalemia?
    a. Fruits such as bananas and apricots
    b. Green, leafy vegetables
    c. Milk and yogurt
    d. Nuts and legumes

17. Which medication does the nurse anticipate administering to antagonize the effects of potassium on the heart for a patient in severe metabolic acidosis?
    a. Sodium bicarbonate
    b. Magnesium sulfate
    c. Furosemide (Lasix)
    d. Calcium gluconate

18. A patient complains of tingling in the fingers as well as feeling depressed. The nurse assesses positive Trousseau's and Chvostek's signs. Which decreased laboratory results does the nurse observe when the patient's laboratory work has returned?
    a. Potassium
    b. Phosphorus
    c. Calcium
    d. Magnesium

19. A patient is admitted with a diagnosis of renal failure. The patient complains of "stomach distress" and describes ingesting several antacid tablets over the past 2 days. Blood pressure is 110/70 mm Hg, face is flushed, and the patient is experiencing generalized weakness. Which is the most likely magnesium level associated with the symptoms the patient is having?
    a. 11 mEq/L
    b. 5 mEq/L
    c. 2 mEq/L
    d. 1 mEq/L

20. What clinical indication of hypophosphate-mia does the nurse assess in a patient?

a. Bone pain

b. Paresthesia

c. Seizures

d. Tetany

21. The nurse is caring for a patient with diabetes type I who is having severe vomiting and diarrhea. What condition that exhibits blood values with a low pH and a low plasma bicarbonate concentration should the nurse assess for?

a. Respiratory acidosis

b. Respiratory alkalosis

c. Metabolic acidosis

d. Metabolic alkalosis

14

Shock and Multiple Organ Dysfunction Syndrome

Learning Objectives

1. Describe shock and its underlying pathophysiology.
2. Compare clinical findings of the compensatory, progressive, and irreversible stages of shock.
3. Describe organ dysfunction that may occur with shock.
4. Describe similarities and differences in shock due to hypovolemic, cardiogenic, neurogenic, anaphylactic, and septic shock states.
5. Identify medical and nursing management priorities in treating patients in shock.
6. Identify vasoactive medications used in treating shock, and describe nursing implications associated with their use.
7. Discuss the importance of nutritional support in all forms of shock.
8. Discuss the role of nurses in psychosocial support of patients experiencing shock and their families.
9. Discuss multiple organ dysfunction syndrome.

SECTION I: ASSESSING YOUR UNDERSTANDING

Activity A *Fill in the blanks.*

1. The basic, underlying characteristic of shock is _____, which results in _____, _____, _____, _____, and _____.

2. Energy metabolism occurs in the cells, where _____ is primarily responsible for cellular energy in the form of _____.

3. To maintain an adequate blood pressure, three components of the circulatory system must respond effectively: the _____, _____, and _____.

4. The formula for calculating cardiac output is: cardiac output is the product of _____ times _____. Peripheral resistance is determined by the _____.

5. Baroreceptors are located in the _____ and _____, whereas chemoreceptors are located in the _____ and _____.

6. With the progression of shock, damage at the _____ and _____ level occurs when the blood pressure drops.

7. Two crystalloids commonly used for fluid replacement in hypovolemic shock are: _____ and _____.

8. A new cardiac marker for ventricular dysfunction, _____, increases when the ventricle is overdistended. It is being used to assess the cardiovascular effects of shock.

Activity B *Briefly answer the following.*

1. Define the term *mean arterial pressure (MAP)*.

_____

_____

2. Name three medical management goals for cardiogenic shock.

_____

_____

3. Name the causes of circulatory shock.

_____

_____

4. Name the causes of neurogenic shock.

_____

_____

Activity C *Match the type of shock listed in Column II with its associated cause listed in Column I. Some answers may be used more than once.*

Column I

____ 1. Valvular damage

____ 2. Peritonitis

____ 3. Burns

____ 4. Bee sting allergy

____ 5. Immunosuppression

____ 6. Spinal cord injury

____ 7. Dysrhythmias

____ 8. Vomiting

____ 9. Pulmonary embolism

____ 10. Penicillin sensitivity

Column II

a. Hypovolemic, owing to an internal fluid shift

b. Hypovolemic, owing to an external fluid loss

c. Cardiogenic

d. Circulatory of a neurogenic nature

e. Circulatory of an anaphylactic nature

f. Circulatory of a septic nature

g. Noncoronary cardiogenic shock

SECTION II: APPLYING YOUR KNOWLEDGE

Activity D *Consider the scenarios and answer the questions.*

CASE STUDY: Hypovolemic Shock

Mr. Mazda is a 57-year-old, 154-lb (70-kg) patient who was received on the nursing unit from the recovery room after having a hemicolectomy for colon cancer. On initial assessment, Mr. Mazda was alert, yet anxious; his skin was cool, pale, and moist; and his abdominal dressings were saturated with bright red blood. Urinary output was 100 mL over 4 hours. The patient was receiving 1,000 mL of lactated Ringer's solution. Vital signs were blood pressure (BP), 80/60 mm Hg; heart rate, 126 beats per minute (bpm); and respirations 40 breaths/min (baseline vital signs were 130/70, 84, and 22, respectively). The nurse assessed that the patient was experiencing hypovolemic shock.

1. The nurse understands that hypovolemic shock will occur with an intravascular volume reduction of 15% to 30%. How much intravascular volume does the nurse determine that Mr. Mazda has lost?

_____

2. The nurse is assessing the patient for the signs of the compensatory stage of shock. What assessment data does the nurse determine is significant for the presence of compensatory shock?

_____

_____

3. The nurse is assessing Mr. Mazda's urinary output hourly. What level of output does the nurse know is indicative of decreased glomerular filtration?

_____

4. What type of fluids does the nurse anticipate administering to this patient?

_____

CASE STUDY: Septic Shock

Mr. Dressler, a 43-year-old Caucasian, was admitted to the medical–surgical unit on the third postoperative day after a vertical bonded gastroplasty for morbid obesity. He had initially transferred to the intensive care unit from the recovery room. Mr. Dressler had a normal postoperative recovery period until his first afternoon on the unit. A registered nurse went into his room to assess 4:00 PM vital signs and noted that his temperature was 102°F, his HR was >90 bpm, his respirations were >20 breaths/min, and his systolic BP was <90 mm Hg. He was shaking with chills, his skin was warm and dry, yet his extremities were cool to the touch. The nurse, assessing that Mr. Dressler was probably experiencing septicemia, immediately notified the physician.

1. The nurse believes that Mr. Dressler may be experiencing a systemic inflammatory response syndrome (SIRS). What does the nurse understand SIRS is?

_____

_____

2. Mr. Dressler's condition may advance to severe sepsis. What additional signs and symptoms should the nurse assess for?

_____

_____

3. The nurse expects that the physician will request body fluid specimens for culture and sensitivity tests. What specimens should the nurse prepare to collect?

_____

_____

4. What common and serious side effects of fluid replacement should the nurse monitor for?

_____

_____

SECTION III: PRACTICING FOR NCLEX

Activity E *Answer the following questions.*

1. The nurse caring for the patient in shock recognizes which physiologic responses that are common to all shock states? (Select all that apply.)
   a. Increased intravascular volume
   b. Activation of the inflammatory response
   c. Hypoperfusion of tissues
   d. Must produce energy through aerobic metabolism
   e. Increase in cellular Activity

2. The nurse is calculating a patient's mean arterial pressure (MAP). What is the patient's MAP, if the blood pressure is 110/70 mm Hg?
   a. 65
   b. 73
   c. 83
   d. 91

3. The nurse is monitoring a patient in the compensatory stage of shock. What lab values does the nurse understand will elevate in response to the release of aldosterone and catecholamines?
   a. T3 and T4
   b. Myoglobin and CK-MB
   c. BUN and creatinine
   d. Sodium and glucose levels

4. The nurse obtains a blood pressure of 120/78 mm Hg from a patient in hypovolemic shock. Since the blood pressure is within normal range for this patient, what stage of shock does the nurse realize this patient is experiencing?
   a. Initial stage
   b. Compensatory stage
   c. Progressive stage
   d. Irreversible stage

5. What can the nurse include in the plan of care to ensure early intervention along the continuum of shock to improve the patient's prognosis? (Select all that apply.)
   a. Assess the patient who is at risk for shock.
   b. Administer vasoconstrictive medications to patients at risk for shock.
   c. Administer prophylactic packed red blood cells to patients at risk for shock.
   d. Administer intravenous fluids.
   e. Monitor for changes in vital signs.

6. The nurse assesses a patient in compensatory shock whose lungs have decompensated. What clinical manifestations would the nurse expect to find? (Select all that apply.)
   a. A heart rate >100 bpm
   b. Crackles
   c. Lethargy and mental confusion
   d. Respirations <15 breaths/min
   e. Compensatory respiratory acidosis

7. The nurse assesses a BP reading of 80/50 mm Hg from a patient in shock. What stage of shock does the nurse recognize the patient is in?
   a. Initial
   b. Compensatory
   c. Progressive
   d. Irreversible

8. The nurse determines that a patient in shock is experiencing a decrease in stroke volume when what clinical manifestation is observed?
   a. Increase in diastolic pressure
   b. Decrease in respiratory rate
   c. Increase in systolic blood pressure
   d. Narrowed pulse pressure

9. The nurse is using continuous central venous oximetry (ScvO$_2$) to monitor the blood oxygen saturation of a patient in shock. What value would the nurse document as normal for the patient?
   a. 40%
   b. 50%
   c. 60%
   d. 70%

10. A patient is in the progressive stage of shock with lung decompensation. What treatment does the nurse anticipate assisting with?
    a. Pericardiocentesis
    b. Thoracotomy with chest tube insertion
    c. Administration of oxygen via venture mask
    d. Intubation and mechanical ventilation

11. The nurse observes a patient in the progressive stage of shock with blood in the nasogastric tube and when connected to suction. What does the nurse understand could be occurring with this patient?
    a. The patient has developed a stress ulcer that is bleeding.
    b. The patient is having a reaction to the vasoconstricting medications.
    c. The patient has a tumor in the esophagus.
    d. The patient has bleeding esophageal varices.

12. When a patient in shock is receiving fluid replacement, what should the nurse monitor frequently? (Select all that apply.)
    a. Urinary output
    b. Mental status
    c. Vital signs
    d. Ability to perform range of motion exercises
    e. Visual acuity

13. The nurse is monitoring the patient in shock. The patient begins bleeding from previous venipuncture sites, in the indwelling catheter, and rectum, and the nurse observes multiple areas of ecchymosis. What does the nurse suspect has developed in this patient?
    a. Stress ulcer
    b. Disseminated intravascular coagulation (DIC)
    c. Septicemia
    d. Stevens-Johnson syndrome from the administration of antibiotics

14. The nurse receives an order to administer a colloidal solution for a patient experiencing hypovolemic shock. What common colloidal solution will the nurse most likely administer?
    a. Blood products
    b. 5% albumin
    c. 6% dextran
    d. 6% hetastarch

15. The nurse is performing glucose checks for sliding scale four times per day for a patient in the progressive stage of shock. What glucose range would the nurse expect to see for the best outcomes in this patient?

  a. 100–120 mg/dL

  b. 120–140 mg/dL

  c. 140–180 mg/dL

  d. 160–190 mg/dL

16. A patient is in the irreversible state of shock and is unresponsive. The family requests to stay with the patient during this time. What is the best response by the nurse?

  a. "You don't want to remember your family member this way."

  b. "We have specific visiting hours that must be adhered to."

  c. "I will make arrangements for your family to be able to stay with the patient."

  d. "The healthcare team needs room to do procedures to help your family member, so it would be best if you stayed in the waiting area."

17. When planning the care of the patient in cardiogenic shock, what does the nurse understand is the primary treatment goal?

  a. Improve the heart's pumping mechanism

  b. Limit further myocardial damage

  c. Preserve the healthy myocardium

  d. Treat the oxygenation needs of the heart muscle

18. What priority intervention can the nurse provide to decrease the incidence of septic shock for patients who are at risk?

  a. Insert indwelling catheters for incontinent patients.

  b. Use strict hand hygiene techniques.

  c. Administer prophylactic antibiotics for all patients at risk.

  d. Have patients wear masks in the health care facility.

19. A patient arrives in the emergency department with complaints of chest pain radiating to the jaw. What medication does the nurse anticipate administering to reduce pain and anxiety as well as reducing oxygen consumption?

  a. Codeine

  b. Demerol

  c. Dilaudid

  d. Morphine

20. A patient presents to the emergency department after being stung by a bee, complaining of difficulty breathing. What vasoconstrictive medication should be given at this time?

  a. Dexamethasone

  b. Prednisone

  c. Benadryl

  d. Epinephrine

CHAPTER 15

Oncology: Nursing Management in Cancer Care

Learning Objectives

1. Compare the function and behavior of normal and cancer cells.
2. Differentiate between benign and malignant tumors.
3. Identify agents and factors that have been found to be carcinogenic.
4. Describe the role of nurses in health education and prevention in decreasing the incidence of cancer.
5. Differentiate among the goals of cancer care: prevention, diagnosis, cure, control, and palliation.
6. Describe the roles of surgery, radiation therapy, chemotherapy, hematopoietic stem cell transplantation, hyperthermia, targeted therapy, and symptom management in treating cancer.
7. Use the nursing process as a framework for the care of patients with cancer.
8. Identify potential complications for the patient with cancer and discuss associated nursing care.
9. Identify assessment parameters and nursing management of patients with oncologic emergencies.

SECTION I: ASSESSING YOUR UNDERSTANDING

Activity A *Fill in the blanks.*

1. In the United States, the three leading causes of cancer deaths in the United States are
_____, _____, and
_____ in men, and _____,
_____, and _____ in
women.

2. _____ and _____ are
two examples of tumor-specific antigens in
the altered cell membranes of malignant cells.

3. The two key ways by which cancer is spread
are the _____ and the _____.

4. About _____% of all cancers are
thought to be related to the environment.

5. The single most lethal chemical carcinogen,
accounting for 30% of all cancer deaths, is
_____.

6. _____, _____,
and _____ are three dietary
substances (cruciferous vegetables) that appear
to reduce cancer risk. _____,
_____, _____,
and _____ tend to increase
the risk of cancer.

7. The two *most common* side effects of chemo-therapy are _____ and _____.

8. Myelosuppression, caused by chemotherapeutic agents, results in _____, _____, _____, _____, and an increased risk of _____ and _____.

9. Three chemotherapeutic agents that are particularly toxic to the renal system are _____, _____, and _____.

Activity B *Briefly answer the following.*

1. Define, in very simple language, the cause of cancer.

_____

_____

2. Name two examples of an inherited cancer susceptibility syndrome.

_____

3. List four of seven cancers that are associated with an increased intake of alcohol.

_____ _____

_____ _____

4. Identify five substances produced by the immune system in response to cancer cells.

_____ _____

_____ _____

_____

5. Toxicity occurs with radiation therapy. For each of the following, list three common side effects.

   a. Skin: _____, _____, and _____.

   b. Oral mucosal membrane: _____, _____, and _____.

   c. Stomach or colon: _____, _____, and _____.

   d. Bone marrow-producing sites: _____, _____, and _____.

6. List five of nine signs that indicate that an extravasation of an infusion of a cancer chemotherapeutic agent has occurred.

_____ _____

_____ _____

_____

Activity C

PART I

Match the term listed in Column II with its associated definition listed in Column I.

Column I

____ 1. Growth of new capillaries from the host tissue

____ 2. Innate process of programmed cell death

____ 3. The use of thermal energy to destroy cancer cells

____ 4. Point at which blood counts are their lowest

____ 5. Target antibodies to destroy specific malignant cells

____ 6. A substance that can cause tissue necrosis

____ 7. A dry oral cavity caused by salivary gland dysfunction

____ 8. Substances produced by the immune system cells to enhance the function of the immune system

Column II

a. Angiogenesis

b. Apoptosis

c. Cytokines

d. Monoclonal antibodies

e. Nadir

f. Radiofrequency ablation

g. Vesicant

h. Xerostomia

PART II

Match the type of neoplasm in Column II with its associated description listed in Column I.

Column I

____ 1. Cells bear little resemblance to the normal cells of the tissue from which they arose.

____ 2. Rate of growth is usually slow.

____ 3. Tumor tissue is encapsulated.

____ 4. Tumor spreads by way of blood and lymph channels to other areas of the body.

____ 5. Growth tends to recur when removed.

Column II

a. Benign

b. Malignant

PART III

Match the drug category listed in Column II with an associated antineoplastic agent listed in Column I. For each drug, list a common side effect in Column I. Some answers may be used more than once.

Column I

____ 1. Cisplatin _____

____ 2. 5-fluorouracil (5-FU) _____

____ 3. Estrogens _____

____ 4. Thiotepa _____

____ 5. Lomustine (CCNU) _____

____ 6. Doxorubicin
_____

____ 7. Ifosfamide
_____

____ 8. Methotrexate
_____

____ 9. Vincristine (VCR)
_____

____ 10. Irinotecan _____

____ 11. Asparaginase
_____

Column II

a. Alkylating agent

b. Nitrosourea

c. Antimetabolite

d. Antitumor antibiotic

e. Plant alkaloid/ mitotic spindle

f. Hormonal agent

g. Miscellaneous agent

h. Topoisomerase 1 inhibitors

SECTION II: APPLYING YOUR KNOWLEDGE

Activity D *Consider the scenarios and answer the questions.*

CASE STUDY: Cancer of the Breast

Kim is a 45-year-old mother of four who, after a needle aspiration biopsy, is diagnosed as having a malignant breast tumor, stage III. She was scheduled for a modified radical mastectomy. On assessment, her breast tissue had a dimpling or "orange-peel" appearance. Nursing diagnoses included: (a) fear and ineffective coping related to the diagnosis and (b) disturbance in self-concept related to the nature of the surgery.

1. The nurse determines by the patient's history that her mother died of breast cancer. What is the correlation with the diagnosis of breast cancer in this patient?

_____

2. What should the nurse assess in order to assist Kim in adapting to the loss of her breast?

_____

3. Kim's husband refuses to participate in any discussion about his wife's diagnosis. What defense mechanism does the nurse determine the husband is using?

_____

4. The nurse assesses Kim's pain postoperatively, with Kim stating the pain is an 8 on a scale of 0–10. What other factors can alter Kim's perception of pain?

_____

5. Kim is scheduled to begin radiation therapy, followed by chemotherapy with 5-FU. What can the nurse tell Kim about the effects of the radiation therapy so that she will be prepared?

_____

_____

6. What measures can the nurse educate Kim to take to assist in protecting her skin between radiation treatments?

_____

7. After radiation therapy, Kim begins a regimen of chemotherapy with 5-FU. Three weeks after treatment begins, Kim develops a fever, sore throat, and cold symptoms. What does the nurse determine that these symptoms could be related to?

_____

CASE STUDY: Cancer of the Lung

Mr. Donato is a 48-year-old accountant who has been a one-pack-a-day smoker for 23 years. He has had a persistent cough for 1 year that is hacking and nonproductive, and has had repeated unresolved upper respiratory tract infections. He went to see his physician because he was fatigued, had been anorexic, and had lost 12 lb over the last 3 months. Diagnostic evaluation led to the diagnosis of a localized tumor with no evidence of metastatic spread. Mr. Donato is scheduled for a lobectomy in 3 days.

1. After this patient receives a diagnosis of cancer, what does the nurse anticipate will be the first reaction in the grieving process?

_____

2. What interventions can the nurse provide to support the patient and family during the grieving process?

_____

_____

3. What assessment data would the nurse determine could indicate a compromised nutritional status?

_____

4. What should the nurse assess for in the postoperative period that may indicate the presence of infection?

_____

SECTION III: PREPARING FOR NCLEX

Activity E *Answer the following questions.*

1. What can the nurse do to meet the challenges in caring for a patient with cancer?

a. Identify own perception of cancer and set realistic goals.

b. Set the same goals for all patients with cancer.

c. Tell the patient about the things the patient has done to cause cancer.

d. Ensure that the patient has the financial means to afford their care.

2. A patient, age 67 years, is admitted for diagnostic studies to rule out cancer. The patient is Caucasian, has been employed as a landscaper for 40 years, and has a 36-year history of smoking a pack of cigarettes daily. What significant risk factors does the nurse recognize this patient has? (Select all that apply.)

a. Age

b. Cigarette smoking

c. Occupation

d. Race

e. Marital status

3. What foods should the nurse suggest that the patient consume less of in order to reduce nitrate intake because of the possibility of carcinogenic action?

a. Eggs and milk

b. Fish and poultry

c. Ham and bacon

d. Green, leafy vegetables

4. A patient will be having an endoscopic procedure with a diagnostic biopsy. What type of biopsy does the nurse explain will remove an entire piece of suspicious tissue?

a. Excisional biopsy

b. Incisional biopsy

c. Needle biopsy

d. Punch biopsy

5. A patient is admitted for an excisional biopsy of a breast lesion. What intervention should the nurse provide for the care of this patient?

   a. Clarify information provided by the physician.

   b. Provide aseptic care to the incision postoperatively.

   c. Provide time for the patient to discuss her concerns.

   d. Counsel the patient about the possibility of losing her breast.

6. A patient is scheduled for cryosurgery for cervical cancer and tells the nurse, "I am not exactly sure what the doctor is going to do." What is the best response by the nurse?

   a. "The physician is going to use medication to inject the area."

   b. "The physician is going to use liquid nitrogen to freeze the area."

   c. "The physician is going to use a laser to remove the area."

   d. "The physician is going to use radiofrequency to ablate the area."

7. The nurse at the clinic explains to the patient that the surgeon will be removing a mole on the patient's back that has the potential to develop into cancer. The nurse informs the patient that this is what type of procedure?

   a. Diagnostic

   b. Palliative

   c. Prophylactic

   d. Reconstructive

8. A patient will be receiving radiation for 6 weeks for the treatment of breast cancer and asks the nurse why it takes so long. What is the best response by the nurse?

   a. "It allows time for you to cope with the treatment."

   b. "It will allow time for the repair of healthy tissue."

   c. "It will decrease the incidence of leukopenia and thrombocytopenia."

   d. "It is not really understood why you have to go for 6 weeks of treatment."

9. A patient with uterine cancer is being treated with internal radiation therapy. What would the nurse's priority responsibility be for this patient?

   a. Explain to the patient that she will continue to emit radiation for approximately 1 week after the implant is removed.

   b. Maintain as much distance as possible from the patient while in the room.

   c. Alert family members that they should restrict their visiting to 5 minutes at any one time.

   d. Wear a lead apron when providing direct patient care.

10. What disadvantages of chemotherapy should the patient be informed about prior to starting the regimen?

    a. It attacks cancer cells during their vulnerable phase.

    b. It functions against disseminated disease.

    c. It causes a systemic reaction.

    d. It targets normal body cells as well as cancer cells.

11. A patient is taking vincristine, a plant alkaloid for the treatment of cancer. What system should the nurse be sure to assess for symptoms of toxicity?

    a. Gastrointestinal system

    b. Nervous system

    c. Pulmonary system

    d. Urinary system

12. The nurse assesses that extravasation of a chemotherapy agent has occurred. What should the initial action of the nurse be?

    a. Apply a warm compress to the area.

    b. Discontinue the infusion.

    c. Inject an antidote, if required.

    d. Place ice over the site of infiltration.

13. What intervention should the nurse provide to reduce the incidence of renal damage when a patient is taking a chemotherapy regimen?

   a. Encourage fluid intake to dilute the urine.

   b. Take measures to acidify the urine and prevent uric acid crystallization.

   c. Withhold medication when the blood urea nitrogen level exceeds 20 mg/dL.

   d. Limit fluids to 1,000 mL daily to prevent accumulation of the drug's end products after cell lysis.

14. What does the nurse understand is the rationale for administering allopurinol for a patient receiving chemotherapy?

   a. It stimulates the immune system against the tumor cells.

   b. It treats drug-related anemia.

   c. It prevents alopecia.

   d. It lowers serum and uric acid levels.

15. A patient is to receive Bacille Calmette-Guerin (BCG), a nonspecific biologic response modifier. Why would the patient receive this form of treatment?

   a. For cancer of the bladder

   b. For cancer of the breast

   c. For cancer of the lungs

   d. For skin cancer

16. What is the best way for the nurse to assess the nutritional status of a patient with cancer?

   a. Weigh the patient daily.

   b. Monitor daily caloric intake.

   c. Observe for proper wound healing.

   d. Assess BUN and creatinine levels.

CHAPTER 16

End-of-Life Care

Learning Objectives

1. Discuss the historical, legal, and sociocultural perspectives of palliative and end-of-life care in the United States.
2. Define palliative care.
3. Compare and contrast the settings where palliative care and end-of-life care are provided.
4. Describe the principles and components of hospice care.
5. Identify barriers to improving care at the end of life.
6. Reflect on personal experience with and attitudes toward death and dying.
7. Apply skills for communicating with terminally ill patients and their families.
8. Provide culturally and spiritually sensitive care to terminally ill patients and their families.
9. Implement nursing measures to manage physiologic responses to terminal illness.
10. Support actively dying patients and their families.
11. Identify components of uncomplicated grief and mourning, and implement nursing measures to support patients and families.

SECTION I: ASSESSING YOUR UNDERSTANDING

Activity A *Fill in the blanks.*

1. Dr. _____, who spearheaded a movement to increase an awareness of the dying process among health care practitioners, published a landmark book, _____, in 1969.

2. _____ refers to providing another person the means to end his or her own life.

3. _____ involves the prescription by a physician of a lethal dose of medication for the purpose of ending someone's life.

4. The two most common primary hospice diagnoses for Medicare patients are _____ and _____.

5. Two types of medications routinely used to treat the underlying obstructed pathology associated with dyspnea are _____ and _____.

6. Three medications that are commonly used to stimulate appetite in anorexic patients are

   _____, _____, and _____.

Activity B *Briefly answer the following.*

1. Name the eight key domains underlying a more comprehensive and humane approach to care of the dying as identified by the National Consensus Project for Quality Palliative Care (NCP, 2009).

   _____

   _____

2. Define the terms *palliative care* and *hospice care*.

   _____

   _____

3. How did Dr. Kübler-Ross's work help the medical and nursing community view the dying process in a more personalized way?

_____

_____

4. What is the difference between the living will and durable power of attorney?

_____

_____

5. What is the American Nurses Association (ANA) position on assisted suicide and nursing?

_____

_____

SECTION II: APPLYING YOUR KNOWLEDGE

Activity C *Consider the scenario and answer the questions.*

Betty Smith is accompanied to the clinic by her daughter for follow-up care related to advanced uterine cancer. Her daughter reports that although she prepares her favorite foods, Betty is not interested in eating anything. The daughter states, "With Mom's declining health, I am going to need help with her care."

1. What medications does the nurse understand that the physician can prescribe to help increase Betty's appetite?

_____

2. Betty is prescribed Decadron for the anorexia. What should the nurse tell Betty and her daughter about the length of time this medication will be used?

_____

3. What suggestions could the nurse make to help the patient and family receive assistance with Betty's care?

_____

SECTION III: PRACTICING FOR NCLEX

Activity D *Answer the following questions.*

1. A patient is diagnosed with a terminal illness and has been given less than 6 months to live. What type of referral should the nurse make to assist this patient and family at home?
   a. A rehabilitation center
   b. Hospice
   c. Adult day care
   d. Physical therapy

2. A patient diagnosed with terminal pancreatic cancer is unaware of the diagnosis and his daughter has requested that he not be told. What awareness context does the nurse determine this is?
   a. Suspected awareness
   b. Mutual pretense awareness
   c. Closed awareness
   d. Open awareness

3. A patient is diagnosed with stage II breast cancer. For the patient to use the Medicare Hospice Benefit, her life expectancy needs to be what length of time?
   a. 2 months
   b. 4 months
   c. 6 months
   d. 8 months

4. A patient with end-stage chronic obstructive pulmonary disease is admitted to a hospice facility and asks the admitting nurse, "How long will I be allowed to stay here?" What is the best response by the nurse?
   a. "You will be able to stay only for approximately 1 month and then you will be discharged."
   b. "You will be able to stay for 2 months before being discharged."
   c. "There is no time limit for your stay. You can stay until you die."
   d. "When your stay reaches 6 months, you will be recertified for a continued stay."

5. A patient authorizes a son to make medical decisions and brings the completed forms for the nurse to place on the chart. What form does the nurse understand this is?

   a. An advance directive

   b. A living will

   c. A standard addendum to a will

   d. A proxy directive

6. A dying patient wants to talk to the nurse. The patient states, "I know I'm dying, aren't I?" What would an appropriate nursing response be?

   a. "This must be very difficult for you."

   b. "Tell me more about what's on your mind."

   c. " I'm so sorry. I know how you must feel."

   d. "You know you're dying?"

7. A terminally ill patient in pain asks the nurse to administer enough pain medication to end the suffering forever. What is the best response by the nurse?

   a. "I can't do that, I will go to jail."

   b. "I am surprised that you would ask me to do something like that."

   c. "I will see if the physician will order enough for that to occur."

   d. "I will notify the physician that the current dose of medication is not relieving your pain."

8. A patient's family member asks the nurse what the purpose of hospice is. What is the best response by the nurse?

   a. "It will hasten the death of the patient."

   b. " It will prolong life in a dignified manner."

   c. " It will use artificial means of life support if the patient requests it."

   d. " It will enable the patient to remain home if that is what is desired."

9. A terminally ill patient is admitted to the hospital. The patient grabs the nurse's hand and asks, "Am I dying?" What response would be best for the nurse to give?

   a. "Why do you think that?"

   b. "Did someone tell you that you are dying?"

   c. "Tell me more about what's on your mind."

   d. "I am not at liberty to disclose that information."

10. A patient near the end of life is experiencing anorexia-cachexia syndrome. What characteristics of the syndrome does the nurse recognize? (Select all that apply.)

    a. Alterations in carbohydrate, fat, and protein metabolism

    b. Endocrine dysfunction

    c. Anemia

    d. Neurologic dysfunction

    e. Bladder incontinence

Perioperative Concepts and Nursing Management

17

Preoperative Nursing Management

Learning Objectives

1. Define the three phases of perioperative patient care.
2. Describe a comprehensive preoperative assessment to identify surgical risk factors.
3. Describe the gerontologic considerations related to preoperative management.
4. Identify health factors that affect patients preoperatively.
5. Identify legal and ethical considerations related to obtaining informed consent for surgery.
6. Describe preoperative nursing measures that decrease the risk for infection and other postoperative complications.
7. Describe the immediate preoperative preparation of the patient.
8. Develop a preoperative education plan designed to promote the patient's recovery from anesthesia and surgery, thus preventing postoperative complications.

SECTION 1: ASSESSING YOUR UNDERSTANDING

Activity A *Fill in the blanks.*

1. The preoperative phase begins _____ and ends when the patient _____.

2. The intraoperative phase begins when the patient _____ and ends when _____.

3. The hazards of surgery for the elderly are directly proportional to _____ and _____.

4. The leading causes of postoperative morbidity and mortality in older adults are _____ and _____ complications.

5. Diabetics undergoing surgery are at risk for four complications: _____, _____, _____, and _____.

6. Aspirin is withheld _____ days prior to surgery, if possible, because it acts by _____.

Activity B *Briefly answer the following.*

1. Informed consent for a surgical procedure is necessary when a procedure meets any of the following: _____, _____, _____, or _____.

2. List three significant nutritional concerns for the elderly surgical patient: _____, _____, and _____.

3. Name three primary goals necessary to promote postoperative mobility: _____, _____, and _____.

4. What are 10 potential risk factors related to surgery?

_____ _____

_____ _____

_____ _____

_____ _____

Activity C *Match the nutrient in Column II with its associated rationale for use in Column I.*

Column I

___ **1.** Essential for normal blood clotting

___ **2.** Allows collagen deposition to occur

___ **3.** Necessary for DNA synthesis

___ **4.** Increases inflammatory response in wounds

___ **5.** Vital for capillary formation

Column II

a. Protein

b. Vitamin C

c. Vitamin A

d. Vitamin K

e. Zinc

Activity D

Medication Administration

For each drug classification, list the potential effects of interaction with anesthetics.

1. Anticoagulants _____

2. Antiseizure agents _____

3. Corticosteroids _____

4. Diuretics _____

5. Insulin _____

6. Phenothiazines _____

7. Tranquilizers _____

8. Monoamine oxidase inhibitors (MAO)

_____

Preoperative Nursing

For each essential preoperative nursing activity, write an appropriate nursing goal. An example is provided.

1. (Example) Restriction of nutrition and fluids
<u>Prevent aspiration</u>

2. Intestinal preparation _____

3. Preoperative skin preparation (cleansing)

_____

4. Urinary catheterization _____

5. Administration of preoperative medications

_____

6. Transportation of patient to presurgical suite

_____

SECTION II: APPLYING YOUR KNOWLEDGE

Activity E *Consider the scenario and answer the questions.*

The nurse is caring for a 42-year-old patient who is scheduled for an inguinal hernia repair with general anesthesia. While performing a preoperative history and physical assessment, the nurse begins to suspect that the patient may have a history of substance abuse. The patient does admit to smoking a pack of cigarettes daily.

1. What important interventions should the nurse instruct the patient to do in order to prevent complications postoperatively?

_____

_____

2. What is the best method for the nurse to obtain information about the patient's possible use of substances?

_____

_____

3. What instructions should regarding smoking should the nurse provide to the patient prior to scheduling the patient for the surgical procedure?

_____

_____

SECTION III: PRACTICING FOR NCLEX

Activity F *Answer the following questions.*

1. The on-call perioperative team is called for an urgent surgery to be performed as soon as they arrive. What surgical procedure is considered urgent?

   a. An appendectomy

   b. An exploratory laparotomy

   c. A repair of multiple stab wounds

   d. A face lift

2. A patient is scheduled for a reduction mammoplasty. What classification of surgery does the nurse understand that this is?

   a. Urgent

   b. Optional

   c. Required

   d. Reconstructive

3. A patient is scheduled for a surgical procedure. For which surgical procedure should the nurse prepare an informed consent form for the surgeon to sign?

   a. An open reduction of a fracture

   b. An insertion of an intravenous catheter

   c. Irrigation of the external ear canal

   d. Urethral catheterization

4. When caring for a patient with alcoholism, when should the nurse assess for symptoms of alcoholic withdrawal?

   a. Within the first 12 hours

   b. About 24 hours postoperatively

   c. On the second or third day

   d. 4 days after a surgical procedure

5. The physician schedules an elective surgical procedure for a patient who smokes cigarettes. When should the nurse recommend that the patient cease smoking before the surgical procedure to minimize risks associate with cigarette smoking?

   a. 1 to 2 months

   b. 3 to 4 months

   c. 2 weeks

   d. 3 weeks

6. The nurse is caring for a patient with liver disease who had a surgical procedure. When should the nurse alert the physician?

   a. When the patient's blood ammonia concentration reaches 180 mg/dL

   b. When a lactate dehydrogenase concentration is 300 units

   c. When a serum albumin concentration is 5.0 g/dL

   d. When a serum globulin concentration reaches 2.8 g/dL

7. A patient with renal failure is scheduled for a surgical procedure. When would surgery be contraindicated for this patient due to laboratory results?

   a. A blood urea nitrogen level of 42 mg/dL

   b. A creatine kinase level of 120 U/L

   c. A serum creatinine level of 0.9 mg/dL

   d. A urine creatinine level of 1.2 mg/dL

8. A patient with uncontrolled diabetes is scheduled for a surgical procedure. What chief life-threatening hazard should the nurse monitor for?

   a. Dehydration

   b. Hypertension

   c. Hypoglycemia

   d. Glucosuria

9. What is the blood glucose level goal for a diabetic patient who will be having a surgical procedure?

   a. 80 to 110 mg/dL

   b. 150 to 240 mg/dL

   c. 250 to 300 mg/dL

   d. 300 to 350 mg/dL

10. The nurse is monitoring a presurgical patient for electrolyte imbalance. Which classification of medication may cause electrolyte imbalance?

   a. Corticosteroids

   b. Diuretics

   c. Phenothiazines

   d. Insulin

11. The nurse assesses an older adult patient who complains of dimmed vision. What does this alert the nurse to plan for?

    a. A safe environment

    b. Restrictions of the patient's unassisted mobility activities

    c. Probable cataract extractions

    d. Referral to an ophthalmologist

12. The nurse is caring for a patient who is obese prior to a surgical procedure. What surgical complications positively correlated with obesity should the nurse monitor for? (Select all that apply.)

    a. Cardiovascular system

    b. Gastrointestinal system

    c. Pulmonary system

    d. Renal system

    e. Nervous system

13. The patient is NPO prior to having a colonoscopy. The patient is to take a daily blood pressure pill prior to the procedure. Until when may water be given prior to the procedure?

    a. Up to 8 hours before surgery

    b. Up to 6 hours before surgery

    c. Up to 4 hours before surgery

    d. Up to 2 hours before surgery

14. The patient asks the nurse why food is withheld before surgery. What is the best response by the nurse?

    a. "Aspiration is a concern and can be a complication if food or fluid is taken close to the surgery time."

    b. "Distention is a severe complication if food or fluid is taken close to the surgery time."

    c. "Infection may occur if food or fluid is taken prior to surgery."

    d. "Obstruction will occur if food or fluid is taken prior to surgery."

15. When does the nurse understand the patient is knowledgeable about the impending surgical procedure?

    a. The patient participates willingly in the preoperative preparation.

    b. The patient discusses stress factors causing the patient to feel depressed.

    c. The patient expresses concern about postoperative pain.

    d. The patient verbalizes fears to family.

16. How does the nurse determine that the patient may have hidden fears about the impending surgical procedure? (Select all that apply.)

    a. The patient tells the nurse of concerns with the outcome of the procedure.

    b. The patient informs the nurse of problems with postoperative nausea in the past and that it was a bad experience.

    c. The patient avoids communication with the nurse.

    d. The patient repeatedly asks questions that have previously been answered.

    e. The patient talks incessantly.

17. What is the best response by the nurse when the patient states, "I'm so nervous about my surgery"?

    a. "Relax. Your recovery period will be shorter if you're less nervous."

    b. "Stop worrying. It only makes you more nervous."

    c. "You needn't worry. Your doctor has done this surgery many times before."

    d. "Would you like to discuss the concerns that you have?"

18. Why is assessment of dentition important in the patient preparing to have a surgical procedure with general anesthesia?

    a. The patient may require referral to the dentist.

    b. Oral hygiene is important for all patients.

    c. Decayed teeth or dental prosthesis can become dislodged during intubation.

    d. The patient can sue if a tooth falls out during surgery.

19. A patient preparing for a surgical procedure is taking corticosteroids for Crohn's disease. What should the patient be monitored for?

a. Obstruction

b. Infection

c. Hypoglycemia

d. Adrenal insufficiency

20. A patient having a surgical procedure takes aspirin 325 mg daily for prevention of platelet aggregation. When should the patient stop taking the aspirin before the surgery?

a. 2 weeks

b. 4 weeks

c. 7 to 10 days

d. 2 to 3 days

CHAPTER 8

Intraoperative Nursing Management

Learning Objectives

1. Describe the interdisciplinary approach to the care of the patient during surgery.
2. Describe the gerontologic considerations related to intraoperative management.
3. Describe the principles of surgical asepsis.
4. Describe the roles of the surgical team members during the intraoperative phase of care.
5. Identify adverse effects of surgery and anesthesia.
6. Identify the surgical risk factors related to age-specific populations and nursing interventions to reduce those risks.
7. Compare types of anesthesia with regard to uses, advantages, disadvantages, and nursing responsibilities.
8. Use the nursing process to optimize patient outcomes during the intraoperative period.
9. Describe the role of the nurse in ensuring patient safety during the intraoperative period.

SECTION I: ASSESSING YOUR UNDERSTANDING

Activity A *Fill in the blanks.*

1. The type of anesthesia most likely to be used for a patient undergoing a colonoscopy is _____, and the most frequently used agents are _____ and _____.

2. The anesthetic most commonly used for general anesthesia by intravenous injection is _____, which can cause _____ as a serious, toxic side effect.

3. Spinal anesthesia is a conduction nerve block that occurs when a local anesthetic is injected into _____.

4. The conduction block anesthesia commonly used in labor is the _____.

5. With malignant hyperthermia, the core body temperature can increase 1°C to 2°C every 5 minutes, reaching or exceeding a body temperature of _____ degrees in a short amount of time.

6. The most commonly used volatile liquid anesthetic agent is _____.

7. A local infiltration anesthetic can last for up to _____.

Activity B *Briefly answer the following.*

1. Differentiate between the *restricted zone, semi-restricted zone,* and the *unrestricted zone.*

   _____

   _____

   _____

2. Explain why anesthesia dosage is reduced with age.

   _____

   _____

3. List four primary responsibilities of a Registered Nurse First Assistant (RNFA).

   _____

   _____

4. List five health hazards associated with the surgical environment: _____,

_____, _____,

_____, and _____.

5. What nursing assessment indicates that a patient has recovered from the effects of spinal anesthesia?

_____

6. List five potential intraoperative complications: _____, _____,

_____, _____,

and _____.

7. Distinguish between the purposes for three types of anesthesia: epidural, general, and local.

_____

_____

8. List 10 potential adverse effects of surgery and anesthesia and their associated causes.

_____

_____

_____

_____

9. Why are the elderly at a higher risk of complications from anesthesia?

_____

_____

10. What risks are to be avoided when lasers are used in the surgical environment?

_____

_____

11. What is meant by *anesthesia awareness*?

_____

_____

Activity C

Inhalation Anesthetic Agents

Match the inhalation anesthetic agent in Column II with its associated nursing implication found in Column I.

Column I

____ 1. Monitor for chest pain and stroke

____ 2. Monitor blood pressure frequently

____ 3. Observe for respiratory depression

____ 4. Monitor respirations closely

____ 5. Monitor for malignant hypothermia

Column II

a. Ethrane

b. Fluothane

c. Forane

d. Nitrous oxide

e. Suprane

Common Intravenous Medications

Match the commonly used intravenous medication in Column II with its associated common usage in Column I.

Column I

____ 1. Sedation with regional anesthesia

____ 2. Hypnotic and anxiolytic; adjunct to induction

____ 3. Epidural infusion for postoperative analgesia

____ 4. Maintenance of relaxation

____ 5. Skeletal muscle relaxation for orthopedic surgery

Column II

a. Fentanyl

b. Midazolam

c. Pancuronium

d. Propofol

e. Succinylcholine

SECTION II: APPLYING YOUR KNOWLEDGE

Activity D *Consider the scenarios and answer the questions.*

CASE STUDY: General Anesthesia

Anne, age 34, is in excellent health and is scheduled for open reduction of a fractured femur. The general anesthetic drugs to be used include enflurane and nitrous oxide.

1. What does the nurse understand are the advantages of enflurane?

   _____

2. What should the nurse make it a priority to monitor for when nitrous oxide is used?

   _____

3. After the patient has been administered Ethrane, what is important for the nurse to monitor for?

   _____

CASE STUDY: Moderate Sedation

A 22-year-old male patient has dislocated his right shoulder while playing basketball. He will be having a closed reduction of his shoulder with moderate sedation in the emergency department.

1. What does moderate sedation involve?

   _____

2. What should the nurse continually assess while performing moderate sedation?

   _____

3. What is the goal of moderate sedation?

   _____

SECTION III: PRACTICING FOR NCLEX

Activity E *Answer the following questions.*

1. What are the circulating nurse's responsibilities, in contrast to the scrub nurse's responsibilities?
   a. Assisting the surgeon
   b. Coordinating the surgical team
   c. Setting up the sterile tables
   d. Passing instruments

2. The circulating nurse is preparing a patient for a surgical procedure. What primary responsibility does the circulating nurse have in the perioperative experience?
   a. Discussing the complications of the surgical procedure with the patient
   b. Coordinating the efforts of the surgical team
   c. Marking the operative site
   d. Passing instruments during the intraoperative phase

3. An unconscious patient with normal pulse and respirations would be considered to be in what stage of general anesthesia?
   a. Beginning anesthesia
   b. Excitement
   c. Surgical anesthesia
   d. Medullary depression

4. Why should the nurse be vigilant with assessment of perioperative risks on the older adult patient? (Select all that apply.)
   a. Ciliary action decreases, reducing the cough reflex.
   b. Fatty tissue increases, prolonging the effects of anesthesia.
   c. Liver size decreases, reducing the metabolism of anesthetics.
   d. Peristalsis increases.
   e. The elasticity of skin increases and decreases the risk of shearing.

5. The nurse should know that, postoperatively, a general anesthetic is primarily eliminated via what organ(s)?
   a. The kidneys
   b. The lungs
   c. The skin
   d. The liver

6. The anesthesiologist is administering a stable and safe nondepolarizing muscle relaxant. What medication does the nurse anticipate will be administered?
   a. Anectine (succinylcholine chloride)
   b. Norcuron (vecuronium bromide)
   c. Pavulon (pancuronium bromide)
   d. Syncurine (decamethonium)

7. What intravenous anesthetic administered by the anesthesiologist has a powerful respiratory depressant effect sufficient to cause apnea and cardiovascular depression?
   a. Amidate
   b. Ketalar
   c. Pentothal
   d. Versed

8. The nurse is completing a postoperative assessment for a patient who has received a depolarizing neuromuscular blocking agent. The nursing assessment includes careful monitoring of which body system?
   a. Cardiovascular system
   b. Endocrine system
   c. Gastrointestinal system
   d. Genitourinary system

9. A patient is complaining of a headache after receiving spinal anesthesia. What does the nurse understand may be the cause of the headache related to the spinal anesthesia? (Select all that apply.)
   a. The patient lying in the supine position
   b. Leakage of spinal fluid from the subarachnoid space
   c. Size of the spinal needle used
   d. Degree of patient hydration
   e. An allergic reaction to the medication used

10. The physician requests lidocaine 2% with epinephrine for use in local infiltration anesthesia. What does the nurse understand is the purpose of adding epinephrine to the lidocaine? (Select all that apply.)
    a. The epinephrine causes vasoconstriction.
    b. The epinephrine prevents rapid absorption of the anesthetic drug.
    c. The epinephrine prolongs the local action of the anesthetic agent.
    d. The lidocaine will not anesthetize the area locally without the epinephrine.
    e. The epinephrine will prevent the patient from having an allergic reaction to the lidocaine.

11. The patient asks the nurse how long the local infiltration anesthetic will last. What is the nurse's best response?
    a. "The anesthetic may last for 1 hour."
    b. "The anesthetic may last for 3 hours."
    c. "The anesthetic may last for 5 hours."
    d. "The anesthetic may last for 7 hours."

12. A patient is scheduled to have a heart valve replacement with a porcine valve. Which patient does the nurse understand may refuse the use of any porcine-based product?
    a. A patient of Catholic faith
    b. A patient of Jewish faith
    c. A patient of Baptist faith
    d. A patient of Lutheran faith

13. The nurse is caring for a patient who is at risk for malignant hyperthermia subsequent to general anesthesia. What is the most common early sign that the nurse should assess for?
    a. Hypertension
    b. Muscle rigidity ("tetanylike" movements)
    c. Oliguria
    d. Tachycardia

14. How would the operating room nurse place a patient in the Trendelenburg position?
    a. Flat on his back with his arms next to his sides
    b. On his back with his head lowered so that the plane of his body meets the horizontal on an angle
    c. On his back with his legs and thighs flexed at right angles
    d. On his side with his uppermost leg adducted and flexed at the knee

15. The patient received ketamine (Ketalar) during a surgical procedure. What intervention by the nurse will assist with an optimal recovery period?
    a. Make sure that the patient is stimulated frequently.
    b. Place the patient in a darkened, quiet part of the recovery area.
    c. The patient does not require a recovery period and may go back to the hospital room.
    d. Speak to the patient in a loud, clear voice.

16. A patient is having a surgical procedure that requires the patient to be in the prone position. What is an expected patient outcome?

a. The patient will not experience anxiety during the preoperative phase.

b. The patient will not experience signs of an allergic reaction.

c. The patient remains free of perioperative positioning injury.

d. The patient will not experience signs and symptoms of infection.

17. The circulating nurse is performing a skin preparation for a patient who is unconscious from general anesthesia when the scrub nurse states, "I know her, she sure has gotten fat!" What is the best response by the circulating nurse?

a. "It is inappropriate to make comments even when patients appear to be unconscious from anesthesia."

b. "She sure has gained weight. I hope that she will heal after the surgery."

c. "Be sure you don't say anything like that when she is coming out of the anesthesia in case she hears you."

d. "If you say anything like that again, I will report you to the nurse manager."

18. The patient is having a repair of a vaginal prolapse. What position does the nurse place the patient in?

a. Left lateral Sim's

b. Prone position

c. Lithotomy position

d. Trendelenburg

19. What medication should the nurse prepare to administer in the event the patient has malignant hyperthermia?

a. Dantrolene sodium (Dantrium)

b. Fentanyl citrate (Sublimaze)

c. Narcan

d. Thiopental sodium (Pentobarbital)

Postoperative Nursing Management

1. Describe the responsibilities of the postanesthesia care nurse in the prevention of immediate postoperative complications.
2. Compare postoperative care of the ambulatory surgery patient with that of the hospitalized surgery patient.
3. Identify common postoperative problems and their management.
4. Describe the gerontologic considerations related to postoperative management.
5. Describe variables that affect wound healing.
6. Demonstrate postoperative dressing techniques.
7. Identify assessment parameters appropriate for the early detection of postoperative complications.

SECTION I: ASSESSING YOUR UNDERSTANDING

Activity A *Fill in the blanks.*

1. The primary nursing objective during the immediate postoperative assessment is to maintain _____ and prevent _____.

2. Five types of shock are _____, _____, _____, _____, and _____.

3. The *most serious* and *most frequent* postoperative complications involve the _____ system.

4. Two potential postoperative complications following abdominal surgery are _____ and _____.

5. The return of peristalsis in the postoperative period can be determined by the presence of _____ and _____, both of which are assessed by the nurse.

6. Pain stimulates _____, which increases _____ and _____.

7. Noxious impulses stimulate _____, which increases _____ and _____.

8. Hypothalamic stress responses increase _____ and _____, which can lead to _____ and _____.

Activity B *Briefly answer the following.*

1. List five areas of concern for a recovery room postanesthesia care unit (PACU) nurse who has just received a patient from the operating room:

   _____, _____, _____, _____, and _____.

2. Distinguish among the three classifications of hemorrhage (primary, intermediary, and secondary) and include the defining characteristics of each.

Primary: _____

Intermediary: _____

Secondary: _____

3. Explain patient-controlled analgesia (PCA).

_____

_____

4. Explain why the postoperative complications of atelectasis and hypostatic pneumonia are reduced as a result of early ambulation.

_____

_____

5. Distinguish between wound *dehiscence* and *evisceration.*

_____

_____

6. What are the eight classic signs of hypovolemic shock?

_____

_____

7. What nursing assessment activities and interventions may detect postoperative deep vein thrombosis and pulmonary embolism?

_____

_____

8. How does the nurse know when the patient is ready for discharge from the PACU?

_____

_____

9. What three postoperative conditions put a patient at risk for common respiratory complications?

_____

_____

10. How do these factors affect the progress of wound healing?

Age _____

Edema _____

Nutritional deficits _____

Oxygen deficits _____

Medications _____

Systemic disorders _____

SECTION II: APPLYING YOUR KNOWLEDGE

Activity C *Consider the scenarios and answer the questions.*

CASE STUDY: Hypopharyngeal Obstruction

Deana is unconscious when she is transferred to the recovery room. She has experienced prolonged anesthesia, and all her muscles are relaxed.

1. What is the primary objective in the immediate postoperative period?

_____

2. What signs would the nurse recognize as indicative of a hypopharyngeal occlusion?

_____

3. What intervention does the nurse provide to treat hypopharyngeal airway obstruction?

_____

CASE STUDY: Wound Healing

Elizabeth is returned from the recovery room to a patient care area after a routine cholecystectomy.

1. What are the three phases of wound healing for this surgical patient?

_____

2. What should the ongoing assessment of the surgical site involve?

_____

3. What clinical manifestations does the nurse anticipate observing in the inflammatory phase of wound healing in the postoperative patient?

_____

4. What interventions can the nurse provide to promote adequate tissue oxygenation during the inflammatory phase of wound healing?

_____

SECTION III: PRACTICING FOR NCLEX

Activity D *Answer the following questions.*

1. What complication in the immediate postoperative period should the nurse understand requires early intervention to prevent?
   a. Laryngospasm
   b. Hyperventilation
   c. Hypoxemia and hypercapnia
   d. Pulmonary edema and embolism

2. Unless contraindicated, how should the nurse position an unconscious patient?
   a. Flat on the back, without elevation of the head, to facilitate frequent turning and minimize pulmonary complications
   b. In semi-Fowler's position, to promote respiratory function and reduce the incidence of orthostatic hypotension when the patient can eventually stand
   c. In Fowler's position, which most closely simulates a sitting position, thus facilitating respiratory as well as gastrointestinal functioning
   d. On the side with a pillow at the patient's back and the chin extended, to minimize the dangers of aspiration

3. The nurse is responsible for monitoring cardiovascular function in a postoperative patient. What method can the nurse use to measure cardiovascular function?
   a. Complete blood count
   b. Central venous pressure
   c. Upper endoscopy
   d. Chest x-ray

4. What measurement should the nurse report to the physician in the immediate postoperative period?
   a. A systolic blood pressure lower than 90 mm Hg
   b. A temperature reading between 97°F and 98°F
   c. Respirations between 20 and 25 breaths/min
   d. A hemoglobin of 13.6

5. What evidence does the nurse understand indicates that a patient is ready for discharge from the recovery room or PACU? (Select all that apply.)
   a. The patient has been extubated but still has an oropharyngeal airway in.
   b. The patient is arousable but falls back to sleep rapidly.
   c. The patient has a blood pressure within 10 mm Hg of the baseline.
   d. The patient has sonorous respirations and occasionally requires chin lift.
   e. The patient rates pain a 9 out of 10 on a 0–10 scale after receiving morphine sulfate.

6. The nurse is preparing to discharge a patient from the PACU using a PACU room scoring guide. With what score can the patient be transferred out of the recovery room?
   a. 5
   b. 6
   c. 7
   d. 8

7. Using the PACU room scoring guide, a nurse would give a patient an admission cardiovascular score of 2 if the patient's blood pressure is what percentage of his or her preanesthetic level?
   a. 20%
   b. 30% to 40%
   c. 40% to 50%
   d. Greater than 50%

8. When vomiting occurs postoperatively, what is the most important nursing intervention?

   a. Measure the amount of vomitus to estimate fluid loss, in order to accurately monitor fluid balance.

   b. Offer tepid water and juices to replace lost fluids and electrolytes.

   c. Support the wound area so that unnecessary strain will not disrupt the integrity of the incision.

   d. Turn the patient's head completely to one side to prevent aspiration of vomitus into the lungs.

9. What abnormal postoperative urinary output should the nurse report to the physician for a 2-hour period?

   a. <30 mL

   b. Between 75 and 100 mL

   c. Between 100 and 200 mL

   d. >200 mL

10. When should the nurse encourage the postoperative patient to get out of bed?

    a. Within 6 to 8 hours after surgery

    b. Between 10 and 12 hours after surgery

    c. As soon as it is indicated

    d. On the second postoperative day

11. What does the nurse recognize as one of the most common postoperative respiratory complications in elderly patients?

    a. Pleurisy

    b. Pneumonia

    c. Hypoxemia

    d. Pulmonary edema

12. The nurse documents the presence of granulation tissue in a healing wound. How should the nurse describe the tissue?

    a. Necrotic and hard

    b. Pale yet able to blanch with digital pressure

    c. Pink to red and soft, bleeding easily

    d. White with long, thin areas of scar tissue

13. A physician's admitting note lists a wound as healing by second intention. What does the nurse expect to find?

    a. A deep, open wound that was previously sutured

    b. A sutured incision with a little tissue reaction

    c. A wound with a deep, wide scar that was previously resutured

    d. A wound in which the edges were not approximated

14. A patient has a wound that has hemorrhaged. What does the nurse understand is the cause of the patient's increased risk of infection?

    a. Reduced amounts of oxygen and nutrients are available

    b. The tissue becomes less resilient

    c. Retrograde bacterial contamination may occur

    d. Dead space and dead cells provide a culture medium

15. The nurse determines that a patient has postoperative abdominal distention. What does the nurse determine that the distention may be directly related to?

    a. A temporary loss of peristalsis and gas accumulation in the intestines

    b. Beginning food intake in the immediate postoperative period

    c. Improper body positioning during the recovery period

    d. The type of anesthetic administered

16. The nurse is concerned that a postoperative patient may have a paralytic ileus. What assessment data may indicate that the patient does have a paralytic ileus?

    a. Abdominal tightness

    b. Abdominal distention

    c. Absence of peristalsis

    d. Increased abdominal girth

17. The nurse determines that a patient is at risk for the development of thrombophlebitis. What interventions can the nurse provide to prevent this? (Select all that apply.)

   a. Assisting the patient with leg exercises

   b. Encouraging early ambulation

   c. Massaging the legs every 4 hours

   d. Avoiding placement of pillows or blanket rolls under the patient's knees

   e. Applying compression stockings only at night

18. What complication is the nurse aware of that is associated with deep venous thrombosis?

   a. Pulmonary embolism

   b. Immobility because of calf pain

   c. Marked tenderness over the anteromedial surface of the thigh

   d. Swelling of the entire leg owing to edema

19. What intervention by the nurse is most effective for reducing hospital-acquired infections?

   a. Administration of prophylactic antibiotics

   b. Aseptic wound care

   c. Control of upper respiratory tract infections

   d. Proper hand-washing techniques

20. The nurse is assessing a postoperative patient's abdominal wound and observes a portion of intestines protruding through the wound. What is the priority intervention for the nurse to provide?

   a. Apply an abdominal binder snugly so that the intestines can be slowly pushed back into the abdominal cavity.

   b. Approximate the wound edges with adhesive tape so that the intestines can be gently pushed back into the abdomen.

   c. Carefully push the exposed intestines back into the abdominal cavity.

   d. Cover the protruding coils of intestines with sterile dressings moistened with sterile saline solution.

Gas Exchange and Respiratory Function

CHAPTER 20

Assessment of Respiratory Function

Learning Objectives

1. Describe the structures and functions of the upper and lower respiratory tracts.
2. Describe ventilation, diffusion, perfusion, and ventilation–perfusion imbalances.
3. Explain proper techniques utilized to perform a comprehensive respiratory assessment.
4. Discriminate between normal and abnormal assessment findings identified by inspection, palpation, percussion, and auscultation of the respiratory system.
5. Recognize and evaluate the major symptoms of respiratory dysfunction by applying concepts from the patient's health history and physical assessment findings.
6. Identify the diagnostic tests and related nursing implications used to evaluate respiratory function.

SECTION I: ASSESSING YOUR UNDERSTANDING

Activity A *Fill in the blanks.*

1. The two centers in the brain that are responsible for the neurologic control of ventilation are _____ and _____.

2. The alveoli begin to lose elasticity at about age ____ years, resulting in decreased gas diffusion.

3. The lungs are enclosed in a serous membrane called the _____.

4. The left lung, in contrast to the right lung, has _____.

5. The divisions of the lung proceed in the following order, beginning at the mainstem bronchi: _____, _____, _____, and _____.

6. _____ are the alveolar cells that secrete surfactant.

7. Gas exchange between the lungs and blood and between the blood and tissues is called _____.

8. The maximum volume of air that can be inhaled after a normal inhalation is known as _____.

9. Tidal volume, which may not significantly change with disease, has a normal value of approximately _____ mL.

10. The exchange of oxygen and carbon dioxide from the alveoli into the blood occurs by _____.

11. The pulmonary circulation is considered a _____, _____.

12. The symbol used to identify the partial pressure of oxygen is _____.

Activity B *Briefly answer the following.*

1. Distinguish between the terms *ventilation* and *respiration*.

_____

_____

2. Describe the function of the epiglottis.

_____

_____

3. List four conditions that cause low compliance or distensibility of the lungs:

_____, _____,

_____, and _____.

4. Define the term *partial pressure*.

_____

_____

5. List six major signs and symptoms of respiratory disease.

_____   _____

_____   _____

_____   _____

6. List four conditions that are influenced by genetic factors that affect respiratory function:

_____, _____,

_____, and _____.

7. Explain the breathing pattern characterized as Cheyne–Stokes respirations.

_____

_____

8. What is the purpose of cilia?_____

_____

9. What are four common phenomena that can alter bronchial diameter?

_____, _____,

_____, _____.

10. What is the difference between diffusion and pulmonary perfusion?_____

_____

SECTION II: APPLYING YOUR KNOWLEDGE

Activity C *Consider the scenarios and answer the questions.*

CASE STUDY: Bronchoscopy

Mr. Kecklin is scheduled for a bronchoscopy for the diagnostic purpose of locating a pathologic process.

1. Because a bronchoscopy was ordered, the nurse knows that the suspected lesion may be located where?

_____

_____

2. The nurse is preparing the patient for a bronchoscopy. What interventions by the nurse are required prior to the procedure?

_____

_____

3. What complications should the nurse be aware may occur during a bronchoscopy?

_____

_____

4. After the bronchoscopy, what should the nurse assess Mr. Kecklin for?

_____

_____

5. What intervention by the nurse should be provided to Mr. Kecklin after his bronchoscopy?

_____

_____

CASE STUDY: Thoracentesis

Mrs. Lomar is admitted to the clinical area for a thoracentesis. The physician wants to remove excess air from the pleural cavity.

1. What interventions by the nurse are required prior to the thoracentesis?

_____

_____

2. Into which position should the nurse assist the patient prior to the thoracentesis?

_____

_____

3. What anatomic site does the nurse anticipate the physician will use for the thoracentesis?

_____

_____

4. What should the nurse assess for after the patient has a thoracentesis?

_____

_____

SECTION III: PRACTICING FOR NCLEX

Activity D *Answer the following questions.*

1. A patient with sinus congestion complains of discomfort when the nurse is palpating the supraorbital ridges. The nurse knows that the patient is referring to which sinus?

a. Frontal

b. Ethmoidal

c. Maxillary

d. Sphenoidal

2. When the nurse is assessing the older adult patient, what gerontologic changes in the respiratory system should the nurse be aware of? (Select all that apply.)

a. Decreased alveolar duct diameter

b. Increased presence of mucus

c. Decreased gag reflex

d. Increased presence of collagen in alveolar walls

e. Decreased presence of mucus

3. A nurse caring for a patient with a pulmonary embolism understands that a high ventilation–perfusion ratio may exist. What does this mean for the patient?

a. Perfusion exceeds ventilation.

b. There is an absence of perfusion and ventilation.

c. Ventilation exceeds perfusion.

d. Ventilation matches perfusion.

4. A nurse understands that a safe but low level of oxygen saturation provides for adequate tissue saturation while allowing no reserve for situations that threaten ventilation. What is a safe but low oxygen saturation level for a patient?

a. 40 mm Hg

b. 75 mm Hg

c. 80 mm Hg

d. 95 mm Hg

5. The nurse is taking a respiratory history for a patient who has come into the clinic with a chronic cough. What information should the nurse obtain from this patient? (Select all that apply.)

a. Financial ability to pay the bill

b. Social support

c. Previous history of lung disease in the patient or family

d. Occupational and environmental influences

e. Previous history of smoking

6. A patient comes to the emergency department complaining of a knifelike pain when taking a deep breath. What does this type of pain likely indicate to the nurse?

a. Bacterial pneumonia

b. Bronchogenic carcinoma

c. Lung infarction

d. Pleurisy

7. The nurse is caring for a patient with a pulmonary disorder. What observation by the nurse is indicative of a very late symptom of hypoxia?

a. Cyanosis

b. Dyspnea

c. Restlessness

d. Confusion

8. The nurse inspects the thorax of a patient with advanced emphysema. What does the nurse expect the chest configuration to be for this patient?

a. Barrel chest

b. Funnel chest

c. Kyphoscoliosis

d. Pigeon chest

9. The nurse is performing chest auscultation for a patient with asthma. How does the nurse describe the high-pitched, sibilant, musical sounds that are heard?

   a. Rales

   b. Crackles

   c. Wheezes

   d. Rhonchi

10. The nurse auscultates crackles in a patient with a respiratory disorder. With what disorder would crackles be commonly heard?

    a. Asthma

    b. Bronchospasm

    c. Collapsed alveoli

    d. Pulmonary fibrosis

11. During a preadmission assessment, for what diagnosis would the nurse expect to find decreased tactile fremitus and hyperresonant percussion sounds?

    a. Bronchitis

    b. Emphysema

    c. Atelectasis

    d. Pulmonary edema

12. The nurse is reviewing the blood gas results for a patient with pneumonia. What arterial blood gas measurement best reflects the adequacy of alveolar ventilation?

    a. PaO_2

    b. $PaCO_2$

    c. pH

    d. SaO_2

13. The nurse is instructing the patient on the collection of a sputum specimen. What should be included in the instructions? (Select all that apply.)

    a. Initially, clear the nose and throat.

    b. Spit surface mucus and saliva into a sterile specimen container.

    c. Take a few deep breaths before coughing.

    d. Use diaphragmatic contractions to aid in the expulsion of sputum.

    e. Rinse with mouthwash prior to providing the specimen.

14. A physician wants a study of diaphragmatic motion because of suspected pathology. What does the nurse anticipate that the physician will most likely order?

    a. Barium swallow

    b. Bronchogram

    c. Fluoroscopy

    d. Tomogram

15. The nurse is instructing a patient who is scheduled for a perfusion lung scan. What should be included in the information about the procedure? (Select all that apply.)

    a. A mask will be placed over the nose and mouth during the test.

    b. The patient will be expected to lie under the camera.

    c. The imaging time will amount to 20 to 40 minutes.

    d. The patient will be expected to be NPO for 12 hours prior to the procedure.

    e. An injection will be placed into the lung during the procedure.

16. The nurse is performing an assessment for a patient with congestive heart failure. The nurse asks if the patient has difficulty breathing in any position other than upright. What is the nurse referring to?

    a. Dyspnea

    b. Orthopnea

    c. Tachypnea

    d. Bradypnea

17. The nurse is interviewing a patient who says he has a dry, irritating cough that is not "bringing anything up." What medication should the nurse question the patient about taking?

    a. Angiotensin converting enzyme (ACE) inhibitors

    b. Aspirin

    c. Bronchodilators

    d. Cardiac glycosides

18. What finding by the nurse may indicate that the patient has chronic hypoxia?

    a. Crackles

    b. Peripheral edema

    c. Clubbing of the fingers

    d. Cyanosis

19. The nurse is assessing a patient in respiratory failure. What finding is a late indicator of hypoxia?

a. Clubbing of fingers

b. Cyanosis

c. Crackles

d. Restlessness

20. The nurse is performing an assessment of a patient who arrived in the emergency department with a barbiturate overdose. The respirations are normal for 3 to 4 breaths followed by a 60-second period of apnea. How does the nurse document the respirations?

a. Cheyne-Stokes

b. Tachypnea

c. Bradypnea

d. Biot's respirations

CHAPTER 21

Respiratory Care Modalities

Learning Objectives

1. Describe the nursing management of patients receiving oxygen therapy, incentive spirometry, small-volume nebulizer therapy, chest physiotherapy, and breathing retraining.
2. Describe the patient education and home care considerations for patients receiving oxygen therapy.
3. Describe the nursing care of a patient with an endotracheal tube and a patient with a tracheostomy.
4. Demonstrate the procedure of tracheal suctioning.
5. Use the nursing process as a framework for care of patients who are mechanically ventilated.
6. Describe the process of weaning the patient from mechanical ventilation.
7. Describe the significance of preoperative nursing assessment and patient education for the patient who is going to have thoracic surgery.
8. Explain the principles of chest drainage and the nursing responsibilities related to the care of the patient with a chest drainage system.
9. Use the nursing process as a framework for care of a patient who has had a thoracotomy.

SECTION I: ASSESSING YOUR UNDERSTANDING

Activity A *Fill in the blanks.*

1. Oxygen transport to the tissues is dependent on four factors: _____, _____, _____, and _____.

2. Oxygen toxicity may occur when oxygen concentration at greater than ____% is administered for _____ (length of time).

3. Hypoxemia usually leads to _____, a decrease in oxygen supply to the tissues.

4. Antioxidants such as _____, _____, and _____ may help defend against oxygen free radicals.

5. In many patients with _____, the stimulus for respiration is a decrease in blood oxygen rather than an elevation in carbon dioxide levels.

6. It is important when a patient is on oxygen to post a _____ to prevent the danger of fire.

7. A _____ is used when a patient requires a low to medium concentration of oxygen for which precise accuracy is not essential.

8. A patient will require a _____ mask, which is the most reliable and accurate method of delivery, when a precise concentration of oxygen is required.

9. A patient in the process of being weaned from the ventilator will have a _____ connected to the endotracheal tube.

10. A patient has a dry suction water seal connected to a chest tube. When the water seal rises above _____ cm level, intrathoracic pressure increases.

11. The sigh mechanism on an assist-control ventilator needs to be adjusted to provide _____ sigh(s) per hour at a rate that is _____ times the tidal volume.

12. The oxygen flow rate for a nasal cannula should not exceed _____ L/min.

13. Cuff pressure for an endotracheal tube should be maintained at _____ mm Hg and should be checked every _____ hours.

14. For a patient to be safely weaned from a ventilator, the vital capacity should be _____ mL/kg; the minute ventilation should be _____ L/min; and the tidal volume should be _____ mL/kg.

15. Decreased gas exchange at the cellular level resulting from a toxic substance is classified as _____.

16. The term used to describe thoracic surgery in which an entire lung is removed is known as _____.

17. The water seal used in a disposable chest drainage system is effective if the water seal chamber is filled to the level of _____ cm H_2O.

Activity B *Briefly answer the following.*

1. List five signs and symptoms of oxygen toxicity:

_____, _____,

_____, _____,

and _____.

2. For a patient with chronic obstructive pulmonary disease (COPD), the stimulus for respiration is _____

_____.

3. Five examples of low-flow oxygen delivery systems are: _____,

_____, _____,

_____, and _____.

4. List three goals of chest physiotherapy (CPT):

_____, _____,

and _____.

5. What function does bilevel positive airway pressure (bi-PAP) ventilation serve for the patient?

_____

_____

_____

6. Explain how positive-pressure ventilators work.

_____

_____

7. Explain what is meant when the patient is said to be "bucking the ventilator."

_____

_____

_____

8. List four nursing diagnoses for a patient receiving mechanical ventilation: _____,

_____, _____,

and _____.

9. List seven postoperative risk factors for atelectasis and pneumonia.

_____   _____

_____   _____

_____   _____

_____

Activity C *Match the term listed in Column II with its associated definition listed in Column I.*

Column I

_____ **1.** Toxic substance interferes with the ability of tissues to use oxygen.

_____ **2.** Result of decreased effective hemoglobin concentration

_____ **3.** Results from inadequate capillary circulation

_____ **4.** Decreased oxygen level in the blood

_____ **5.** A decrease in the arterial oxygen tension in the blood

_____ **6.** Decrease in oxygen supply to the tissues

Column II

a. Hypoxia

b. Hypoxemia

c. Anemic hypoxia

d. Histotoxic hypoxia

e. Circulatory hypoxia

f. Hypoxemic hypoxia

SECTION II: APPLYING YOUR KNOWLEDGE

Activity D *Consider the scenarios and answer the questions.*

CASE STUDY: Pneumonectomy: Preoperative Concerns

Mrs. Miley, an older adult patient, is admitted to the clinical area in preparation for a scheduled pneumonectomy for the treatment of lung cancer.

1. What assessment data is important for the nurse to obtain during the admission history and physical examination?

_____

_____

2. The nurse evaluates the laboratory work for the patient preoperatively and determines that the creatinine level is elevated. Which body system requires assessment related to the results of this lab test?

_____

3. What is the best way for the nurse to assess Mrs. Miley's functional lung capacity?

_____

_____

CASE STUDY: Pneumonectomy: Postoperative Concerns

Mrs. Miley is returned to the clinical area after being in the intensive care unit (ICU). She is recovering from a right pneumonectomy.

1. While developing the plan of care for the patient, what does the nurse determine is the priority postoperative nursing objective?

_____

2. The patient has a central venous pressure catheter inserted by the physician. What can the catheter readings help the nurse to detect?

_____

3. While performing a respiratory assessment on Mrs. Miley, the nurse hears crackles in the lower lung bases and observes that the patient has dyspnea when turning over for the assessment. What does the nurse recognize these symptoms may indicate?

_____

4. The nurse is assessing the patient for signs of impending respiratory insufficiency. What symptoms does the nurse recognize would indicate this in the patient?

_____

CASE STUDY: Patient with Mechanical Ventilation

Mr. Brown, a 25-year-old man with a drug overdose, has been maintained on a volume-cycled ventilator for 3 weeks.

1. What priority nursing assessment would be indicated for this patient?

_____

2. What assessment findings by the nurse would indicate that the patient may be experiencing hypoxia and hypoxemia?

_____

3. The nurse is revising the plan of care for Mr. Brown. What nursing intervention would allow the goal of maintaining optimal gas exchange to be accomplished?

_____

_____

4. The nurse wants to determine early whether Mr. Brown is "bucking" his ventilator so that preventative measures can be taken. What clinical manifestations would be important for the nurse to recognize?

_____

_____

CASE STUDY: Weaning from Ventilator

Mr. O'Day, a 71-year-old trauma victim, is to be weaned from his ventilator.

1. Before weaning, what should Mr. O'Day's ventilatory capacity be?

_____

_____

_____

2. Mr. O'Day is scheduled to be extubated. What assessment criteria should he meet prior to extubation?

_____

_____

_____

3. What does the nurse recognize as an optimal PaO_2 range for the patient weaning from oxygen?

_____

SECTION III: PRACTICING FOR NCLEX

Activity E *Answer the following questions.*

1. The nurse is admitting a patient with COPD. The decrease of what substance in the blood gas analysis would indicate to the nurse that the patient is experiencing hypoxemia?

a. PaO_2

b. pH

c. PCO_2

d. HCO_3

2. A patient is brought into the emergency department with carbon monoxide poisoning after escaping a house fire. What should the nurse monitor this patient for?

a. Anemic hypoxia

b. Histotoxic hypoxia

c. Hypoxic hypoxia

d. Stagnant hypoxia

3. A patient with emphysema is placed on continuous oxygen at 2 L/min at home. Why is it important for the nurse to educate the patient and family that they must have No Smoking signs placed on the doors?

a. Oxygen is combustible.

b. Oxygen is explosive.

c. Oxygen prevents the dispersion of smoke particles.

d. Oxygen supports combustion.

4. A patient has been receiving 100% oxygen therapy by way of a nonrebreather mask for several days. Now the patient complains of tingling in the fingers and shortness of breath, is extremely restless, and describes a pain beneath the breastbone. What should the nurse suspect?

a. Oxygen-induced hypoventilation

b. Oxygen toxicity

c. Oxygen-induced atelectasis

d. Hypoxia

5. A patient is to receive an oxygen concentration of 70%. What is the best way for the nurse to deliver this concentration?

a. A nasal cannula

b. An oropharyngeal catheter

c. A partial rebreathing mask

d. A Venturi mask

6. A patient with COPD requires oxygen administration. What method of delivery does the nurse know would be best for this patient?

a. A nasal cannula

b. An oropharyngeal catheter

c. A nonrebreathing mask

d. A Venturi mask

7. The nurse is educating the patient in the use of a mini-nebulizer. What should the nurse encourage the patient to do? (Select all that apply.)

    a. Hold the breath at the end of inspiration for a few seconds.

    b. Cough frequently.

    c. Take rapid, deep breaths.

    d. Frequently evaluate progress.

    e. Prolong the expiratory phase after using the nebulizer.

8. A patient is being educated in the use of incentive spirometry prior to having a surgical procedure. What should the nurse be sure to include in the education?

    a. Have the patient lie in a supine position during the use of the spirometer.

    b. Encourage the patient to try to stop coughing during and after using the spirometer.

    c. Inform the patient that using the spirometer is not necessary if the patient is experiencing pain.

    d. Encourage the patient to take approximately 10 breaths per hour, while awake.

9. The nurse is educating a patient with COPD about the technique for performing pursed lip breathing. What does the nurse inform the patient is the importance of using this technique?

    a. It prolongs exhalation.

    b. It increases the respiratory rate to improve oxygenation.

    c. It will assist with widening the airway.

    d. It will prevent the alveoli from overexpanding.

10. A patient is being mechanically ventilated with an oral endotracheal tube in place. The nurse observes that the cuff pressure is 25 mm Hg. The nurse is aware of what complications that can be caused by this pressure? (Select all that apply.)

    a. Tracheal aspiration

    b. Hypoxia

    c. Tracheal ischemia

    d. Tracheal bleeding

    e. Pressure necrosis

11. A patient in the ICU has been orally intubated and on mechanical ventilation for 2 weeks after having a severe stroke. What action does the nurse anticipate the physician will take now that the patient has been intubated for this length of time?

    a. The patient will be extubated and another endotracheal tube will be inserted.

    b. The patient will be extubated and a nasotracheal tube will be inserted.

    c. The patient will have an insertion of a tracheostomy tube.

    d. The patient will begin the weaning process.

12. A new ICU nurse is observed by her preceptor entering a patient's room to suction the tracheostomy after performing the task 15 minutes before. What should the preceptor educate the new nurse to do to ensure that the patient needs to be suctioned?

    a. Auscultate the lung for adventitious sounds.

    b. Have the patient inform the nurse of the need to be suctioned.

    c. Assess the CO_2 level to determine if the patient requires suctioning.

    d. Have the patient cough.

13. The nurse is using an in-line suction kit to suction a patient who is intubated and on a mechanical ventilator. What benefits does in-line suction have for the patient? (Select all that apply.)

    a. Decreases hypoxemia

    b. Decreases patient anxiety

    c. Sustains positive end expiratory pressure (PEEP)

    d. Increases oxygen consumption

    e. Prevents aspiration

14. A patient is diagnosed with mild obstructive sleep apnea after having a sleep study performed. What treatment modality will be the most effective for this patient?

    a. Surgery to remove the tonsils and adenoids

    b. Medications to assist the patient with sleep at night

    c. Continuous positive airway pressure

    d. Bi-level positive airway pressure

15. The nurse hears the patient's ventilator alarm sound and attempts to find the cause. What is the priority action of the nurse when the cause of the alarm is not able to be determined?

   a. Call respiratory therapy and wait until they arrive to determine what is happening.

   b. Disconnect the patient from the ventilator and manually ventilate the patient with a manual resuscitation bag until the problem is resolved.

   c. Stop the ventilator by pressing the off button, wait 15 seconds, and then turn it on again to see if the alarm stops.

   d. Suction the patient since the patient may be obstructed by secretions.

16. A patient with emphysema informs the nurse, "The surgeon will be removing about 30% of my lung so that I will not be so short of breath and will have an improved quality of life." What surgery does the nurse understand the surgeon will perform?

   a. A sleeve resection

   b. A lung volume reduction

   c. A wedge resection

   d. Lobectomy

17. The nurse is assessing a patient with chest tubes connected to a drainage system. What should the first action be when the nurse observes excessive bubbling in the water seal chamber?

   a. Notify the physician.

   b. Place the head of the patient's bed flat.

   c. Milk the chest tube.

   d. Disconnect the system and get another.

18. The nurse is transporting a patient with chest tubes to a treatment room. The chest tube becomes disconnected and falls between the bed rail. What is the priority action by the nurse?

   a. Immediately reconnect the chest tube to the drainage apparatus.

   b. Clamp the chest tube close to the connection site.

   c. Cut the contaminated tip of the tube and insert a sterile connector and reattach.

   d. Call the physician.

19. The nurse suctions a patient through the endotracheal tube for 20 seconds and observes dysrhythmias on the monitor. What does the nurse determine is occurring with the patient?

   a. The patient is hypoxic from suctioning.

   b. The patient is having a stress reaction.

   c. The patient is having a myocardial infarction.

   d. The patient is in a hypermetabolic state.

20. The nurse assesses a patient with a heart rate of 42 and a blood pressure of 70/46. What type of hypoxia does the nurse determine this patient is displaying?

   a. Anemic hypoxia

   b. Circulatory hypoxia

   c. Histotoxic hypoxia

   d. Hypoxic hypoxia

CHAPTER 22

Management of Patients With Upper Respiratory Tract Disorders

Learning Objectives

1. Describe nursing management of patients with upper airway disorders.
2. Compare and contrast the upper respiratory tract infections according to cause, incidence, clinical manifestations, management, and the significance of preventive health care.
3. Use the nursing process as a framework for care of patients with upper airway infection.
4. Describe nursing management of the patient with epistaxis.
5. Use the nursing process as a framework for care of patients undergoing laryngectomy.

SECTION I: ASSESSING YOUR UNDERSTANDING

Activity A *Fill in the blanks.*

1. The most common cause of laryngitis is _____, with symptoms including _____, _____, and _____.

2. Medication therapy for allergic and nonallergic rhinitis focuses on _____.

3. _____ remain the most common treatment for rhinitis and are administered for sneezing, pruritus, and rhinorrhea.

4. Rhinosinusitis is classified by duration of symptoms as _____, _____, and _____.

5. _____ is the most common major suppurative complication of sore throat.

6. The most serious complication of a tonsillectomy is _____.

Activity B *Briefly answer the following.*

1. Explain how rhinitis can lead to rhinosinusitis.

_____

_____

_____

2. Name four bacterial organisms that account for more than 60% of all cases of acute rhinosinusitis: _____, _____, _____, and _____.

3. If untreated, chronic rhinosinusitis can lead to severe complications. List four: _____, _____, _____, and _____.

4. List four possible nursing diagnoses for a patient with an upper airway infection:

_____, _____,

_____, and _____.

5. List five potential complications of an upper airway infection: _____,

_____, _____,

_____, and _____.

6. List the clinical manifestations that are used to diagnose obstructive sleep apnea.

_____

_____

_____

7. List three types of alaryngeal communication:

_____, _____,

and _____.

Activity C *Match the term listed in Column II with its associated definition for surgical options for laryngeal cancer listed in Column I.*

Column I

____ **1.** Removal of the mucosa of the edge of the vocal cord

____ **2.** Excision of the vocal cord for lesions in the middle third of the vocal cord

____ **3.** Complete removal of the larynx

____ **4.** Portion of the larynx is removed, along with one vocal cord, and the tumor.

____ **5.** Microelectrodes are used for surgical resection of smaller laryngeal tumors.

Column II

a. Partial laryngectomy

b. Vocal cord stripping

c. Total laryngectomy

d. Laser surgery

e. Cordectomy

SECTION II: APPLYING YOUR KNOWLEDGE

Activity D *Consider the scenarios and answer the questions.*

CASE STUDY: Tonsillectomy and Adenoidectomy

Isabel, a 14-year-old girl, has just undergone a tonsillectomy and adenoidectomy. The staff nurse assists her with transport from the recovery area to her room.

1. The nurse observes Isabel swallowing frequently. What may this assessment finding indicate to the nurse?

_____

2. The nurse assesses Isabel and her vital signs. What specific postoperative complication should the nurse monitor for?

_____

3. What recommended postoperative position should the nurse ensure that Isabel maintains?

_____

_____

4. Isabel is to be discharged the same day of her tonsillectomy. What education should the nurse provide to Isabel and her family?

_____

CASE STUDY: Epistaxis

Gilberta, a 14-year-old high school student, is being sent with her parents to the emergency department of a local hospital for uncontrolled epistaxis.

1. What should the school nurse instruct Gilberta and her parents to do to control the bleeding during transport to the hospital?

_____

_____

_____

2. What emergency medical treatment does the nurse anticipate will be used when Gilberta arrives?

_____

3. The nurse can advise the parents that nasal packing used to control bleeding can be left in place for how long?

_____

CASE STUDY: Cancer of the Larynx

Brenda, a 64-year-old with a long-term history of smoking, recently retired from the chemical laboratory department of a large company. After months of complaining of a persistent cough, sore throat, pain, and burning in the throat, Brenda was admitted to the hospital with a diagnosis of cancer of the larynx.

1. The nurse is assessing Brenda upon admission and understands that which technique should be used to assess for laryngeal carcinoma?

_____

2. Brenda asks the nurse what her treatment will be for stage I cancer of the larynx. What is the best response by the nurse?

_____

_____

3. What information should the nurse give to Brenda about the importance of attending all of her follow-up visits to the physician?

_____

_____

CASE STUDY: Laryngectomy

Jerome, a 52-year-old widower, is admitted for a laryngectomy owing to a malignant tumor.

1. Before developing a care plan, the nurse needs to know whether Jerome's voice will be preserved. What surgical procedure does the nurse understand will not cause damage to the voice box?

_____

2. Jerome is scheduled for a total laryngectomy. What education should the nurse provide to the patient in the preoperative phase of surgery?

_____

_____

_____

3. The nurse is educating Jerome about the presence of a nasogastric catheter after surgery. The nurse should inform him that he will begin receiving oral feedings about how long after the surgery?

_____

4. Jerome asks the nurse when the laryngectomy tube will be removed. What should the nurse tell him?

_____

SECTION III: PRACTICING FOR NCLEX

Activity E *Answer the following questions.*

1. A patient comes to the clinic with a cold and wants something to help relieve the symptoms. What should the nurse include in educating the patient about the uncomplicated common cold? (Select all that apply.)

   a. Tell the patient to take prescribed antibiotics to decrease the severity of symptoms.

   b. Inform the patient about the symptoms of secondary infection.

   c. Suggest that the patient take adequate fluids and get plenty of rest.

   d. Inform the patient that the virus is contagious for 2 days before symptoms appear and during the first part of the symptomatic phase.

   e. Inform the patient that taking an antihistamine will help to decrease the duration of the cold.

2. A patient has herpes simplex infection that developed after having the common cold. What medication does the nurse anticipate will be administered for this infection?

   a. An antiviral agent such as acyclovir

   b. An antibiotic such as amoxicillin

   c. An antihistamine such as Benadryl

   d. An ointment such as bacitracin

3. A patient has been diagnosed with acute rhinosinusitis caused by a bacterial organism. What antibiotic of choice for treatment of this disorder does the nurse anticipate educating the patient about?

   a. Amoxicillin-clavulanate (Augmentin)

   b. Cephalexin (Keflex)

   c. Azithromycin (Zithromax)

   d. Clarithromycin (Biaxin)

4. The nurse is educating a patient diagnosed with acute bacterial rhinosinusitis about interventions that may assist with symptom control. What should the nurse include in this information? (Select all that apply.)

   a. Take an over-the-counter nasal decongestant.

   b. Take an over-the-counter antihistamine.

   c. Ensure an adequate fluid intake.

   d. Increase the humidity in the home.

   e. Apply local heat to promote drainage.

5. A patient comes to the clinic with complaints of a sore throat and is diagnosed with acute pharyngitis. What does the nurse understand is the cause of acute pharyngitis?

   a. Group A, beta-hemolytic streptococci

   b. Gram-negative *Klebsiella*

   c. *Pseudomonas aeruginosa*

   d. *Staphylococcus aureus*

6. A patient diagnosed 2 weeks ago with acute pharyngitis comes to the clinic stating that the sore throat got better for a couple of days and is now back along with an earache. What complications should the nurse be aware of related to acute pharyngitis? (Select all that apply.)

   a. Mastoiditis

   b. Otitis media

   c. Peritonsillar abscess

   d. Pericarditis

   e. Encephalitis

7. The nurse is educating the patient diagnosed with acute pharyngitis on methods to alleviate discomfort. What interventions should the nurse include in the information? (Select all that apply.)

   a. Apply an ice collar.

   b. Stay on bed rest during the febrile stage of the illness.

   c. Gargle with an alcohol-based mouthwash.

   d. Try a liquid or soft diet during the acute stage of the disease.

   e. Drink warm or hot liquids during the acute stage of the disease.

8. A patient comes to the clinic and is diagnosed with tonsillitis and adenoiditis. What bacterial pathogen does the nurse know is commonly associated with tonsillitis and adenoiditis?

   a. Gram-negative *Klebsiella*

   b. *Pseudomonas aeruginosa*

   c. Group A, beta-hemolytic streptococcus

   d. *Staphylococcus aureus*

9. A patient comes to the clinic complaining of a possible upper respiratory infection. What should the nurse inspect that would indicate that an upper respiratory infection may be present?

   a. The nasal mucosa

   b. The buccal mucosa

   c. The frontal sinuses

   d. The tracheal mucosa

10. A patient playing softball was hit in the nose by the ball and has been determined to have an uncomplicated fractured nose with epistaxis. The nurse should prepare to assist the physician with what tasks?

   a. Preparing the patient for a septoplasty

   b. Applying nasal packing

   c. Administering nasal lavage

   d. Applying steroidal nasal spray

11. A patient prescribed a medication for hypertension started taking it 3 days ago and arrives in the emergency department with an edematous face and tongue and having a difficult time speaking. What medication is the nurse aware of that may produce this type of side effect?

   a. Metoprolol succinate (Toprol XL)

   b. Amlodipine (Norvasc)

   c. Enalapril (Vasotec)

   d. Valsartan (Diovan)

12. The nurse is assessing a patient who smokes 2 packs of cigarettes per day and has a strong family history of cancer. What early sign of cancer of the larynx does the nurse look for in this patient?

   a. Burning of the throat when hot liquids are ingested

   b. Enlarged cervical nodes

   c. Dysphagia

   d. Affected voice sounds

13. A patient is diagnosed as being in the early stage of laryngeal cancer of the glottis with only 1 vocal cord involved. For what type of surgical intervention will the nurse plan to provide education?

   a. Total laryngectomy

   b. Cordectomy

   c. Vocal cord stripping

   d. Partial laryngectomy

14. A patient with an advanced laryngeal tumor is to have radiation therapy. The patient tells the nurse, "If I am going to have radiation, I won't need surgery." What is the best response by the nurse?

   a. "That is correct. The radiation will eradicate the tumor and you won't have to have further treatment."

   b. "Radiation is used to shrink the tumor size and is an adjunct to surgery."

   c. "All patients have to have radiation before they have surgery. It is protocol."

   d. "You really don't have to have radiation but you won't have to have such invasive surgery if you have the radiation first."

15. The nurse is caring for a patient who had a total laryngectomy and has drains in place. When does the nurse understand that the drains will most likely be removed?

   a. When the patient has less than 30 mL for 2 consecutive days

   b. When the patient states that there is discomfort and requests removal

   c. When the drainage tube comes out

   d. In 1 week when the patient no longer has serous drainage

CHAPTER 23

Management of Patients With Chest and Lower Respiratory Tract Disorders

Learning Objectives

1. Identify patients at risk for atelectasis and the nursing interventions related to its prevention and management.
2. Compare the various pulmonary infections with regard to causes, clinical manifestations, nursing management, complications, and prevention.
3. Use the nursing process as a framework for care of the patient with pneumonia.
4. Describe nursing measures to prevent aspiration.
5. Relate pleurisy, pleural effusion, and empyema to pulmonary infection.
6. Relate the therapeutic management techniques of acute respiratory distress syndrome to the underlying pathophysiology of the syndrome.
7. Describe risk factors and measures appropriate for prevention and management of pulmonary embolism.
8. Describe preventive measures appropriate for controlling and eliminating occupational lung disease.
9. Discuss the modes of therapy and related nursing management of patients with lung cancer.
10. Describe the complications of chest trauma and their clinical manifestations and nursing management.

SECTION I: ASSESSING YOUR UNDERSTANDING

Activity A *Fill in the blanks.*

1. The diagnosis of hospital-acquired pneumonia is usually associated with the presence of one of three conditions: _____, _____, and _____.

2. The mortality rate with ARDS is as high as ____%. The major cause of death is usually _____.

3. The 5-year survival rate for lung cancer is _____%.

4. _____, _____, and _____ are hallmarks of the severity of atelectasis.

5. When a nonfunctioning nasogastric tube allows the gastric contents to accumulate in the stomach, a condition known as _____ may result.

6. Three common pathogens that cause aspiration pneumonia are _____, _____, and _____.

7. Pneumonia tends to occur in patients with one or more of these five underlying disorders: _____, _____, _____, _____, and _____.

8. Three severe complications of pneumonia are _____, _____, and _____.

9. Four respiratory system mechanisms that can lead to acute respiratory failure (ARF) are _____, _____, _____, and _____.

Activity B *Briefly answer the following.*

1. Atelectasis, which refers to closure or collapse of alveoli, may be chronic or acute in nature. List 10 possible causes of atelectasis in the postoperative patient.

_____ _____

_____ _____

_____ _____

_____ _____

_____ _____

2. Name seven possible clinical manifestations of atelectasis.

_____ _____

_____ _____

_____ _____

_____

3. Identify eight nursing measures that can be used to prevent atelectasis.

_____ _____

_____ _____

_____ _____

_____ _____

4. Explain the meaning of the term *superinfection*.

_____

_____

5. Describe the characteristic and diagnostic feature of ARDS.

_____

_____

6. Define the etiology of cor pulmonale.

_____

_____

7. List at least six etiologic factors and nursing assessments for patients with ARDS.

_____ _____

_____ _____

_____ _____

Activity C *Match the classification of tuberculosis in Column II with its associated definition listed in Column I.*

Column I	Column II
____ 1. Disease; not clinically active	a. Class 0
	b. Class 1
____ 2. Latent infection; no disease (e.g., positive PPD)	c. Class 2
	d. Class 3
____ 3. Suspected disease; diagnosis pending	e. Class 4
	f. Class 5
____ 4. Exposure; no evidence of infection	
____ 5. No exposure; no infection	
____ 6. Disease; clinically active	

SECTION II: APPLYING YOUR KNOWLEDGE

Activity D *Consider the scenarios and answer the questions.*

CASE STUDY: Community-Acquired Pneumonia

Theresa, a 20-year-old college student, lives in a small dormitory with 30 other students. Four weeks into the spring semester, she was diagnosed as having bacterial pneumonia and was admitted to the hospital.

1. What intervention can the nurse provide to decrease the viscosity of the secretions?

_____

2. The nurse is assessing Theresa during the admission process. What manifestations of bacterial pneumonia does the nurse expect to find?

_____

_____

3. The nurse assesses Theresa for arterial hypoxemia. What does the nurse understand is the reason why this complication develops?

4. The nurse is assessing vital signs and lung sounds every 4 hours. What complications should the nurse monitor for?

CASE STUDY: Tuberculosis

Mr. Carrera, a 67-year-old retired baker and pastry chef, is admitted to the clinical area for confirmation of suspected tuberculosis. He is anorexic and fatigued and suffers from "indigestion." His temperature is slightly elevated every afternoon.

1. Mr. Carrera's Mantoux tuberculin test yields an induration area of 6 to 10 mm. What does the nurse interpret these findings to indicate?

2. Mr. Carrera has undergone a series of additional tests and a diagnosis is confirmed. What test does the nurse know provides confirmation that the patient has tuberculosis?

3. Mr. Carrera is started on a multiple-drug regimen. Which medication does the nurse understand may interfere with the metabolism of the beta blocker he is taking?

CASE STUDY: Acute Respiratory Distress Syndrome

Anne, 71 years of age and single, is admitted to the unit with a diagnosis of ARDS. She was receiving treatment at home for viral pneumonia and had appeared to be improving until yesterday.

1. The nurse is assessing Anne for clinical manifestations associated with ARDS. What symptoms does the nurse know positively correlate with ARDS?

2. The nurse is performing a neurological assessment for Anne. What symptoms observed by the nurse indicate that Anne is developing cerebral hypoxia?

3. The nurse observes that Anne is receiving oxygen by way of a nasal cannula at 6 L/min. What does the nurse determine Anne's FiO_2 would be?

CASE STUDY: Pulmonary Embolism

Sandy, a 37-year-old woman recovering from multiple fractures sustained in a car accident, was admitted to the intensive care unit for treatment of a pulmonary embolism. Before admission, she was short of breath after walking up a flight of stairs.

1. Sandy asks the nurse what could have caused this, since she was getting better from the accident and getting plenty of rest. What is the best response by the nurse?

2. What symptom does Sandy exhibit that most frequently occurs in the presence of a pulmonary embolism?

3. With a diagnosis of pulmonary embolism, what decrease in function should the nurse assess for?

SECTION III: PRACTICING FOR NCLEX

Activity E *Answer the following questions.*

1. The nurse is planning for the care of a patient with acute tracheobronchitis. What nursing interventions should be included in the plan of care? (Select all that apply.)
   a. Increasing fluid intake to remove secretions
   b. Encouraging the patient to remain in bed
   c. Using cool-vapor therapy to relieve laryngeal and tracheal irritation
   d. Giving 3 L fluid per day
   e. Administering a narcotic analgesic for pain

2. The nurse knows that a sputum culture is necessary to identify the causative organism for acute tracheobronchitis. What causative fungal organism would the nurse suspect?

   a. *Aspergillus*

   b. *Haemophilus*

   c. *Mycoplasma pneumoniae*

   d. *Streptococcus pneumoniae*

3. The nurse is conducting a community program about prevention of respiratory illness. What illness does the nurse know is the most common cause of death in the United States?

   a. Atelectasis

   b. Pulmonary embolus

   c. Pneumonia

   d. Tracheobronchitis

4. A patient comes to the clinic with fever, cough, and chest discomfort. The nurse auscultates crackles in the left lower base of the lung and suspects that the patient may have pneumonia. What does the nurse know is the most common organism that causes community-acquired pneumonia?

   a. *Staphylococcus aureus*

   b. *Mycobacterium tuberculosis*

   c. *Pseudomonas aeruginosa*

   d. *Streptococcus pneumoniae*

5. A patient has a Mantoux skin test prior to being placed on an immunosuppressant for the treatment of Crohn's disease. What results would the nurse determine is not significant for holding the medication?

   a. 0 to 4 mm

   b. 5 to 6 mm

   c. 7 to 8 mm

   d. 9 mm

6. The nurse is educating a patient who will be started on an antituberculosis medication regimen. The patient asks the nurse, "How long will I have to be on these medications?" What should the nurse tell the patient?

   a. 3 months

   b. 3 to 5 months

   c. 6 to 12 months

   d. 13 to 18 months

7. The nurse is caring for a patient with pleurisy. What symptoms does the nurse recognize are significant for this patient's diagnosis?

   a. Dullness or flatness on percussion over areas of collected fluid

   b. Dyspnea and coughing

   c. Fever and chills

   d. Stabbing pain during respiratory movement

8. The nurse is auscultating the patient's lung sounds to determine the presence of pulmonary edema. What adventitious lung sounds are significant for pulmonary edema?

   a. Crackles in the lung bases

   b. Low-pitched rhonchi during expiration

   c. Pleural friction rub

   d. Sibilant wheezes

9. A patient taking isoniazid (INH) therapy for tuberculosis demonstrates understanding when making which statement?

   a. "I am going to have a tuna fish sandwich for lunch."

   b. "It is all right if I drink a glass of red wine with my dinner."

   c. "It is all right if I have a grilled cheese sandwich with American cheese."

   d. "It is fine if I eat sushi with a little bit of soy sauce."

10. A patient who wears contact lenses is to be placed on rifampin for tuberculosis therapy. What should the nurse tell the patient?

    a. "Only wear your contact lenses during the day and take them out in the evening before bed."

    b. "You should switch to wearing your glasses while taking this medication."

    c. "The physician can give you eye drops to prevent any problems."

    d. "There are no significant problems with wearing contact lenses."

11. The nurse is caring for a patient with suspected ARDS with a pO_2 of 53. The patient is placed on oxygen via face mask and the PO_2 remains the same. What does the nurse recognize as a key characteristic of ARDS?

    a. Unresponsive arterial hypoxemia

    b. Diminished alveolar dilation

    c. Tachypnea

    d. Increased PaO_2

12. A patient is admitted to the hospital with pulmonary arterial hypertension. What assessment finding by the nurse is a significant finding for this patient?

    a. Ascites

    b. Dyspnea

    c. Hypertension

    d. Syncope

13. The nurse is assessing a patient who has been admitted with possible ARDS. What findings would distinguish ARDS from cardiogenic pulmonary edema?

    a. Elevated white blood count

    b. Elevated troponin levels

    c. Elevated myoglobin levels

    d. Elevated B-type natriuretic peptide (BNP) levels

14. A patient with pulmonary hypertension has a positive vasoreactivity test. What medication does the nurse anticipate administering to this patient?

    a. Calcium channel blockers

    b. Angiotensin converting enzyme inhibitor

    c. Beta blockers

    d. Angiotensin receptor blockers

15. The nurse assesses a patient for a possible pulmonary embolism. What frequent sign of pulmonary embolus does the nurse anticipate finding on assessment?

    a. Cough

    b. Hemoptysis

    c. Syncope

    d. Tachypnea

16. The nurse is administering anticoagulant therapy with heparin. What International Normalized Ratio (INR) would the nurse know is within therapeutic range?

    a. 0.5 to 1.0

    b. 1.5 to 2.5

    c. 2.0 to 2.5

    d. 3.0 to 3.5

17. The nurse is planning the care for a patient at risk of developing pulmonary embolism. What nursing interventions should be included in the care plan? (Select all that apply.)

    a. Encouraging a liberal fluid intake

    b. Assisting the patient to do leg elevations above the level of the heart

    c. Instructing the patient to dangle the legs over the side of the bed for 30 minutes, four times a day

    d. Using elastic stockings, especially when decreased mobility would promote venous stasis

    e. Applying a sequential compression device

18. A patient who had a colon resection 3 days ago is complaining of discomfort in the left calf. How should the nurse assess Homan's sign to determine if the patient may have a thrombus formation in the leg?

    a. Dorsiflex the foot while the leg is elevated to check for calf pain.

    b. Elevate the patient's legs for 20 minutes and then lower them slowly while checking for areas of inadequate blood return.

    c. Extend the leg, plantar flex the foot, and check for the patency of the dorsalis pedis pulse.

    d. Lower the patient's legs and massage the calf muscles to note any areas of tenderness.

19. The nurse is having an information session with a women's group at the YMCA about lung cancer. What frequent and commonly experienced symptom should the nurse be sure to include in the session?

    a. Copious sputum production

    b. Coughing

    c. Dyspnea

    d. Severe pain

20. A patient arrives in the emergency department after being involved in a motor vehicle accident. The nurse observes paradoxical chest movement when removing the patient's shirt. What does the nurse know that this finding indicates?

    a. Pneumothorax

    b. Flail chest

    c. ARDS

    d. Tension pneumothorax

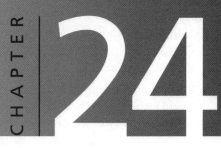
Management of Patients With Chronic Pulmonary Disease

1. Describe the pathophysiology of chronic obstructive pulmonary disease (COPD).
2. Discuss the major risk factors for developing COPD and nursing interventions to minimize or prevent these risk factors.
3. Use the nursing process as a framework for care of patients with COPD.
4. Develop an education plan for patients with COPD.
5. Describe the pathophysiology of bronchiectasis and relate it to signs and symptoms of bronchiectasis.
6. Identify medical and nursing management of bronchiectasis.
7. Describe the pathophysiology of asthma.
8. Discuss the medications used in asthma management.
9. Describe asthma self-management strategies.
10. Describe the pathophysiology of cystic fibrosis.

SECTION I: ASSESSING YOUR UNDERSTANDING

Activity A *Fill in the blanks.*

1. In 2011, COPD and associated respiratory diseases were estimated to affect 24 million adults and was the _____ leading cause of death in the United States (National Heart, Lung and Blood Institute [NHLBI], 2011).

2. _____ also contributes to respiratory symptoms and COPD (GOLD, 2010).

3. Patients with COPD are at risk for _____ and _____, which in turn increase the risk of acute and chronic respiratory failure.

4. _____ is used to evaluate airflow obstruction, which is determined by the ratio of FEV_1 to forced vital capacity (FVC).

5. A _____ is a surgical option for select patients with bullous emphysema.

6. The *single most cost-effective* intervention to reduce the risk of developing COPD or slow its progression is _____.

7. Primary causes for an acute exacerbation of COPD are _____ and _____.

8. To help prevent infections in patients with COPD, the nurse should recommend vaccination against two bacterial organisms: _____ and _____.

9. The strongest predisposing factor for asthma is _____; the three most common symptoms are _____, _____, and _____.

10. Complications of asthma may include _____, _____, _____, and _____.

11. The median survival age for individuals diagnosed with cystic fibrosis is now _____ years.

Activity B *Briefly answer the following.*

1. Describe the results of chronic airway inflammation in COPD.

_____

_____

_____

2. Define the term *emphysema*.

_____

_____

_____

3. Name a genetic risk factor for COPD.

_____

4. List the three *primary symptoms* associated with the progressive stage of COPD.

_____

_____

5. List five of the nine major factors that determine the clinical course and survival of patients with COPD.

_____

_____

6. Name three ways that bronchodilators relieve bronchospasm.

_____

_____

Activity C *Match the drug category listed in Column II with an associated medication in Column I.*

Column I

____ 1. Proventil

____ 2. Atrovent

____ 3. Combivent

____ 4. Theo-Dur

____ 5. Singulair

____ 6. Cromolyn Sodium

Column II

a. Mast cell stabilizer

b. Leukotriene modifier

c. Anticholinergic agent

d. Methylxanthine

e. Combination short-acting beta 2-adrenergic agonist agent

f. Beta 2-adrenergic agonist agent

SECTION II: APPLYING YOUR KNOWLEDGE

Activity D *Consider the scenario and answer the questions.*

CASE STUDY: Emphysema

Lois, who has had emphysema for 25 years, is admitted to the hospital with a diagnosis of bronchitis.

1. The nurse observes that Lois has a "barrel chest." What does the nurse understand causes the shape of the chest?

_____

2. The nurse recognizes the need to be alert for what major presenting symptom of emphysema?

_____

3. The nurse is assessing the results of Lois's arterial blood gas. Which blood gas analysis will correlate with the diagnosis of emphysema?

_____

4. Lois is being medicated with a bronchodilator to reduce airway obstruction. What side effects should the nurse observe for that could be caused by the bronchodilator?

_____

_____

5. The nurse is educating Lois on diaphragmatic breathing. The nurse understands that this type of breathing will help Lois in what ways?

_____

_____

6. The physician prescribes oxygen therapy for Lois. What delivery system does the nurse know will be most effective?

_____

_____

SECTION III: PRACTICING FOR NCLEX

Activity E *Answer the following questions.*

1. A patient comes to the clinic for the third time in 2 months with chronic bronchitis. What clinical symptoms does the nurse anticipate assessing for this patient?

a. Chest pain during respiration

b. Sputum and a productive cough

c. Fever, chills, and diaphoresis

d. Tachypnea and tachycardia

2. The nurse is assigned to care for a patient with COPD with hypoxemia and hypercapnia. When planning care for this patient, what does the nurse understand is the main goal of treatment?

a. Providing sufficient oxygen to improve oxygenation

b. Avoiding the use of oxygen to decrease the hypoxic drive

c. Monitoring the pulse oximetry to assess need for early intervention when PCO_2 levels rise

d. Increasing pH

3. A nurse notes that the FEV_1/FVC ratio is less than 70% for a patient with COPD. What stage should the nurse document the patient is in?

a. 0

b. I

c. II

d. III

4. Upon assessment, the nurse suspects that a patient with COPD may have bronchospasm. What manifestations validate the nurse's concern? (Select all that apply.)

a. Compromised gas exchange

b. Decreased airflow

c. Wheezes

d. Jugular vein distention

e. Ascites

5. The physician orders a beta-2 adrenergic agonist agent (bronchodilator) that is short-acting and administered only by inhaler. What medication does the nurse anticipate will be administered?

a. Alupent

b. Brethine

c. Foradil

d. Isuprel

6. A patient with end-stage COPD and heart failure asks the nurse about lung reduction surgery. What is the best response by the nurse?

a. "You are not a candidate because you have heart failure."

b. "You would have a difficult time recovering from the procedure."

c. "At this point, do you really want to go through something like that?"

d. "You and your physician should discuss the options that are available for treatment."

7. The nurse should be alert for a complication of bronchiectasis that results from a combination of retained secretions and obstruction and that leads to the collapse of alveoli. What complication should the nurse monitor for?

a. Atelectasis

b. Emphysema

c. Pleurisy

d. Pneumonia

8. A patient is prescribed a mast cell stabilizer for the treatment of asthma. Which commonly used medication will the nurse educate the patient about?

   a. Albuterol

   b. Budesonide

   c. Cromolyn sodium

   d. Theophylline

9. The nurse is caring for a patient with status asthmaticus in the intensive care unit (ICU). What does the nurse anticipate observing for the blood gas results related to hyperventilation for this patient?

   a. Metabolic acidosis

   b. Metabolic alkalosis

   c. Respiratory acidosis

   d. Respiratory alkalosis

10. A child is having an asthma attack and the parent can't remember which inhaler to use for quick relief. The nurse accesses the child's medication information and tells the parent to use which inhalant?

    a. Cromolyn sodium

    b. Theo-Dur

    c. Serevent

    d. Proventil

11. The nurse is educating a patient with asthma about preventative measures to avoid having an asthma attack. What does the nurse inform the patient is a priority intervention to prevent an asthma attack?

    a. Using a long-acting steroid inhaler when an attack is coming

    b. Avoiding exercise and any strenuous activity

    c. Preparing a written action plan

    d. Staying in the house if it is too cold or too hot

12. The nurse is assigned to care for a patient in the ICU who is diagnosed with status asthmaticus. Why does the nurse include fluid intake as being an important aspect of the plan of care? (Select all that apply.)

    a. To combat dehydration

    b. To assist with the effectiveness of the corticosteroids

    c. To loosen secretions

    d. To facilitate expectoration

    e. To relieve bronchospasm

13. A patient is being treated for status asthmaticus. What danger sign does the nurse observe that can indicate impending respiratory failure?

    a. Respiratory acidosis

    b. Respiratory alkalosis

    c. Metabolic acidosis

    d. Metabolic alkalosis

14. A patient with cystic fibrosis is admitted to the hospital with pneumonia. When should the nurse administer the pancreatic enzymes that the patient has been prescribed?

    a. After meals and at bedtime

    b. Before meals

    c. With meals

    d. Three times a day regardless of meal time

15. The nurse is instructing the patient with asthma in the use of a newly prescribed leukotriene receptor antagonist. What should the nurse be sure to include in the education?

    a. The patient should take the medication with meals since it may cause nausea.

    b. The patient should take the medication separately without other medications.

    c. The patient should take the medication an hour before meals or 2 hours after a meal.

    d. The patient should take the medication with a small amount of liquid.

Cardiovascular and Circulatory Function

CHAPTER 25

Assessment of Cardiovascular Function

Learning Objectives

1. Describe the relationship between the anatomic structures and the physiologic function of the cardiovascular system.
2. Incorporate assessment of cardiac risk factors into the health history and physical assessment of the patient with cardiovascular disease.
3. Explain the proper techniques to perform a comprehensive cardiovascular assessment.
4. Discriminate between normal and abnormal assessment findings identified by inspection, palpation, percussion, and auscultation of the cardiovascular system.
5. Recognize and evaluate the major manifestations of cardiovascular dysfunction by applying concepts from the patient's health history and physical assessment findings.
6. Discuss the clinical indications, patient preparation, and other related nursing implications for common tests and procedures used to assess cardiovascular function and diagnose cardiovascular diseases.
7. Compare the various methods of hemodynamic monitoring (e.g., central venous pressure, pulmonary artery pressure, and arterial pressure monitoring) with regard to indications for use, potential complications, and nursing responsibilities.

SECTION I: ASSESSING YOUR UNDERSTANDING

Activity A *Fill in the blanks.*

1. Postural (orthostatic) hypotension is a sustained decrease of at least _____ mm Hg in systolic BP or _____ mm Hg in diastolic BP within 3 minutes of moving from a lying or sitting to a standing position (Freeman et al. 2011).

2. _____, _____, and _____ are measured to evaluate a person's risk of developing coronary artery disease (CAD), especially if there is a family history of premature heart disease, or to diagnose a specific lipoprotein abnormality.

3. Homocysteine, an amino acid, is linked to the development of _____ because it can damage the endothelial lining of arteries and promote thrombus formation.

4. A chest x-ray is obtained to determine the _____, _____, and _____ of the heart.

5. After having a cardiac catheterization, the patient is to remain in the bed for _____ to _____ hours.

6. The three factors that determine stroke volume are _____, _____, and _____.

7. Three major cardiovascular risk factors are _____, _____, and _____.

8. If CAD is present, the American Heart Association (AHA) recommends the following laboratory measurements: low-density lipoprotein (LDL), _____; blood pressure (BP), _____; serum glucose concentration, _____; and a body mass index (BMI) of _____.

9. The two most specific enzymes traditionally used to analyze an acute myocardial infarction (MI) are _____ and _____; two new biomarkers, _____ and _____, are early indicators of a myocardial infarction (MI).

Activity B *Briefly answer the following.*

1. List the five categories of cardiovascular disease (CVD): _____, _____, _____, _____, and _____.

2. Distinguish between the functions of the atrioventricular and the semilunar valves.

_____
_____
_____
_____

3. Briefly explain depolarization as it relates to cardiac physiology.

_____
_____
_____

4. Estimate the cardiac output, per beat, for an adult heart rate of 76 beats per minute (bpm) with an average stroke volume of 70 mL per beat.

_____

5. Describe Starling's law of the heart.

_____
_____
_____

6. List four physiologic effects on the cardiovascular system that are associated with the aging process: _____, _____, _____, and _____.

7. To assess the apical pulse, the nurse would find the following location:

_____.

8. List several purposes of cardiac catheterization.

_____
_____
_____

9. Describe selective angiography.

_____
_____

10. Discuss the implications of a low central venous pressure reading.

_____
_____

11. Identify four of seven possible complications of pulmonary artery monitoring: _____, _____, _____, and _____.

Activity C

PART I

Match the anatomic term in Column II with its associated function in Column I.

Column I

____ 1. Separates the right and left atria

____ 2. Is located at the juncture of the superior vena cava and the right atrium

____ 3. Supports the heart in the mediastinum

____ 4. Sits between the right ventricle and the pulmonary artery

____ 5. Distributes venous blood to the lungs

____ 6. Is embedded in the right atrial wall near the tricuspid valve

Column II

a. Parietal pericardium

b. Pulmonary artery

c. Bicuspid valve

d. Pulmonic valve

e. Sinotrial node

f. Atrioventricular node

PART II

Match the terminology associated with coronary atherosclerosis in Column II with its function/characteristic listed in Column I.

Column I

_____ 1. A principal blood lipid

_____ 2. A risk factor that causes pulmonary damage

_____ 3. The functional lesion of atherosclerosis

_____ 4. Biochemical substances, soluble in fat, that accumulate within a blood vessel

_____ 5. A risk factor that is endocrine in origin

_____ 6. A risk factor associated with a type A personality

_____ 7. A risk factor related to weight gain

_____ 8. A recommended dietary restriction that is a risk factor for heart disease

_____ 9. A symptom of myocardial ischemia

_____ 10. Myocardial manifestation of CAD

_____ 11. A lifestyle habit that is considered a modifiable risk factor for heart disease

Column II

a. Atheroma
b. Obesity
c. Chest pain
d. Cholesterol
e. Inactivity
f. Lipids
g. Smoking
h. Dysrhythmias
i. Diabetes
j. Fat
k. Stress

Activity D *Compare the following two figures found in Table 25-2, Assessing Chest Pain, in the main text, depicting the pain pathway of musculoskeletal disorders and pericarditis. Answer the associated questions.*

	Pericarditis	Musculoskeletal Disorders
Duration of pain:	_____	_____
Precipitating events and aggravating factors:	_____	_____
	_____	_____
	_____	_____
	_____	_____
Alleviating factors:	_____	_____
	_____	_____
	_____	_____

SECTION II: APPLYING YOUR KNOWLEDGE

Activity E *Consider the scenario and answer the questions.*

CASE STUDY: Cardiac Assessment for Chest Pain

Mr. Anderson is a 45-year-old executive with a major oil firm. Lately he has experienced frequent episodes of chest pressure that are relieved with rest. He has requested a complete physical examination. The nurse conducts an initial cardiac assessment.

1. The nurse immediately inspects the patient's skin and observes a bluish tinge around his lips. What does the nurse know that this indicates?

   _____

2. The nurse takes a baseline blood pressure measurement after the patient has rested for 10 minutes in a supine position. Which reading reflects a reduced pulse pressure?

   a. 140/90 mm Hg

   b. 140/100 mm Hg

   c. 140/110 mm Hg

   d. 140/120 mm Hg

3. Five minutes after the initial blood pressure measurement is taken, the nurse assesses additional readings with the patient in a sitting and then in a standing position. Which reading is indicative of an abnormal postural response?

   a. lying, 140/110; sitting, 130/110; standing, 135/106 mm Hg

   b. lying, 140/110; sitting, 135/112; standing, 130/115 mm Hg

   c. lying, 140/110; sitting, 135/100; standing, 120/90 mm Hg

   d. lying, 140/110; sitting, 130/108; standing, 125/108 mm Hg

4. The nurse returns Mr. Anderson to the supine position and measures for jugular vein distention. The finding that would indicate an abnormal increase in the volume of the venous system would be obvious distention of the veins when the patient is positioned at what angle?

   _____

5. The nurse auscultates the apex of the heart. Over what area should the nurse place the stethoscope?

   _____

SECTION III: PRACTICING FOR NCLEX

Activity F *Answer the following questions.*

1. The nurse is caring for a patient with a diagnosis of pericarditis. Where does the nurse understand the inflammation is located?

   a. The thin fibrous sac encasing the heart

   b. The inner lining of the heart and valves

   c. The heart's muscle fibers

   d. The exterior layer of the heart

2. The nurse is assessing heart sounds in a patient with heart failure. An abnormal heart sound is detected early in diastole. How would the nurse document this?

   a. S_1

   b. S_2

   c. S_3

   d. S_4

3. The nurse is performing an assessment of the patient's heart. Where would the nurse locate the apical pulse if the heart is in a normal position?

   a. Left 2nd intercostal space at the midclavicular line

   b. Right 2nd intercostal space at the midclavicular line

   c. Right 3rd intercostal space at the midclavicular line

   d. Left 5th intercostal space at the midclavicular line

4. A patient's heart rate is observed to be 140 bpm on the monitor. The nurse knows that the patient is at risk for what complication?

   a. Myocardial ischemia

   b. A pulmonary embolism

   c. Right-sided heart failure

   d. A stroke

5. The nurse is administering a beta blocker to a patient in order to decrease automaticity. Which medication will the nurse administer?

   a. Cardizem

   b. Lopressor

   c. Cordarone

   d. Rythmol

6. The patient has a heart rate of 72 bpm with a regular rhythm. Where does the nurse determine the impulse arises from?

   a. The AV node

   b. The Purkinje fibers

   c. The sinoatrial node

   d. The ventricles

7. The nurse is assessing a patient's electrocardiogram (ECG). What phase does the nurse determine is the resting phase before the next depolarization?

   a. Phase 1

   b. Phase 2

   c. Phase 3

   d. Phase 4

8. The nurse is reviewing the results of the patient's echocardiogram and observes that the ejection fraction is 35%. The nurse anticipates that the patient will receive treatment for what condition?

   a. Pulmonary embolism

   b. Myocardial infarction

   c. Pericarditis

   d. Heart failure

9. The nurse is educating a patient at risk for atherosclerosis. What nonmodifiable risk factors does the nurse identify for the patient?

   a. Stress

   b. Obesity

   c. Positive family history

   d. Hyperlipidemia

10. The nurse is assessing a patient's blood pressure. What does the nurse document as the difference between the systolic and the diastolic pressure?

    a. Pulse pressure

    b. Auscultatory gap

    c. Pulse deficit

    d. Korotkoff sound

11. The nurse is assessing a patient who complains of feeling "light-headed." When obtaining orthostatic vital signs, what does the nurse determine is a significant finding?

    a. A heart rate of 20 bpm above the resting rate

    b. An unchanged systolic pressure

    c. An increase of 10 mm Hg blood pressure reading

    d. An increase of 5 mm Hg in diastolic pressure

12. The nurse observes a certified nursing assistant (CNA) obtaining a blood pressure reading with a cuff that is too small for the patient. The nurse informs the CNA that using a cuff that is too small can affect the reading results in what way?

    a. The results will be falsely decreased.

    b. The results will be falsely elevated.

    c. It will give an accurate reading.

    d. It will be significantly different with each reading.

13. A 52-year-old female patient is going through menopause and asks the nurse about estrogen replacement for its cardioprotective benefits. What is the best response by the nurse?

    a. "That's a great idea. You don't want to have a heart attack."

    b. "Current research determines that the replacement of estrogen will protect a woman after she goes into menopause."

    c. "Current evidence indicates that estrogen is ineffective as a cardioprotectant; estrogen is actually potentially harmful and is no longer a recommended therapy."

    d. "You need to research it and determine what you want to do."

14. A patient tells the nurse, "I was straining to have a bowel movement and felt like I was going to faint. I took my pulse and it was so slow." What does the nurse understand occurred with this patient?

a. The patient may have had a myocardial infarction.

b. The patient had a vagal response.

c. The patient was anxious about being constipated.

d. The patient may have an abdominal aortic aneurysm.

15. A patient had a cardiac catheterization and is now in the recovery area. What nursing interventions should be included in the plan of care? (Select all that apply.)

a. Assessing the peripheral pulses in the affected extremity

b. Checking the insertion site for hematoma formation

c. Evaluating temperature and color in the affected extremity

d. Assisting the patient to the bathroom after the procedure

e. Assessing vital signs every 8 hours

Management of Patients With Dysrhythmias and Conduction Problems

Learning Objectives

1. Correlate the components of the normal electrocardiogram (ECG) with physiologic events of the heart.
2. Define the ECG as a waveform that represents the cardiac electrical event in relation to the lead (placement of electrodes).
3. Analyze elements of an ECG rhythm strip: ventricular and atrial rate, ventricular and atrial rhythm, QRS complex and shape, QRS duration, P wave and shape, PR interval, and P:QRS ratio.
4. Identify the ECG criteria, causes, and management of several dysrhythmias, including conduction disturbances.
5. Use the nursing process as a framework for care of patients with dysrhythmias.
6. Compare the different types of pacemakers, their uses, possible complications, and nursing implications.
7. Describe the nursing management of patients with implantable cardiac devices.
8. Describe the key points of using a defibrillator.
9. Describe the purpose of an implantable cardioverter defibrillator, the types available, and the nursing implications.
10. Describe invasive methods to diagnose and treat recurrent dysrhythmias and discuss the nursing implications.

SECTION I: ASSESSING YOUR UNDERSTANDING

Activity A *Fill in the blanks.*

1. The term _____ is used to describe an irregular or erratic heart rhythm.

2. The ability of the cardiac muscle to initiate an electrical impulse is called _____.

3. The ability of the cardiac muscle to transmit electrical impulses is called _____.

4. The term _____ is used to describe the electrical stimulation of the heart.

5. The ventricles relax in the _____ stage of conduction.

6. _____ treats dysrhythmias by destroying causative cells.

7. The total time for ventricular depolarization and repolarization is represented on an electrocardiogram (ECG) reading as the

   _____.

8. The PR interval on an ECG strip that reflects normal sinus rhythm would be between _____ and _____.

9. A dysrhythmia common in normal hearts and described by patients as "my heart skipped a beat" is _____.

10. A "sawtooth" P wave is seen on an ECG strip with _____.

11. Sinus tachycardia occurs when the ventricular and atrial rate are greater than _____.

Activity B *Briefly answer the following.*

1. What are the four sites of origin for impulses that are used to name dysrhythmias?

_____

_____

2. Describe the normal electrical conduction through the heart.

_____

_____

_____

3. Name five causes of sinus tachycardia.

_____

_____

4. What rate and rhythm are characteristic of ventricular tachycardia?

_____

_____

5. List three potential collaborative problems that a nurse would choose for a patient with dysrhythmias.

_____

_____

6. What is the difference between cardioversion and defibrillation?

_____

_____

_____

7. How are the electrode paddles placed on the patient's chest for defibrillation?

_____

_____

_____

8. Describe the difference between on-demand and fixed-rate or asynchronous pacemaker.

_____

_____

_____

9. Describe the "maze procedure" used in cardiac conduction surgery.

_____

_____

_____

Activity C *Match the description in Column II with the key term in Column I.*

Column I	Column II
____ 1. P wave	a. End of T wave to beginning of next P wave
____ 2. QRS complex	
____ 3. T wave	b. Atrial depolarization
____ 4. U wave	c. Normal range 0.32 to 0.40
____ 5. PR interval	d. Ventricular depolarization
____ 6. ST segment	
____ 7. QT interval	e. Early ventricular depolarization
____ 8. TP interval	f. Ventricular repolarization
	g. Normal range 0.12 to 0.20
	h. Repolarization of the Purkinje fibers

SECTION II: APPLYING YOUR KNOWLEDGE

Activity D

Graph Analysis

Analyze the following ECG graphs and answer the questions.

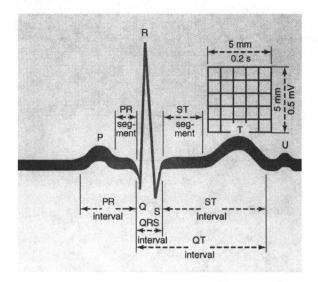

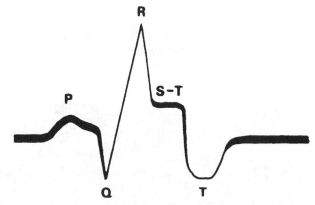

Each small box on the graph above represents 0.04 seconds on the horizontal axis and 1 mm or 0.1 mV on the vertical axis. The PR interval is measured from the beginning of the P wave to the beginning of the QRS complex; the QRS complex is measured from the beginning of the Q wave to the end of the S wave; the QT interval is measured from the beginning of the Q wave to the end of the T wave.

1. Look at the above graphic recording of cardiac electrical activity. For each action below, choose a wave deflection that corresponds to it, and write the appropriate letter or letters on the line provided:

   a. ____ ventricular muscle repolarization

   b. ____ time required for an impulse to travel through the atria and the conduction system to the Purkinje fibers

   c. ____ atrial muscle depolarization

   d. ____ ventricular muscle depolarization

   e. ____ early ventricular repolarization of the ventricles

2. Consider the above graphic recording, and identify three alterations that are consistent with myocardial ischemia and infarction hours to days after the attack:

   a. _____

   b. _____

   c. _____

Graphic Recordings

Analyze the graphic recording for each of the following dysrhythmias and describe the altered deflection.

1.

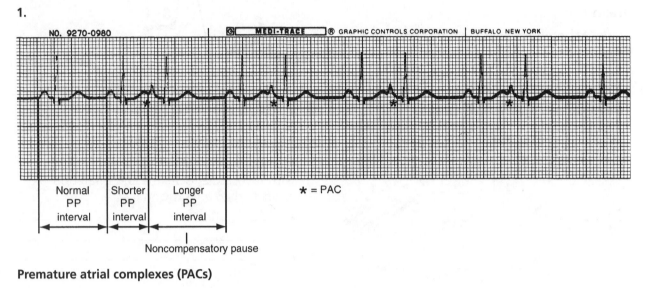

★ = PAC

Premature atrial complexes (PACs)

_____

_____

_____

2.

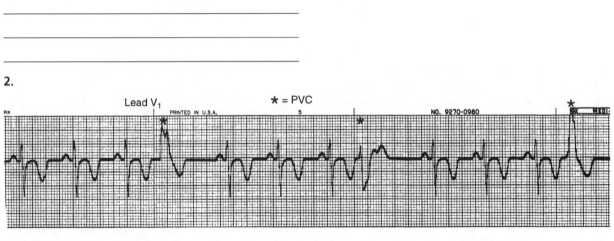

Multifocal PVCs in quadrigeminy

_____

_____

_____

3.

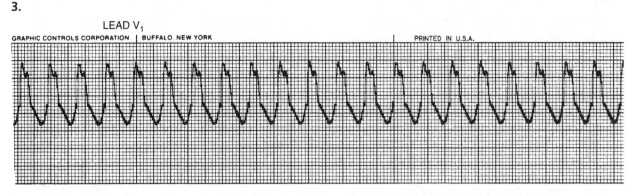

LEAD V$_1$

GRAPHIC CONTROLS CORPORATION | BUFFALO. NEW YORK | PRINTED IN U.S.A.

Ventricular tachycardia

_____

_____

_____.

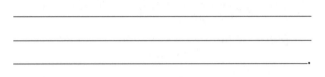 **Activity E** *Consider the scenario and answer the questions.*

CASE STUDY: Permanent Pacemaker

Mr. Woo is a 58-year-old Asian man who is scheduled for permanent pacemaker insertion as treatment for a tachydysrhythmia that does not respond to medication therapy. He is scheduled for an endocardial implant. Answer the following questions related to pacemaker management.

1. Mr. Woo's pacemaker is set at 72 bpm. His heart rate is 76 bpm. Is this expected? Explain the rationale for your answer.

_____

_____

2. What should the nurse monitor for at the incision site for potential complications?

_____

3. What common initial postoperative complication should the nurse monitor for after Mr. Woo has an insertion of a permanent pacemaker?

_____

4. What should the nurse document about Mr. Woo's pacemaker on the chart?

_____

_____

5. What nursing interventions and expected patient outcomes would be used to meet the goals of patient care?

_____

_____

_____

_____

SECTION III: PRACTICING FOR NCLEX

Activity F *Answer the following questions.*

1. A patient comes to the Emergency department with complaints of chest pain after using cocaine. The nurse assesses the patient and obtains vital signs with results as follows: blood pressure 140/92, heart rate 128, respiratory rate 26, and an oxygen saturation of 98%. What rhythm on the monitor does the nurse anticipate viewing?

a. Sinus bradycardia

b. Ventricular tachycardia

c. Normal sinus rhythm

d. Sinus tachycardia

2. The nurse is attempting to determine the ventricular rate and rhythm of a patient's telemetry strip. What should the nurse examine to determine this part of the analysis?

a. PP interval

b. QT interval

c. RR interval

d. TP interval

3. The nurse is monitoring a patient in the post-anesthesia care unit (PACU) following a coronary artery bypass graft, observing a regular ventricular rate of 82 beats/min and "sawtooth" P waves with an atrial rate of approximately 300 beat/min. How does the nurse interpret this rhythm?

a. Atrial fibrillation

b. Atrial flutter

c. Ventricular tachycardia

d. Ventricular fibrillation

4. A patient with mitral valve stenosis and coronary artery disease (CAD) is in the telemetry unit with pneumonia. The nurse assesses a 6-second rhythm strip and determines that the ventricular rhythm is highly irregular at 88, with no discernible P waves. What does the nurse determine this rhythm to be?

a. Atrial flutter

b. Ventricular flutter

c. Sinus tachycardia

d. Nonparoxysmal junctional tachycardia

5. A patient with hypertension has a newly diagnosed atrial fibrillation. What medication does the nurse anticipate administering to prevent the complication of atrial thrombi?

a. Adenosine (Adenocard)

b. Amiodarone (Pacerone)

c. Warfarin (Coumadin)

d. Atropine

6. The nurse in the intensive care unit (ICU) hears an alarm sound in the patient's room. Arriving in the room, the patient is unresponsive, without a pulse, and a flat line on the monitor. What is the first action by the nurse?

a. Begin cardiopulmonary resuscitation (CPR)

b. Administer epinephrine

c. Administer atropine 0.5 mg

d. Defibrillate with 360 joules (monophasic defibrillator)

7. The nurse is defibrillating a patient in ventricular fibrillation with paddles on a monophasic defibrillator. How much paddle pressure should the nurse apply when defibrillating?

a. 5 to 10 lbs

b. 10 to 15 lbs

c. 15 to 20 lbs

d. 20 to 25 lbs

8. A patient with dilated cardiomyopathy is having frequent episodes of ventricular fibrillation. What choice would be best to sense and terminate these episodes?

a. Implantable cardioverter defibrillator

b. Pacemaker

c. Atropine

d. Epinephrine

9. The nurse is observing the monitor of a patient with a first-degree atrioventricular (AV) block. What is the nurse aware characterizes this block?

a. A variable heart rate, usually fewer than 60 bpm

b. An irregular rhythm

c. Delayed conduction, producing a prolonged PR interval

d. P waves hidden with the QRS complex

10. The nurse is assessing vital signs in a patient with a permanent pacemaker. What should the nurse document about the pacemaker?

a. Date and time of insertion

b. Location of the generator

c. Model number

d. Pacer rate

11. A patient has had an implantable cardioverter defibrillator inserted. What should the nurse be sure to include in the education of this patient prior to discharge? (Select all that apply.)

   a. Avoid magnetic fields such as metal detection booths.

   b. Call for emergency assistance if feeling dizzy.

   c. Record events that trigger a shock sensation.

   d. The patient may have a throbbing pain that is normal

   e. The patient will have to schedule monthly chest x-rays to make sure the device is patent.

12. A patient is 2 days postoperative after having a permanent pacemaker inserted. The nurse observes that the patient is having continuous hiccups as the patient states, "I thought this was normal." What does the nurse understand is occurring with this patient?

   a. Fracture of the lead wire

   b. Lead wire dislodgement

   c. Faulty generator

   d. Sensitivity is too low

13. A patient who had a myocardial infarction is experiencing severe chest pain and alerts the nurse. The nurse begins the assessment but suddenly the patient becomes unresponsive, no pulse, with the monitor showing a rapid, disorganized ventricular rhythm. What does the nurse interpret this rhythm to be?

   a. Ventricular tachycardia

   b. Atrial fibrillation

   c. Third-degree heart block

   d. Ventricular fibrillation

14. A patient has a persistent third-degree heart block and has had several periods of syncope. What priority treatment should the nurse anticipate for this patient?

   a. Insertion of a pacemaker

   b. Administration of atropine

   c. Administration of epinephrine

   d. Insertion of an implantable cardioverter defibrillator (ICD)

15. A patient has had several episodes of recurrent tachydysrhythmias over the last 5 months and medication therapy has not been effective. What procedure should the nurse prepare the patient for?

   a. Insertion of an ICD

   b. Insertion of a permanent pacemaker

   c. Catheter ablation therapy

   d. Maze procedure

CHAPTER 27

Management of Patients With Coronary Vascular Disorders

Learning Objectives

1. Describe the pathophysiology, clinical manifestations, and treatment of coronary atherosclerosis.
2. Describe the pathophysiology, clinical manifestations, and treatment of angina pectoris.
3. Use the nursing process as a framework for care of patients with angina pectoris.
4. Describe the pathophysiology, clinical manifestations, and treatment of myocardial infarction.
5. Use the nursing process as a framework for care of a patient with acute coronary syndrome.
6. Describe percutaneous coronary interventional and coronary artery revascularization procedures.
7. Describe the nursing care of a patient who has had a percutaneous coronary interventional procedure for treatment of coronary artery disease.
8. Use the nursing process as a framework for care of a patient who has undergone cardiac surgery.

SECTION I: ASSESSING YOUR UNDERSTANDING

Activity A *Fill in the blanks.*

1. A thrombus is a dangerous complication of atherosclerosis because it can lead to _____ and _____.

2. A person at increased risk for heart disease is encouraged to stop _____ through any means possible.

3. _____ use by women who smoke is inadvisable because these medications significantly increase the risk for CAD and sudden cardiac death.

4. Hypertension is defined as blood pressure measurements that repeatedly exceed _____ mm Hg.

5. The patient with suspected MI should immediately receive _____, _____, _____, and _____.

6. The leading cause of death in the United States for men and women of all ethnic and racial groups is _____.

7. The most common cause of cardiovascular disease is _____.

8. The most frequently occurring sign of myocardial ischemia is _____.

9. More than 50% of people with coronary artery disease have the risk factor of _____.

10. Management of coronary heart disease requires a therapeutic range of cholesterol and lipoproteins. An acceptable blood level of total cholesterol is _____ with an LDL/HDL ratio of _____. The desired level of LDL should be _____, and the HDL level should be greater than _____. Triglycerides should be less than _____.

11. The American Heart Association (AHA) recommends that an average American diet contain about _____% fat.

12. The key, diagnostic indicator for MI seen on an electrocardiogram (ECG) is _____ _____.

13. The vessel most commonly used for coronary artery bypass grafting (CABG) is the _____.

14. A possible complication of rupture or hemorrhage of the lipid core into the plaque is _____.

Activity B *Briefly answer the following.*

1. List four of the seven modifiable risk factors that are considered major causes of coronary artery disease: _____, _____, _____, and _____.

2. A positive diagnosis of metabolic syndrome occurs when three of the following six conditions are met:

_____ _____

_____ _____

_____ _____

3. List three collaborative problems for a patient with angina: _____, _____, and _____.

4. List four symptoms seen in postpericardiotomy syndrome: _____, _____, _____, and _____.

5. Describe an atheroma:

_____

_____

_____

6. What does the phrase *door to balloon time* mean?

_____

_____

Activity C *Match the medication affecting lipoprotein metabolism in Column II with the associated classification in Column I.*

Column I

____ 1. HMG-CoA reductase inhibitor

____ 2. Nicotinic acid

____ 3. Fibric acids

____ 4. Bile acid sequestrants

____ 5. Cholesterol absorption inhibitor

____ 6. Omega-3-acid-ethyl esters

Column II

a. Fish oil capsule

b. TriCor

c. Colestid

d. Zetia

e. Niacor

f. Pravachol

SECTION II: APPLYING YOUR KNOWLEDGE

Activity D *Consider the scenarios and answer the questions.*

CASE STUDY: Angina Pectoris

Ermelina, a 64-year-old retired secretary, is admitted to the medical–surgical area for management of chest pain caused by angina pectoris.

1. The patient asks the nurse, "What is causing this pain?" What is the best response by the nurse?

_____

_____

2. The patient is diagnosed with chronic stable angina. The nurse can anticipate that her pain may follow what type of pattern?

_____

3. Ermelina has nitroglycerin at her bedside to take PRN. The nurse knows that nitroglycerin acts in what ways?

_____

_____

_____

4. Ermelina took a nitroglycerin tablet at 10:00 AM, after her morning care. It did not relieve her pain, so, 5 minutes later, she repeated the dose. Ten minutes later and still in pain, she calls the nurse. What is the priority intervention by the nurse?

_____

_____

CASE STUDY: Decreased Myocardial Tissue Perfusion

Mr. Lillis, a 46-year-old bricklayer, is brought to the ED by ambulance with a suspected diagnosis of MI. He appears ashen, is diaphoretic and tachycardiac, and has severe chest pain. The nursing diagnosis is decreased cardiac output, related to decreased myocardial tissue perfusion.

1. The nurse is aware that there is a critical time period for this patient. When should the nurse be most vigilant in monitoring this patient?

_____

2. The nurse is interpreting the results of the ECG. What findings does the nurse understand are indicative of initial myocardial injury?

_____

3. The nurse evaluates a series of laboratory tests within the first few hours. What laboratory results are positive indicators of MI?

_____

4. The nurse should closely monitor the patient for a complication of an MI that leads to sudden death during the first 48 hours. Which complication should the nurse monitor for?

_____

SECTION III: PREPARING FOR NCLEX

Activity E *Answer the following questions.*

1. The nurse is reviewing the results of a total cholesterol level for a patient who has been taking simvastatin (Zocor). What results display the effectiveness of the medication?
   a. 160–190 mg/dL
   b. 210–240 mg/dL
   c. 250–275 mg/dL
   d. 280–300 mg/dL

2. The nurse is discussing risk factors for developing CAD with a patient in the clinic. Which results would indicate that the patient is not at significant risk for the development of CAD?
   a. Cholesterol, 280 mg/dL
   b. Low density lipoprotein (LDL), 160 mg/dL
   c. High-density lipoprotein (HDL), 80 mg/dL
   d. A ratio of LDL to HDL, 4.5 to 1.0

3. A patient asks the nurse how long he will have to wait after taking nitroglycerin before experiencing pain relief. What is the best answer by the nurse?
   a. 3 minutes
   b. 15 minutes
   c. 30 minutes
   d. 60 minutes

4. The nurse is educating the patient about administering nitroglycerin prior to discharge from the hospital. What information should the nurse include in the instructions?
   a. Take a nitroglycerin and if the pain is not relieved, drive to the nearest emergency department.
   b. Take 2 nitroglycerins and if the pain is not relieved, go to the emergency department.
   c. Take a nitroglycerin and repeat every 5 minutes if the pain is not relieved until a total of 3 are taken. If pain is not relieved, activate the emergency medical system.
   d. Take 2 nitroglycerins every 10 minutes until a total of 6 pills are taken. If pain is not relieved, activate the emergency medical system.

5. The nurse administers propranolol hydro-chloride to a patient with a heart rate of 64 beats per minute (bpm). One hour later, the nurse observes the heart rate on the mon-itor to be 36 bpm. What medication should the nurse prepare to administer that is an antidote for the propranolol?

a. Digoxin

b. Atropine

c. Protamine sulfate

d. Sodium nitroprusside

6. The nurse is administering a calcium channel blocker to a patient who has symptomatic sinus tachycardia at a rate of 132 bpm. What is the anticipated action of the drug for this patient?

a. Decreases the sinoatrial node automaticity

b. Increases the atrioventricular node conduction

c. Increases the heart rate

d. Creates a positive inotropic effect

7. What ECG findings does the nurse observe in a patient who has had an MI? (Select all that apply.)

a. An absent P wave

b. An abnormal Q wave

c. T-wave inversion

d. ST-segment elevation

e. Prolonged P-R interval

8. The nurse is educating a patient diagnosed with angina pectoris about the difference between the pain of angina and an MI. How should the nurse describe the pain experi-enced during an MI? (Select all that apply.)

a. It is relieved by rest and inactivity.

b. It is substernal in location.

c. It is sudden in onset and prolonged in duration.

d. It is viselike and radiates to the shoulders and arms.

e. It subsides after taking nitroglycerin.

9. The nurse is reviewing the laboratory results for a patient having a suspected MI. What cardiac-specific isoenzyme does the nurse observe for myocardial cell damage?

a. Alkaline phosphatase

b. Creatine kinase (CK-MB)

c. Myoglobin

d. Troponin

10. The nurse is caring for a patient who is hav-ing chest pain associated with an MI. What medication should the nurse administer intravenously to reduce pain and anxiety?

a. Meperidine hydrochloride

b. Hydromorphone hydrochloride

c. Morphine sulfate

d. Codeine sulfate

11. A patient with CAD is having a cardiac cath-eterization. What indicator is present for the patient to have a percutaneous transluminal coronary angioplasty (PTCA)?

a. The patient has compromised left ventricu-lar function.

b. The patient has had angina longer than 3 years.

c. The patient has at least a 70% occlusion of a major coronary artery.

d. The patient has an ejection fraction of 65%.

12. The nurse is assessing a postoperative patient who had a PTCA. Which possible complica-tions should the nurse monitor for? (Select all that apply.)

a. Abrupt closure of the artery

b. Arterial dissection

c. Coronary artery vasospasm

d. Aortic dissection

e. Nerve root pressure

13. A patient in the recovery room after cardiac surgery begins to have extremity paresthesia, peaked T waves, and mental confusion. What type of electrolyte imbalance does the nurse suspect this patient is having?

a. Calcium

b. Magnesium

c. Potassium

d. Sodium

14. A patient has had cardiac surgery and is being monitored in the intensive care unit (ICU). What complication should the nurse monitor for that is associated with an alteration in preload?

a. Cardiac tamponade

b. Elevated central venous pressure

c. Hypertension

d. Hypothermia

15. A patient who had CABG is exhibiting signs of cardiac failure. What medications does the nurse anticipate administering for this patient? (Select all that apply.)

a. Diuretics

b. Digoxin

c. Inotropic agents

d. Dialysis

e. Nitroprusside

Management of Patients With Structural, Infectious, and Inflammatory Cardiac Disorders

Learning Objectives

1. Define valvular disorders of the heart and describe the pathophysiology, clinical manifestations, and management of patients with mitral and aortic disorders.
2. Describe types of cardiac valve repair and replacement procedures used to treat valvular problems and care needed by patients who undergo these procedures.
3. Describe the pathophysiology, clinical manifestations, and management of patients with cardiomyopathies.
4. Describe the pathophysiology, clinical manifestations, and management of patients with infections of the heart.
5. Use the nursing process as a framework of care for the patient with a cardiomyopathy and the patient with pericarditis.

SECTION I: ASSESSING YOUR UNDERSTANDING

Activity A *Fill in the blanks.*

1. Often the first and only sign of mitral valve prolapse is an extra heart sound, referred to as a _____.

2. Mitral regurgitation involves blood flowing back from the _____ into the _____ during systole.

3. When valves do not open completely, a condition called _____ occurs, and blood flow through the valve is reduced.

4. _____ is beneficial for mitral valve stenosis in younger patients, for aortic valve stenosis in older patients, and for patients with complex medical conditions that place them at high risk for complications of more extensive surgical procedures.

5. Surgical repair of chordae tendineae is called _____.

6. If dysrhythmias occur with mitral valve prolapse, the nurse advises the patient to avoid _____, _____, and _____.

7. A nurse, using auscultation to identify aortic regurgitation, would place the stethoscope _____ and would expect to hear _____.

8. With aortic stenosis, the patient should receive _____ to prevent endocarditis.

9. Prompt treatment of streptococcal pharyngitis with _____ can prevent almost all attacks of _____.

10. Infective endocarditis is usually caused by the following bacteria: _____, _____, _____, and _____.

11. Patients with myocarditis may be extremely sensitive to _____ (medication) and should therefore be monitored for serum levels to prevent _____.

Activity B *Briefly answer the following.*

1. Describe the basic dysfunction of mitral valve prolapse.

   _____
   _____
   _____

2. List four potential complications or collaborative problems for patients with cardiomyopathy.

   _____
   _____

3. Identify five common indicators for heart transplantation.

   _____
   _____

4. Briefly describe the pathophysiology of infective endocarditis, beginning with the formation of a vegetation.

   _____
   _____
   _____

5. Briefly describe the pathophysiology of myocarditis.

   _____
   _____
   _____
   _____

6. Describe the anatomic landmark for auscultation of a pericardial friction rub.

   _____
   _____

7. List six underlying causes of pericarditis.

   _____
   _____

Activity C *Match the pathophysiology listed in Column II with the valvular disorder listed in Column I.*

Column I	Column II
____ 1. Mitral valve prolapse	a. Leaflet malformation prevents complete closure.
____ 2. Mitral stenosis	b. Can be caused by rheumatic endocarditis.
____ 3. Mitral regurgitation	c. Characterized by a significantly widened pulse pressure.
____ 4. Aortic valve stenosis	d. Blood seeps backward into left atrium.
____ 5. Aortic regurgitation	e. Thickening and contracture of mitral valve cusps.

SECTION II: APPLYING YOUR KNOWLEDGE

Activity D *Consider the scenarios and answer the questions.*

CASE STUDY: Infective Endocarditis

Mr. Fontana, a 60-year-old executive, is admitted to the hospital with a diagnosis of infective endocarditis. Pertinent history includes a previous diagnosis of mitral valve prolapse. A physical examination at his physician's office before admission revealed complaints of anorexia, joint pain, intermittent fever, and a 10-lb weight loss in the past 2 months.

1. While examining Mr. Fontana's eyes during the admission assessment, the nurse notes conjunctival hemorrhages with pale centers. How should the nurse document this finding?

   _____
   _____

2. The nurse is assessing the patient for central nervous system (CNS) manifestations of the infectious disease. What symptoms should the nurse report as significant?

_____

_____

_____

3. The nurse receives the blood culture results and notes that the *Streptococcus viridans* organism has been identified. How long does the nurse anticipate that the patient will remain on antibiotic intravenous infusion?

_____

CASE STUDY: Acute Pericarditis

Mr. Russell is a 46-year-old Caucasian who developed symptoms of acute pericarditis secondary to a viral infection. Diagnosis was based on the characteristic sign of a friction rub and pain over the pericardium.

1. The patient is experiencing pericardial pain. To alleviate this discomfort, what position could the nurse assist the patient with maintaining?

_____

_____

2. When planning Mr. Russell's care, what should the nurse understand are the objectives of pericarditis management?

_____

_____

_____

3. The nurse is auscultating Mr. Russell's chest for a pericardial friction rub. Where will the nurse auscultate in order to locate the rub?

_____

SECTION III: PRACTICING FOR NCLEX

Activity E *Answer the following questions.*

1. A patient at the clinic describes shortness of breath, periods of feeling "lightheaded," and feeling fatigued despite a full night's sleep. The nurse obtains vital signs and auscultates a systolic click. What does the nurse suspect from the assessment findings?

a. Mitral valve prolapse

b. Mitral regurgitation

c. Aortic stenosis

d. Aortic regurgitation

2. The nurse is educating a patient about the care related to a new diagnosis of mitral valve prolapse. What statement made by the patient demonstrates understanding?

a. "I will avoid caffeine, alcohol, and smoking."

b. "I will take antibiotics before getting my teeth cleaned."

c. "I shouldn't get a tattoo but I can get my tongue pierced."

d. "This disorder will progress and I will need a heart transplant."

3. The nurse is auscultating the heart sounds of a patient with mitral stenosis. The pulse rhythm is weak and irregular. What rhythm does the nurse expect to see on the electrocardiogram (ECG)?

a. First-degree atrioventricular block

b. Ventricular tachycardia

c. Atrial fibrillation

d. Sinus dysrhythmia

4. The nurse suspects a diagnosis of mitral valve regurgitation when what type of murmur is heard on auscultation?

a. Mitral click

b. High-pitched blowing sound at the apex

c. Low-pitched diastolic murmur at the apex

d. Diastolic murmur at the left sternal border

5. The nurse is assessing a patient and feels a pulse with quick, sharp strokes that suddenly collapse. The nurse knows that this type of pulse is diagnostic for which disorder?

   a. Mitral insufficiency

   b. Tricuspid insufficiency

   c. Tricuspid stenosis

   d. Aortic regurgitation

6. A patient has been diagnosed with fused mitral leaflets, causing a backward flow of blood. What type of procedure does the nurse know is commonly performed for this type of problem?

   a. Annuloplasty

   b. Commissurotomy

   c. Valve replacement

   d. Chordoplasty

7. A patient has received a heterograft or a tricuspid valve replacement. What statement made by the patient demonstrates understanding of the valve replacement?

   a. "The xenograft will last for the rest of my life, at least 20 years."

   b. "I will have to take an antirejection drug for the duration of the xenograft."

   c. "I will not take long-term anticoagulation because I want to get pregnant."

   d. "My valve comes from a cadaver."

8. A patient is admitted with suspected cardiomyopathy. What diagnostic test would be most helpful with the identification of this disorder?

   a. Serial enzyme studies

   b. Cardiac catheterization

   c. Echocardiogram

   d. Phonocardiogram

9. A patient has had a successful heart transplant for end-stage heart disease. What immunosuppressant will be necessary for this patient to take to prevent rejection?

   a. Procardia

   b. Cyclosporine

   c. Calan

   d. Vancocin

10. A patient is diagnosed with rheumatic endocarditis. What bacterium is the nurse aware causes this inflammatory response?

    a. Group A, beta-hemolytic streptococcus

    b. *Pseudomonas aeruginosa*

    c. *Serratia marcescens*

    d. *Staphylococcus aureus*

11. A patient admitted to the hospital is suspected to have rheumatic endocarditis. What diagnostic test does the nurse anticipate will be ordered?

    a. Throat culture

    b. Echocardiogram

    c. Electrocardiogram

    d. Complete blood count

12. The nurse determines that a patient has a characteristic symptom of pericarditis. What symptom does the nurse recognize as significant for this diagnosis?

    a. Dyspnea

    b. Constant chest pain

    c. Fatigue lasting more than 1 month

    d. Uncontrolled restlessness

13. What medication order would the nurse question for a patient being treated for pericarditis?

    a. Colchicine

    b. Indocin

    c. Ibuprofen

    d. Prednisone

14. The nurse is caring for a patient diagnosed with pericarditis. What serious complication should this patient be monitored for?

    a. Cardiac tamponade

    b. Decreased venous pressure

    c. Hypertension

    d. Left ventricular hypertrophy

15. The nurse is obtaining a history from a patient diagnosed with hypertrophic cardiomyopathy. What information obtained from the patient is indicative of this form of cardiomyopathy?

    a. A history of alcoholism

    b. A history of amyloidosis

    c. A parent has the same disorder

    d. A long-standing history of hypertension

Management of Patients With Complications From Heart Disease

1. Describe the management of patients with heart failure.
2. Use the nursing process as a framework for care of patients with heart failure.
3. Develop an education plan for patients with heart failure.
4. Describe the medical and nursing management of patients with pulmonary edema.
5. Describe the medical and nursing management of patients with thromboembolism, pericardial effusion, and cardiac arrest.

SECTION I: ASSESSING YOUR UNDERSTANDING

Activity A *Fill in the blanks.*

1. Two factors that determine preload are _____ and _____.
   Two factors that determine afterload are _____ and _____.

2. Three noninvasive tests are used to assess cardiac hemodynamics: _____ for right ventricular preload, _____ for left ventricular afterload, and _____ for left ventricular preload.

3. The most common thromboembolitic problem among patients with heart failure is

   _____.

4. For cardiopulmonary resuscitation, the recommended chest compression rate is _____ times/min. The compression to ventilation ratio of _____ is recommended without stopping for ventilation.

5. Four common etiologic factors that cause myocardial dysfunction include

   _____, _____, _____, and _____.

6. Name three types of cardiomyopathy:

   _____, _____, and _____. Of these, _____ is the most common.

7. The primary clinical manifestations of pulmonary congestion in left-sided heart failure are _____, _____, _____, _____, and a probable _____.

8. The primary systemic clinical manifestations of right-sided heart failure are _____, _____, _____, _____, _____, and _____.

9. _____, _____, _____, and _____ are four types of drugs normally prescribed for systolic heart failure.

10. Coronary atherosclerosis results in tissue ischemia, which causes myocardial dysfunction, because _____ and _____ result from _____.

Activity B *Briefly answer the following.*

1. Decipher the formula CO = HR × SV.

   _____

   _____

2. Distinguish between the terms *preload* and *afterload*.

   Preload: _____

   _____

   Afterload: _____

   _____

3. List four common side effects of diuretics:

   _____   _____

   _____   _____

4. List six symptoms indicative of hypokalemia.

   _____   _____

   _____   _____

   _____   _____

5. Identify six causes of cardiogenic shock.

   _____   _____

   _____   _____

   _____   _____

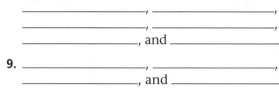

Activity C *Match the type of ventricular heart failure listed in Column II with its associated pathophysiology in Column I.*

Column I

___ 1. Fatigability

___ 2. Dependent edema

___ 3. Pulmonary congestion predominates

___ 4. Distended neck veins

___ 5. Ascites

___ 6. Dyspnea from fluid in alveoli

___ 7. Orthopnea

___ 8. Hepatomegaly

___ 9. Cough that may be blood-tinged

___ 10. Nocturia

Column II

a. Left-sided heart failure

b. Right-sided heart failure

SECTION II: APPLYING YOUR KNOWLEDGE

Activity D *Consider the scenario and answer the questions.*

CASE STUDY: Pulmonary Edema

Mr. Wolman is to be discharged from the hospital to home. He is 79 years old, lives with his wife, and has just recovered from mild pulmonary edema secondary to congestive heart failure.

1. What would the rationale be for the nurse advising Mr. Wolman to rest frequently at home?

   _____

   _____

2. What position should the nurse inform the patient to sleep in when he goes home? Why?

   _____

   _____

3. Mr. Wolman will be discharged with a prescription of digoxin 0.25 mg once daily. What education should the nurse include regarding symptoms of toxicity?

   _____

   _____

4. Mr. Wolman also takes Lasix (40 mg) twice a day. What foods should the nurse suggest that would be a supplement for potassium?

   _____

SECTION III: PRACTICING FOR NCLEX

Activity E *Answer the following questions.*

1. The nurse is assessing a patient who reports no symptoms of heart failure at rest but is symptomatic with increased physical activity. Under what classification does the nurse understand this patient would be categorized?

   a. I

   b. II

   c. III

   d. IV

2. The nurse observes that a patient has 2+ pitting edema in the lower extremities. What does the nurse know that the presence of pitting edema indicates regarding fluid retention?

   a. A weight gain of 4 lbs

   b. A weight gain of 6 lbs

   c. A weight gain of 8 lbs

   d. A weight gain of 10 lbs

3. A patient has been experiencing increasing shortness of breath and fatigue. The physician has ordered a diagnostic test in order to determine what type of heart failure the patient is having. What diagnostic test does the nurse anticipate being ordered?

   a. A chest x-ray

   b. An echocardiogram

   c. An electrocardiogram

   d. A ventriculogram

4. A patient is seen in the emergency department (ED) with heart failure secondary to dilated cardiomyopathy. What key diagnostic test does the nurse assess to determine the severity of the patient's heart failure?

   a. Blood urea nitrogen (BUN)

   b. Complete blood count (CBC)

   c. B-type natriuretic peptide (BNP)

   d. Serum electrolytes

5. A patient has missed 2 doses of digitalis (Digoxin). What laboratory results would indicate to the nurse that the patient is within therapeutic range?

   a. 0.25 mg/mL

   b. 4.0 mg/mL

   c. 2.0 mg/mL

   d. 3.2 mg/mL

6. A patient is admitted to the intensive care unit (ICU) with left-sided heart failure. What clinical manifestations does the nurse anticipate finding when performing an assessment? (Select all that apply.)

   a. Jugular vein distention

   b. Ascites

   c. Pulmonary crackles

   d. Dyspnea

   e. Cough

7. The nurse is assigned to care for a patient with heart failure. What classification of medication does the nurse anticipate administering that will improve symptoms as well as increase survival?

   a. ACE inhibitor

   b. Calcium channel blocker

   c. Diuretic

   d. Bile acid sequestrants

8. A patient taking an ACE inhibitor has developed a dry, hacking cough. Because of this side effect, the patient no longer wants to take that medication. What medication that has similar hemodynamic effects does the nurse anticipate the physician ordering?

   a. Valsartan (Diovan)

   b. Furosemide (Lasix)

   c. Metoprolol (Lopressor)

   d. Isosorbide dinitrate (Dilatrate)

9. A patient in severe pulmonary edema is being intubated by the respiratory therapist. What priority action by the nurse will assist in the confirmation of tube placement in the proper position in the trachea?

   a. Observe for mist in the endotracheal tube.

   b. Listen for breath sounds over the epigastrium.

   c. Call for a chest x-ray.

   d. Attach a pulse oximeter probe and obtain values.

10. The nurse is performing a respiratory assessment for a patient in left-sided heart failure. What does the nurse understand is the best determinant of the patient's ventilation and oxygenation status?

   a. Pulse oximetry

   b. Listening to breath sounds

   c. End-tidal CO_2

   d. Arterial blood gases

11. The nurse hears the alarm sound on the telemetry monitor and observes a flat line. The patient is found unresponsive, without a pulse, and no respiratory effort. What is the first action by the nurse?

   a. Administer epinephrine 1:10,000 10 mL IV push.

   b. Deliver breaths with a bag-valve mask.

   c. Defibrillate the patient with 360 joules.

   d. Call for help and begin chest compressions.

12. A patient in cardiogenic shock after a myocardial infarction is placed on an intra-aortic balloon pump. What does the nurse understand is the mechanism of action of the balloon pump?

   a. The balloon keeps the vessels open so that blood will adequately deliver to the myocardium.

   b. The balloon inflates at the beginning of diastole and deflates before systole to augment the pumping action of the heart.

   c. The balloon delivers an electrical impulse to correct dysrhythmias the patient experiences.

   d. The balloon will inflate at the beginning of systole and deflate before diastole to provide a long-term solution to a failing myocardium.

13. The nurse is preparing to administer hydralazine and isosorbide dinitrate (Dilatrate). When obtaining vital signs, the nurse notes that the blood pressure is 90/60. What is the priority action by the nurse?

   a. Hold the medication and call the physician.

   b. Administer the medication and check the blood pressure in 30 minutes.

   c. Administer a saline bolus of 250 mL and then administer the medication.

   d. Administer the hydralazine and hold the dinitrate.

14. A patient seen in the clinic has been diagnosed with stage A heart failure (according to the staging classification of the American College of Cardiology [ACC]). What education will the nurse provide to this patient?

   a. Information about ACE inhibitors and risk factor reduction

   b. Information about diuretic therapy and risk factor reduction

   c. Information about beta blockers, ACE inhibitors, and diuretics

   d. Information about implantable cardioverter/defibrillators

15. The physician writes orders for a patient to receive an angiotensin II receptor blocker for treatment of heart failure. What medication does the nurse administer?

   a. Digoxin (Lanoxin)

   b. Valsartan (Diovan)

   c. Metolazone (Zaroxolyn)

   d. Carvedilol (Coreg)

Assessment and Management of Patients With Vascular Disorders and Problems of Peripheral Circulation

Learning Objectives

1. Identify anatomic and physiologic factors that affect peripheral blood flow and tissue oxygenation.
2. Use appropriate parameters for assessment of peripheral circulation.
3. Use the nursing process as a framework of care for patients with vascular insufficiency of the extremities.
4. Compare the various diseases of the arteries and their causes, pathophysiologic changes, clinical manifestations, management, and prevention.
5. Describe the prevention and management of venous thromboembolism.
6. Compare strategies to prevent venous insufficiency, leg ulcers, and varicose veins.
7. Use the nursing process as a framework of care for patients with leg ulcers.
8. Describe the relationship between lymphangitis and lymphedema.

SECTION I: ASSESSING YOUR UNDERSTANDING

Activity A *Fill in the blanks.*

1. Arterioles offer resistance to blood flow by altering their diameter, and are often referred to as _____.

2. The hallmark symptom of peripheral arterial occlusive disease is _____.

3. _____ is a sensitive marker of cardiovascular inflammation, both systemically and locally.

4. Venous stasis, postthrombotic syndrome, is characterized by _____, _____, _____, and _____.

5. The strongest risk factor for the development of atherosclerotic lesions is _____.

Activity B *Briefly answer the following.*

1. List the six clinical symptoms associated with acute arterial embolism, also known as the six Ps.

   _____ _____

   _____ _____

   _____ _____

2. List the classic triad (Virchow's) of factors associated with the development of venous thromboembolism.

   _____

   _____

3. What is the most important factor in regulating the caliber of blood vessels, which determines resistance to flow?

   _____

   _____

   _____

4. Describe the etiology of pain associated with the condition known as *intermittent claudication.*

   _____

   _____

   _____

5. Describe the clinical picture of a patient presenting with a dissected aorta.

   _____

   _____

6. In what ways can patients with peripheral vascular disease maintain foot and leg care?

   _____

   _____

7. Name four major complications of venous thrombosis.

   _____

   _____

Activity C *Match the type of vessel insufficiency listed in Column II with its associated symptom listed in Column I.*

Column I

___ 1. Intermittent claudication

___ 2. Paresthesia

___ 3. Dependent rubor

___ 4. Cold, pale extremity

___ 5. Ulcers of lower legs and ankles

___ 6. Muscle fatigue and cramping

___ 7. Diminished or absent pulses

___ 8. Reddish-blue discoloration with dependency

Column II

a. Arterial insufficiency

b. Venous insufficiency

SECTION II: APPLYING YOUR KNOWLEDGE

Activity D *Consider the scenario and answer the questions.*

CASE STUDY: Peripheral Arterial Occlusive Disease

Fred, a 43-year-old construction worker, has a history of hypertension. He smokes two packs of cigarettes a day, is nervous about the possibility of being unemployed, and has difficulty coping with stress. His current concern is calf pain during minimal exercise, which decreases with rest.

1. What does the nurse know is the hallmark symptom of peripheral arterial occlusion disease?

   _____

2. The patient is having ankle–brachial index (ABI) determined. The right posterior tibial reading is 75 mm Hg and the brachial systolic pressure is 150 mm Hg. What would the ABI be for this patient?

   _____

3. The nurse is educating Fred about managing his condition. What methods can the nurse suggest to increase arterial blood supply?

_____

_____

_____

4. What is the best method for the nurse to assess Fred's peripheral pulses to obtain consistent results with other health care practitioners?

_____

_____

_____

SECTION III: PRACTICING FOR NCLEX

Activity E *Answer the following questions.*

1. What does the nurse understand is the most important factor in regulating the caliber of blood vessels, which determines resistance to flow?

   a. Hormonal secretion
   b. Independent arterial wall activity
   c. The influence of circulating chemicals
   d. The sympathetic nervous system

2. The nurse is assessing a patient with suspected acute venous insufficiency. What clinical manifestations would indicate this condition to the nurse? (Select all that apply.)

   a. Cool and cyanotic skin
   b. Initial absence of edema
   c. Sharp pain that may be relieved by the elevation of the extremity
   d. Full superficial veins
   e. Brisk capillary refill of the toes

3. The nurse is caring for a patient with peripheral arterial insufficiency. What can the nurse suggest to help relieve leg pain during rest?

   a. Elevating the limb above heart level
   b. Lowering the limb so that it is dependent
   c. Massaging the limb after application of cold compresses
   d. Placing the limb in a plane horizontal to the body

4. A patient is suspected to have a thoracic aortic aneurysm. What diagnostic test(s) does the nurse anticipate preparing the patient for? (Select all that apply.)

   a. Computed tomography
   b. Transesophageal echocardiography
   c. X-ray
   d. Electroencephalogram
   e. Electrocardiogram (ECG)

5. A nurse suspects the presence of an abdominal aortic aneurysm. What assessment data would the nurse correlate with a diagnosis of abdominal aortic aneurysm? (Select all that apply.)

   a. A pulsatile abdominal mass
   b. Low back pain
   c. Lower abdominal pain
   d. Decreased bowel sounds
   e. Diarrhea

6. A patient with impaired renal function is scheduled for a multidetector computer tomography (MDCT) scan. What preprocedure medication may the nurse administer to this patient?

   a. Oral N-acetylcysteine
   b. Oral iodine
   c. Dipyridamole (Persantine)
   d. Epinephrine

7. A patient is having an angiography to detect the presence of an aneurysm. After the contrast is administered by the interventionist, the patient begins to complain of nausea and difficulty breathing. What medication is a priority to administer at this time?

   a. Metoprolol (Lopressor)
   b. Epinephrine
   c. Hydrocortisone (Solu-Cortef)
   d. Cimetidine (Tagamet)

8. The nurse is assisting a patient with peripheral arterial disease to ambulate in the hallway. What should the nurse include in the education of the patient during ambulation?

   a. "As soon as you feel pain, we will go back and elevate your legs."

   b. "If you feel pain during the walk, keep walking until the end of the hallway is reached."

   c. "Walk to the point of pain, rest until the pain subsides, then resume ambulation."

   d. "If you feel any discomfort, stop and we will use a wheelchair to take you back to your room."

9. The nurse is assessing a patient two days postoperatively who is suspected of having deep vein obstruction. The patient is complaining of pain in the left lower extremity and there is a 2-cm difference in the right and left leg circumference. What intervention can the nurse provide to promote arterial flow to the lower extremities?

   a. Administer a diuretic to decrease the edema in the left lower extremity.

   b. Assist with active range-of-motion (ROM) exercises to the left lower extremity.

   c. Apply cool compresses to the left lower extremity.

   d. Apply a heating pad to the patient's abdomen.

10. The nurse is monitoring a patient who is on heparin anticoagulant therapy. What should the nurse determine the therapeutic range of the international normalized ratio (INR) should be?

    a. 2.0–3.0

    b. 4.0–5.0

    c. 5.0–6.0

    d. 7.0–8.0

11. The nurse is caring for a patient who has started anticoagulant therapy with warfarin (Coumadin). When does the nurse understand that therapeutic benefits will begin?

    a. Within 12 hours

    b. Within the first 24 hours

    c. In 2 days

    d. In 3 to 5 days

12. The nurse is caring for a patient with venous insufficiency. What should the nurse assess the patient's lower extremities for?

    a. Rudor

    b. Cellulitis

    c. Dermatitis

    d. Ulceration

13. The nurse is educating a patient with chronic venous insufficiency about prevention of complications related to the disorder. What should the nurse include in the information given to the patient? (Select all that apply.)

    a. Avoid constricting garments.

    b. Elevate the legs above the heart level for 30 minutes every 2 hours.

    c. Sit as much as possible to rest the valves in the legs.

    d. Sleep with the foot of the bed elevated about 6 inches.

    e. Sit on the side of the bed and dangle the feet.

14. The physician prescribed a Tegapore dressing to treat a venous ulcer. What should the nurse expect that the ABI will be if the circulatory status is adequate?

    a. 0.10

    b. 0.25

    c. 0.35

    d. 0.50

15. A patient with diabetes is being treated for a wound on the lower extremity that has been present for 30 days. What option for treatment is available to increase diffusion of oxygen to the hypoxic wound?

    a. Surgical debridement

    b. Enzymatic debridement

    c. Hyperbaric oxygen

    d. Vacuum-assisted closure device

16. The nurse is performing wound care for a patient with a necrotic sacral wound. The prescribed treatment is isotonic saline solution with fine mesh gauze and a dry dressing to cover. What type of debridement is the nurse performing?

    a. Surgical debridement

    b. Nonselective debridement

    c. Enzymatic debridement

    d. Selective debridement

Assessment and Management of Patients With Hypertension

Learning Objectives

1. Define normal blood pressure and categories of abnormal pressures.
2. Identify risk factors for hypertension.
3. Explain the differences between normal blood pressure and hypertension and discuss the significance of hypertension.
4. Describe treatment approaches for hypertension, including lifestyle modifications and medication therapy.
5. Use the nursing process as a framework for care of the patient with hypertension.
6. Describe hypertensive crises and their treatment.

SECTION I: ASSESSING YOUR UNDERSTANDING

Activity A Fill in the blanks.

1. Blood pressure is the product of _____ multiplied by _____.

2. Cardiac output is the product of _____ multiplied by _____.

3. Approximately _____% of adults have hypertension.

4. A risk factor assessment, as advocated by the Seventh Report of the Joint National Committee on Prevention, Detection, Evaluation, and Treatment of High Blood Pressure (JNC 7), is needed to classify and guide the treatment of hypertensive people at risk for _____.

5. The desired goal for the systolic blood pressure for a person with diabetes or chronic kidney disease is _____.

6. An estimated _____% of patients discontinue their medications within 1 year of beginning to take them.

7. Patients may experience _____ if antihypertensive medications are suddenly stopped.

8. _____ and _____ are the two classes of hypertensive crisis that require immediate intervention.

Activity B Briefly answer the following.

1. What is the correlation between cigarette smoking and high blood pressure?

_____

_____

_____

2. What is a major concern for medical and nursing management of hypertension?

_____

3. What conditions may trigger a hypertensive emergency or urgency?

_____

_____

_____

4. For a patient diagnosed with hypertension, what lifestyle modifications will assist with the management of the disease process?

_____

_____

_____

5. A patient is instructed to adhere to a DASH diet. What does the diet recommend?

_____

_____

_____

Activity C *Match the hypertension medication listed in Column II with its associated action listed in Column I.*

Column I

____ **1.** Blocks reabsorption of sodium and water in kidneys

____ **2.** Stimulates alpha$_2$-adrenergic receptors

____ **3.** Stimulates dopamine and alpha$_2$-adrenergic receptors

____ **4.** Blocks beta-adrenergic receptors

____ **5.** Inhibits aldosterone

____ **6.** Displaces norepinephrine from storage sites

Column II

a. Inderal

b. Tenex

c. Aldactone

d. Lasix

e. Aldomet

f. Corlopam

SECTION II: APPLYING YOUR KNOWLEDGE

Activity D *Consider the scenario and answer the questions.*

CASE STUDY: Secondary Hypertension

Georgia, a 30-year-old woman, is diagnosed as having secondary hypertension when serial blood pressure recordings show her average reading to be 170/100 mm Hg. Her hypertension is the result of renal dysfunction.

1. How will Georgia's kidney help maintain her hypertensive state?

_____

_____

2. The nurse informs Georgia that she should make an appointment to see her ophthalmologist. Why is it important that Georgia adhere to follow-up with an ophthalmologist?

_____

_____

_____

3. Georgia is prescribed furosemide (Lasix) 20 mg once every day. What does the nurse understand about the action of Lasix?

_____

_____

4. What health education can the nurse suggest to Georgia to reduce complications and improve disease outcomes?

_____

_____

_____

SECTION III: PRACTICING FOR NCLEX

Activity E *Answer the following questions.*

1. A patient is being seen at the clinic on a monthly basis for assessment of blood pressure. The patient has been checking her blood pressure at home as well and has reported a systolic pressure of 158 and a diastolic pressure of 64. What does the nurse suspect this patient is experiencing?

   a. Isolated systolic hypertension

   b. Secondary hypertension

   c. Primary hypertension

   d. Hypertensive urgency

2. The nurse is assessing a patient with severe hypertension. When performing a focused assessment of the eyes, what does the nurse understand may be observed related to the hypertension?

   a. Cataracts

   b. Glaucoma

   c. Retinal detachment

   d. Papilledema

3. A patient with hypertension is waking up several times a night to urinate. The nurse knows that what laboratory studies may indicate pathologic changes in the kidneys due to the hypertension? (Select all that apply.)

   a. Creatinine

   b. Blood urea nitrogen (BUN)

   c. Complete blood count (CBC)

   d. Urine for culture and sensitivity

   e. AST and ALT

4. A patient with long-standing hypertension is admitted to the hospital with hypertensive urgency. The physician orders a chest x-ray, which reveals an enlarged heart. What diagnostic test does the nurse anticipate preparing the patient for to determine left ventricular enlargement?

   a. Cardiac catheterization

   b. Echocardiography

   c. Stress test

   d. Tilt-table test

5. A patient with hypertension has been able to maintain a blood pressure of 130/70 mm Hg for 1 year while reducing dietary sodium and taking hydrochlorothiazide (HCTZ) and atenolol (Tenormin). What treatment plan will the nurse educate the patient about?

   a. Continuing the medication and reducing dietary sodium

   b. Discontinuing the HCTZ and atenolol and continuing to reduce sodium intake

   c. Gradual reducing the HCTZ and the atenolol and continuing to reduce sodium intake

   d. Gradually reducing the atenolol and continuing the HCTZ

6. A patient is taking amiloride (Midamor) and lisinopril (Zestril) for the treatment of hypertension. What laboratory studies should the nurse monitor while the patient is taking these two medications together?

   a. Magnesium level

   b. Potassium level

   c. Calcium level

   d. Sodium level

7. A patient has severe coronary artery disease (CAD) and hypertension. Which medication order should the nurse consult with the physician about that is contraindicated for a patient with severe CAD?

   a. Clonidine (Catapres)

   b. Amiloride (Midamor)

   c. Bumetanide (Bumex)

   d. Methyldopa (Aldomet)

8. A patient has been diagnosed with prehypertension and has been encouraged to exercise regularly and begin a weight loss program. After what period of time does the nurse tell the patient to return for a follow-up visit?

   a. 2 months

   b. 6 months

   c. 1 year

   d. 2 years

9. The nurse is assessing the blood pressure for a patient who has hypertension and the nurse does not hear an auscultatory gap. What outcome may be documented in this circumstance?

   a. A low diastolic reading

   b. A high systolic pressure reading

   c. A normal reading

   d. A high diastolic or low systolic reading

10. The nurse is performing an assessment on a patient to determine the effects of hypertension on the heart and blood vessels. What specific assessment data will assist in determining this complication? (Select all that apply.)

    a. Heart rate

    b. Respiratory rate

    c. Heart rhythm

    d. Character of apical and peripheral pulses

    e. Lung sounds

11. The nurse is planning the care of a patient admitted to the hospital with hypertension. What objective will help to meet the needs of this patient?

    a. Lowering and controlling the blood pressure without adverse effects and without undue cost

    b. Making sure that the patient adheres to the therapeutic medication regimen

    c. Instructing the patient to enter a weight loss program and begin an exercise regimen

    d. Scheduling the patient for all follow-up visits and making phone calls to the home to ensure adherence

12. A patient informs the nurse, "I can't adhere to the dietary sodium decrease that is required for the treatment of my hypertension." What can the nurse educate the client about regarding this statement?

    a. If dietary sodium isn't restricted, the patient will be unable to control the blood pressure and will be at risk for stroke.

    b. The patient can speak to the physician about increasing the dosage of medication instead of reducing the added salt.

    c. It takes 2 to 3 months for the taste buds to adapt to changes in salt intake.

    d. The patient should use other methods of flavoring foods.

13. A patient is flying overseas for 1 week for business and packed antihypertensive medications in a suitcase. After arriving at the intended destination, the patient found that the luggage had been stolen. If the patient cannot take the medication, what condition becomes a concern?

    a. Isolated systolic hypertension

    b. Rebound hypertension

    c. Angina

    d. Left ventricular hypertrophy

14. A patient is brought to the emergency department with complaints of a bad headache and an increase in blood pressure. The blood pressure reading obtained by the nurse is 260/180 mm Hg. What is the therapeutic goal for reduction of the mean blood pressure?

    a. Reduce the blood pressure by 20% to 25% within the first hour of treatment.

    b. Reduce the blood pressure to about 140/80 mm Hg.

    c. Rapidly reduce the blood pressure so the patient will not suffer a stroke.

    d. Reduce the blood pressure by 50% within the first hour of treatment.

15. A patient arrives at the clinic for a follow-up visit for treatment of hypertension. The nurse obtains a blood pressure reading of 180/110 but finds no evidence of impending or progressive organ damage when performing the assessment on the patient. What situation does the nurse understand this patient is experiencing?

    a. Hypertensive emergency

    b. Primary hypertension

    c. Secondary hypertension

    d. Hypertensive urgency

Hematologic Function

CHAPTER 32

Assessment of Hematologic Function and Treatment Modalities

Learning Objectives

1. Describe the process of hematopoiesis.
2. Describe the processes involved in maintaining hemostasis.
3. Discuss the significance of the health history to the assessment of hematologic health.
4. Describe the significance of physical assessment and diagnostic test findings to the diagnosis of hematologic dysfunction.
5. Identify therapies for blood disorders, including the nursing implications for the administration of blood components.

SECTION I: ASSESSING YOUR UNDERSTANDING

Activity A *Fill in the blanks.*

1. The volume of blood in humans is about _____ L.

2. Blood cell formation (hematopoiesis) occurs in the _____.

3. Red bone marrow activity is confined in adults to the _____, _____, _____, and _____.

4. The principal function of the erythrocyte, which is composed primarily of _____, is to _____.

5. Each 100 mL of blood should normally contain _____ g of hemoglobin.

6. Women of childbearing years need an additional _____ daily of iron to replace that loss during menstruation.

7. The nurse advises a patient who is iron deficient to take extra vitamin _____, which is known for increasing iron absorption.

8. Plasma proteins consist primarily of _____ and _____.

9. The two most common areas used for bone marrow aspirations in an adult are _____ and _____.

Activity B *Briefly answer the following.*

1. When a patient suffers a trauma, that patient is at risk for excess blood loss. What protective mechanism is activated to prevent excess blood loss?

   _____

   _____

   _____

2. Describe why the stroma of the bone marrow is important.

   _____

   _____

3. Name five substances that the bone marrow requires for normal erythrocyte production, and describe what can result if any of these factors are deficient.

   _____

   _____

   _____

4. When the physician informs the nurse that the patient has a "shift to the left," what does this mean?

   _____

   _____

5. Describe how natural killer (NK) cells serve as an important part of the body's immune defense system.

   _____

   _____

   _____

6. When the nurse must administer blood or blood components, what knowledge is required?

   _____

   _____

Activity C *Match the key term listed in Column II with its associated definition listed in Column I.*

Column I

____ **1.** The fluid portion of blood

____ **2.** Another term for platelets

____ **3.** The mature form of white blood cells (WBCs)

Column II

a. Bone marrow

b. Monocytes

c. Hemostasis

d. RES

e. Plasma

f. Phagocytosis

Column I

____ **4.** The process of continually replacing blood cells

____ **5.** The site of blood cell formation

____ **6.** Makes up 95% of the mass of the red blood cell (RBC)

____ **7.** The ingestion and digestion of bacteria by neutrophils

____ **8.** The largest classification of leukocytes

____ **9.** A clotting factor present in plasma

____ **10.** A plasma protein primarily responsible for the maintenance of fluid balance

____ **11.** The site of activity for most macrophages

____ **12.** The process of stopping bleeding from a severed blood vessel

____ **13.** A protein that forms the basis of blood clotting

____ **14.** Integral component of the immune system

____ **15.** The term for red blood cell

____ **16.** The letters used for the term reticulo-endothelial system

____ **17.** The balance between clot formation and clot dissolution

____ **18.** A term used to describe T lymphocytes

Column II

g. Lymphocytes

h. Albumin

i. T cells

j. Thrombocytes

k. Spleen

l. Neutrophils

m. Hemostasis

n. Erythrocyte

o. Hematopoiesis

p. Hemoglobin

q. Fibrinogen

r. plasminogen

SECTION II: APPLYING YOUR KNOWLEDGE

Activity D *Consider the scenario and answer the questions.*

CASE STUDY: Blood Transfusion

Jerry has been admitted to the hospital with a diagnosis of gastrointestinal bleeding and has a hemoglobin of 8 g/dL. He has been type- and cross-matched for two units of packed RBCs and is to receive his first unit.

1. The nurse is performing a pretransfusion history. What information should be obtained prior to the transfusion?

   _____

   _____

   _____

2. The nurse is preparing to administer 1 unit of packed RBCs to Jerry. What should the nurse check prior to initiating the transfusion?

   _____

   _____

   _____

3. The nurse begins the transfusion of packed cells after obtaining vital signs. Fifteen minutes after the infusion begins, Jerry informs the nurse that he is itching all over. How does the nurse respond?

   _____

   _____

SECTION III: PRACTICING FOR NCLEX

Activity E *Answer the following questions.*

1. The physician believes that the patient has a deficiency in the leukocyte responsible for cell-mediated immunity. What should the nurse check the WBC count for?

   a. Basophils

   b. Monocytes

   c. Plasma cells

   d. T lymphocytes

2. An older adult patient presents to the physician's office with a complaint of exhaustion. The nurse, aware of the most common hematologic condition affecting the elderly, knows that which laboratory values should be assessed?

   a. WBC count

   b. RBC count

   c. Thrombocyte count

   d. Levels of plasma proteins

3. A nurse is caring for a patient who has had a bone marrow aspiration with biopsy. What complication should the nurse be aware of and monitor the patient for?

   a. Hemorrhage

   b. Infection

   c. Shock

   d. Splintering of bone fragments

4. A patient with chronic kidney disease is being examined by the nurse practitioner for anemia. The nurse has reviewed the laboratory data for hemoglobin and RBC count. What other test results would the nurse anticipate observing?

   a. Decreased level of erythropoietin

   b. Decreased total iron-binding capacity

   c. Increased mean corpuscular volume

   d. Increased reticulocyte count

5. A female patient has a hemoglobin of 6.4 g/dL and is preparing to have a blood transfusion. Why would it be important for the nurse to obtain information about the patient's history of pregnancy prior to the transfusion?

   a. A high number of pregnancies can increase the risk of reaction.

   b. If the patient has never been pregnant, it increases the risk of reaction.

   c. Obtaining information about gravidity and parity is routine information for all female patients.

   d. If the patient has been pregnant, she may have developed allergies.

6. A patient will need a blood transfusion for the replacement of blood loss from the gastrointestinal tract. The patient states, "That stuff isn't safe!" What is the best response from the nurse?

   a. "I agree that you should be concerned with the safety of the blood, but it is important that you have this transfusion."

   b. "The blood is carefully screened, so there is no possibility of you contracting any illness or disease from the blood."

   c. "I understand your concern. The blood is carefully screened but is not completely risk free."

   d. "You will have to decide if refusing the blood transfusion is worth the risk to your health."

7. A patient with chronic anemia has had many blood transfusions over the last 3 years. What type of transfusion reaction should the nurse monitor for that is commonly found in patients who frequently receive blood transfusions?

   a. Allergic reactions

   b. Acute hemolytic reaction

   c. Circulatory overload

   d. Febrile nonhemolytic reactions

8. The nurse is administering a blood transfusion to a patient over 4 hours. After 2 hours, the patient complaints of chills and has a fever of 101°F, an increase from a previous temperature of 99.2°F. What does the nurse recognize is occurring with this patient?

   a. The patient is having an allergic reaction to the blood.

   b. The patient is experiencing vascular collapse.

   c. The patient is having decrease in tissue perfusion from a shock state.

   d. The patient is having a febrile nonhemolytic reaction.

9. The nurse is administering 2 units of packed RBCs to an older adult patient who has a bleeding duodenal ulcer. The patient begins to experience difficulty breathing and the nurse assesses crackles in the lung bases, jugular vein distention, and an increase in blood pressure. What action by the nurse is necessary if the reaction is severe? (Select all that apply.)

   a. Continue the infusion but slow the rate down.

   b. Place the patient in an upright position with the feet dependent.

   c. Administer diuretics as prescribed.

   d. Discontinue the transfusion.

   e. Administer oxygen.

10. A patient receiving plasma develops transfusion-related acute lung injury (TRALI) 4 hours after the transfusion. What type of aggressive therapy does the nurse anticipate the patient will receive to prevent death from the injury? (Select all that apply.)

    a. Serial chest x-rays

    b. Oxygen

    c. Fluid support

    d. Intubation and mechanical ventilation

    e. Intra-aortic balloon pump

11. A patient who has long-term packed RBC transfusions has developed symptoms of iron toxicity that affect liver function. What immediate treatment should the nurse anticipate preparing the patient for that can help prevent organ damage?

    a. Iron chelation therapy

    b. Oxygen therapy

    c. Therapeutic phlebotomy

    d. Anticoagulation therapy

12. A patient develops a hemolytic reaction to a blood transfusion. What actions should the nurse take after this occurs? (Select all that apply.)

   a. Administer diphenhydramine (Benadryl).

   b. Begin iron chelation therapy.

   c. Obtain appropriate blood specimens.

   d. Collect a urine sample to detect hemoglobin.

   e. Document the reaction according to policy.

13. The nurse is preparing a patient for a bone marrow aspiration and biopsy from the site of the posterior superior iliac crest. What position will the nurse place the patient in?

   a. Lateral position with one leg flexed

   b. Lithotomy position

   c. Supine with head of the bed elevated 30 degrees

   d. Jackknife position

14. A patient with chronic kidney disease has chronic anemia. What pharmacologic alternative to blood transfusion may be used for this patient?

   a. GM-CSF (Leukine)

   b. Erythropoietin (Epogen)

   c. Eltrombopag (Promacta)

   d. Thrombopoietin (TPO)

15. A patient is undergoing platelet pheresis at the outpatient clinic. What does the nurse know is the most likely clinical disorder the patient is being treated for?

   a. Essential thrombocythemia

   b. Extreme leukocytosis

   c. Sickle cell anemia

   d. Renal transplantation

33

Management of Patients With Nonmalignant Hematologic Disorders

Learning Objectives

1. Differentiate between the hypoproliferative and the hemolytic anemias and compare and contrast the physiologic mechanisms, clinical manifestations, medical management, and nursing interventions for each.
2. Use the nursing process as a framework for care of patients with anemia.
3. Use the nursing process as a framework for care of patients with sickle cell crises.
4. Discuss treatment of secondary polycythemias.
5. Describe the processes involved in neutropenia and lymphopenia and the general principles of medical and nursing management of patients with these disorders.
6. Describe the medical and nursing management of patients with bleeding and thrombotic disorders.
7. Use the nursing process as a framework for care of patients with disseminated intravascular coagulation.

SECTION I: ASSESSING YOUR UNDERSTANDING

Activity A *Fill in the blanks.*

1. _____ is a condition in which the hemoglobin concentration is lower than normal, reflecting the presence of fewer than the normal number of erythrocytes within the circulatory system.

2. A healthy person can often tolerate as much as a _____ % gradual reduction in hemoglobin without pronounced symptoms or significant incapacity.

3. General complications of severe anemia include _____, _____, and _____.

4. The overall prevalence of anemia increases with age, from _____ % in persons aged 65–69, to _____ % in persons over age 85.

5. A _____ assessment should be performed for patients with known megaloblastic anemia.

6. _____ and _____ should not be taken with iron preparations, because they greatly diminish the absorption of iron.

7. _____ is a rare disease caused by a decrease in or damage to marrow stem cells, damage to the microenvironment within the marrow, or replacement of the marrow with fat.

8. Chronic use of _____ to reduce gastric acid production can inhibit B_{12} absorption, as can the use of _____ in managing diabetes.

9. Assessment of patients who have or are at risk for megaloblastic anemia includes inspection of the _____, _____, and _____.

10. _____ is a severe hemolytic anemia that results from inheritance of the sickle hemoglobin gene, which causes the hemoglobin molecule to be defective.

11. _____ is a controversial treatment strategy that treats DIC by interrupting the thrombosis process.

Activity B *Briefly answer the following.*

1. Name five factors that influence the development of anemia-associated symptoms.

_____

_____

_____

2. When the patient has anemia, what medical management goal will the nurse assist the patient and health care team in achieving?

_____

3. Describe how anemia impacts the older adult patient.

_____

_____

_____

4. When the nurse is educating the patient and family about a healthy diet for the treatment of iron deficiency anemia, who and what should be included?

_____

_____

_____

5. List the four most common causes of iron deficiency anemia in men and postmenopausal women.

_____

_____

6. What chemical agents may be responsible for producing bone marrow aplasia?

_____

_____

_____

7. Name the diagnostic findings present in patients who have sickle cell trait versus those present in patients who have sickle cell anemia.

_____

_____

_____

_____

8. Name at least five types of situations in which the transfusion of red blood cells (RBCs) is highly effective.

_____

_____

9. List at least seven triggers that may lead to the development of disseminated intravascular coagulation (DIC).

_____

_____

_____

Activity C *Match the type of anemia in Column I with the classification in Column II. Answers will be used more than once.*

Column I	Column II
____ 1. Aplastic anemia	a. Hypoproliferative anemias
____ 2. Sickle cell anemia	
____ 3. Folic acid deficiency	b. Megaloblastic anemias
____ 4. Thalassemia major	c. Hemolytic anemias
____ 5. Iron deficiency	
____ 6. B_{12} deficiency	

SECTION II: APPLYING YOUR KNOWLEDGE

Activity D *Consider the scenario and answer the questions.*

George is a 75-year-old patient with urosepsis being treated in the intensive care unit (ICU). The nurse assesses George and finds that he has blood in his urine and stool, and is oozing blood from his central line site and his gums.

1. What does the nurse suspect may be occurring with George?

   _____

2. What medications should the nurse avoid administering to George?

   _____

   _____

   _____

3. The nurse is monitoring George's vital signs every 15 minutes. What other monitoring is essential to include along with the vital signs?

   _____

   _____

4. What medication does the nurse anticipate infusing?

   _____

SECTION III: PRACTICING FOR NCLEX

Activity E *Answer the following questions.*

1. The nurse is assessing a patient who comes to the clinic complaining of feeling constantly tired and very weak. The patient also has a very sore tongue, and upon observing the patient's oral cavity, the nurse notices the tongue is beefy red. What type of anemia does the nurse know these symptoms indicate?
   a. Iron deficiency anemia
   b. Megaloblastic anemia
   c. Sickle cell anemia
   d. Aplastic anemia

2. The nurse observes a co-worker who always seems to be eating a cup of ice. The nurse encourages the co-worker to have an examination and diagnostic workup with the physician. What type of anemia is the nurse concerned the co-worker may have?
   a. Iron deficiency anemia
   b. Megaloblastic anemia
   c. Sickle cell anemia
   d. Aplastic anemia

3. The nurse is performing an assessment for a client with anemia admitted to the hospital to have blood transfusions administered. Why would the nurse need to include a nutritional assessment for this patient?
   a. It is part of the required assessment information.
   b. It is important for the nurse to determine what type of foods the patient will eat.
   c. It may indicate deficiencies in essential nutrients.
   d. It will determine what type of anemia the patient has.

4. The nurse is assessing a patient who is a strict vegetarian. What type of anemia is the nurse aware that this patient is at risk for?
   a. Iron deficiency anemia
   b. Aplastic anemia
   c. Megaloblastic anemia
   d. Sickle cell anemia

5. A patient describes numbness in the arms and hands with a tingling sensation. The patient also frequently stumbles when walking. What vitamin deficiency does the nurse determine may cause some of these symptoms?
   a. Thiamine
   b. Folate
   c. B_{12}
   d. Iron

6. The nurse is educating a patient with iron deficiency anemia about food sources high in iron and how to enhance the absorption of iron when eating these foods. What can the nurse inform the client would enhance the absorption?

   a. Eating calf's liver with a glass of orange juice

   b. Eating leafy green vegetables with a glass of water

   c. Eating apple slices with carrots

   d. Eating a steak with mushrooms

7. A patient with end-stage kidney disease (ESKD) has developed anemia. What laboratory finding does the nurse understand to be significant in this stage of anemia?

   a. Potassium level of 5.2 mEq/L

   b. Magnesium level of 2.5 mg/dL

   c. Calcium level of 9.4 mg/dL

   d. Creatinine level of 6 mg/100 mL

8. A patient with ESRD is taking recombinant erythropoietin for the treatment of anemia. What laboratory study does the nurse understand will have to be assessed at least monthly related to this medication?

   a. Potassium level

   b. Creatinine level

   c. Hemoglobin level

   d. Folate levels

9. A patient had gastric bypass surgery 3 years ago and now, experiencing fatigue, visits the clinic to determine the cause. The patient takes pantoprazole (Protonix) for the treatment of frequent heartburn. What type of anemia is this patient at risk for?

   a. Aplastic anemia

   b. Iron deficiency anemia

   c. Sickle cell anemia

   d. Pernicious anemia

10. The nurse is preparing the patient for a test to determine the cause of vitamin B_{12} deficiency. The patient will receive a small oral dose of radioactive vitamin B_{12} followed by a large parenteral dose of nonradioactive dose of B_{12}. What test is the patient being prepared for?

    a. Bone marrow aspiration

    b. Schilling test

    c. Bone marrow biopsy

    d. Magnetic resonance imaging (MRI) study

11. Which patient does the nurse recognize as being most likely to be affected by sickle cell disease?

    a. A 14-year-old African American boy

    b. A 26-year-old Eastern European Jewish woman

    c. An 18-year-old Chinese woman

    d. A 28-year-old Israeli man

12. A patient with sickle cell disease is brought to the emergency department by a parent. The patient has a fever of 101.6°F, heart rate of 116, and a respiratory rate of 32. The nurse auscultates bilateral wheezes in both lung fields. What does the nurse suspect this patient is experiencing?

    a. Pneumocystis pneumonia

    b. Acute chest syndrome

    c. An exacerbation of asthma

    d. Pulmonary edema

13. A patient with sickle cell anemia is to begin treatment for the disease with hydroxyurea (Hydrea). What does the nurse inform the patient will be the benefits of treatment with this medication? (Select all that apply.)

    a. Fewer painful episodes of sickle cell crisis

    b. Lower incidence of acute chest syndrome

    c. Decreased need for blood transfusions

    d. Decreased need for other analgesic medications

    e. Ability to reverse the damage done from sickling of cells

14. A patient with sickle cell disease comes to the emergency department complaining of severe pain in the back, right hip, and right arm. What intervention is important for the nurse to provide?

   a. Administer aspirin

   b. Administer ibuprofen

   c. Start an intravenous line with dextrose 5% in 0.24 normal saline

   d. Begin oxygen at 2 L/M

15. A patient is taking prednisone 60 mg per day for the treatment of an acute exacerbation of Crohn's disease. The patient has developed lymphopenia with a lymphocyte count of less than 1,500 mm^3. What should the nurse monitor the client for?

   a. The onset of a bacterial infection

   b. Bleeding

   c. Abdominal pain

   d. Diarrhea

34

Management of Patients With Hematologic Neoplasms

Learning Objectives

1. Distinguish between hematologic clonal disorders and frank malignancy.
2. Compare the leukemias in terms of their incidence, physiologic alterations, clinical manifestations, management, and prognosis.
3. Use the nursing process as a framework for care of patients with acute leukemia.
4. Compare the myeloproliferative disorders in terms of their incidence, clinical manifestations, management, complications, and prognosis.
5. Describe nursing management of patients with lymphoma or multiple myeloma.

SECTION I: ASSESSING YOUR UNDERSTANDING

Activity A *Fill in the blanks.*

1. The development of hematologic neoplasms is complex. Understanding the processes and the rationale for treatments is important so that nurses may appropriately _____, _____, _____, and _____ with patients who have hematologic neoplasms.

2. Hematopoietic malignancies are often classified by the _____ involved.

3. Multiple myeloma is a malignancy of the most mature form of _____, the plasma cell.

4. The common feature of the _____ is an unregulated proliferation of leukocytes in the bone marrow.

5. The leukemias are commonly classified according to the stem cell line involved, either _____ or _____.

6. The leukemias are also classified as _____ or _____.

7. In acute myeloid leukemia (AML), any age group can be affected, although it infrequently occurs before age _____ and the incidence rises with age, with a peak incidence at age _____ years.

8. Complications of AML include _____ and _____, the major causes of death from this condition.

9. Chronic myeloid leukemia (CML) arises from a mutation in the myeloid _____.

10. Myelodysplastic syndromes (MDSs) are a group of clonal disorders of the myeloid stem cell that cause _____ in one or more types of cell lines.

Activity B *Briefly answer the following.*

1. What do the signs and symptoms of AML result from?

_____

_____

2. If a bone marrow analysis is performed on a patient with AML, what results are seen?

_____

_____

3. What is the goal of treatment in acute lymphocytic leukemia (ALL)?

_____

_____

_____

4. Why is caring for a patient with MDS difficult?

_____

5. What are the potential long-term complications of therapy for a patient with Hodgkin lymphoma?

_____

_____

_____

Activity C *Match the name of the clonal stem cell disorder in Column I with the characteristics of the disorder in Column II.*

Column I

____ 1. Acute myeloid leukemia

____ 2. Chronic myeloid leukemia

____ 3. Acute lymphocytic leukemia

____ 4. Chronic lymphocytic leukemia

____ 5. Polycythemia vera

____ 6. Essential thrombocythemia

____ 7. Hodgkin lymphoma

____ 8. Non-Hodgkin lymphoma

____ 9. Multiple myeloma

Column II

a. Proliferative disorder of the myeloid stem cells

b. Malignant disease of the most mature form of B lymphocyte, the plasma cell

c. Arises from a mutation in the myeloid stem cell

d. Results from an uncontrolled proliferation of immature cells derived from the lymphoid stem cell

e. Stem cell disease within the bone marrow

f. Unicentric in origin and is initiated in a single node

g. Derived from a malignant clone of B lymphocytes

h. Results from a defect in the hematopoietic stem cell that differentiates into all myeloid cells

i. Heterogeneous group of cancers that originate from the neoplastic growth of lymphoid tissue

SECTION II: APPLYING YOUR KNOWLEDGE

Activity D *Consider the scenario and answer the questions.*

CASE STUDY: Multiple Myeloma

Carl White, a 67-year-old man, has been seeing his family physician for complaints of back pain. He has been treated for low back strain without relief. The physician performs laboratory studies, which reveal an elevated protein level. A bone marrow biopsy is performed, with results positive for multiple myeloma.

1. When discussing the characteristics of Carl's bone pain, what does the nurse determine is congruent with his diagnosis of multiple myeloma?

   _____

   _____

   _____

2. When the nurse is reviewing Carl's laboratory results, a hemoglobin of 7.4 g/dL and a hematocrit of 34% is noted. What does the nurse suspect is causing these blood levels?

   _____

   _____

   _____

3. Carl is not a candidate for autologous hematopoietic stem cell transplantation (HSCT). What would be a primary treatment for him?

   _____

4. Why would nonsteroidal anti-inflammatory drugs (NSAIDs) be used with caution to control Carl's pain?

   _____

   _____

   _____

SECTION III: PRACTICING FOR NCLEX

Activity E *Answer the following questions.*

1. A patient with AML is having aggressive chemotherapy to attempt to achieve remission. The patient is aware that hospitalization will be necessary for several weeks. What type of therapy will the nurse explain that the patient will receive?

   a. Induction therapy

   b. Supportive therapy

   c. Antimicrobial therapy

   d. Standard therapy

2. A patient with AML is having HSCT with radiation therapy. With which complication does the nurse know that the donor's lymphocytes recognize the patient's body as foreign and set up reactions to attack the foreign host?

   a. Acute respiratory distress syndrome

   b. Graft-versus-host disease

   c. Remission

   d. Bone marrow depression

3. The nurse is performing an assessment on a patient with AML and observes multiple areas of ecchymosis and petechiae. What laboratory study should the nurse be concerned about?

   a. WBC count of 4,200 cells/mcL

   b. Hematocrit of 38%

   c. Platelet count of 9,000/mm^3

   d. Creatinine level of 1.0 mg/dL

4. A patient with AML has a neutrophil count that persists at less than 100/mm^3. What should the nurse cautiously monitor this patient for?

   a. Abdominal cramps

   b. Hypotension

   c. Seizure activity

   d. Infection

5. The nurse is caring for a patient with AML with high uric acid levels. What medication does the nurse anticipate administering that will prevent crystallization of uric acid and stone formation?

   a. Allopurinol (Zyloprim)

   b. Filgrastim (Neupogen)

   c. Hydroxyurea (Myleran)

   d. Asparaginase (Elspar)

6. The nurse is caring for a patient with CML who is taking imatinib mesylate (Gleevec). In what phase of the leukemia does the nurse understand that this medication is most useful to induce remission?

   a. Chronic

   b. Transformation

   c. Accelerated

   d. Blast crisis

7. The nurse is educating a patient taking imatinib mesylate (Gleevec) for treatment of leukemia. What should the nurse be sure to include when educating the patient on the best way to take the medication to optimize absorption?

   a. Take the medication with a source of vitamin C to enhance absorption.

   b. Take antacids if needed for gastrointestinal (GI) upset 2 hours after taking Gleevec.

   c. Take the medication with food to enhance absorption.

   d. Take the medication with acetaminophen to prevent decreased absorption and GI upset.

8. Which patient assessed by the nurse is most likely to develop MDS?

   a. A 24-year-old female taking oral contraceptives

   b. A 40-year-old patient with a history of hypertension

   c. A 52-year-old patient with acute kidney injury

   d. A 72-year-old patient with a history of cancer

9. The nurse is administering packed RBC transfusions for a patient with MD). The patient has had several transfusions and is likely to receive several more. What is a priority for the nurse to monitor related to the transfusions?

   a. Creatinine and blood urea nitrogen (BUN) levels

   b. Iron levels

   c. Magnesium levels

   d. Potassium levels

10. The nurse is assessing a patent with polycythemia vera. What skin assessment data would the nurse determine is a normal finding for this patient?

    a. Pale skin and mucous membranes

    b. Bronze skin tone

    c. Ruddy complexion

    d. Jaundice skin and sclera

11. A patient with polycythemia vera has a high RBC count and is at risk for the development of thrombosis. What treatment is important to reduce blood viscosity and to deplete the patient's iron stores?

    a. Blood transfusions

    b. Radiation

    c. Chelation therapy

    d. Phlebotomy

12. A patient with polycythemia vera is complaining of severe itching. What triggers does the nurse know can cause this distressing symptom? (Select all that apply.)

    a. Temperature change

    b. Allergic reaction to the RBC increase

    c. Alcohol consumption

    d. Exposure to water of any temperature

    e. Aspirin

13. The nurse is caring for a patient with Hodgkin lymphoma in the hospital and preparing discharge planning education. Knowing that this patient is at risk for the development of a second malignancy, what education would be beneficial to reduce the risk factors? (Select all that apply.)

   a. Reduce exposure to excessive sunlight

   b. Smoking cessation

   c. Decrease alcohol intake

   d. Decrease intake of antipyretic medications such as acetaminophen

   e. Decrease fat intake

14. A patient is taking hydroxyurea for the treatment of primary myelofibrosis. While the patient is taking this medication, what will the nurse monitor to determine effectiveness?

   a. Leukocyte and platelet count

   b. BUN and creatinine levels

   c. Aspartate aminotransferase (AST) and alanine transaminase (ALT) levels

   d. Hemoglobin and hematocrit

15. The nurse is caring for a patient who will begin taking long-term biphosphate therapy. Why is it important for the nurse to encourage the patient to receive a thorough evaluation of dentition, including panoramic dental x-rays?

   a. The patient is at risk for tooth decay.

   b. The patient will develop gingival hyperplasia.

   c. The patient can develop osteonecrosis of the jaw.

   d. The patient can develop loosening of the teeth.

Immunologic Function

CHAPTER 35

Assessment of Immune Function

1. Describe the body's general immune responses.
2. Discuss the stages of the immune response.
3. Differentiate between cellular and humoral immune responses.
4. Describe the effects of selected variables on function of the immune system.
5. Use assessment parameters for determining the status of patients' immune function.

SECTION I: ASSESSING YOUR UNDERSTANDING

Activity A *Fill in the blanks.*

1. The immune system is essentially composed of _____, _____, and _____.

2. White blood cells (WBCs) involved in immunity are primarily produced in the _____.

3. T lymphocytes, descendants of stem cells, mature in the _____.

4. Granulocytes, which fight invasion by releasing histamine, do not include _____.

5. The leukocytes that arrive first at a site where inflammation occurs are _____.

6. WBCs that function as phagocytes are called _____.

7. The body's first line of defense is the _____.

8. The primary cells responsible for recognition of foreign antigens are _____.

9. Antibodies are believed to be a type of _____.

10. A deficient immune system response that is congenital in origin would be classified as a _____ disorder.

11. During the _____ stage of an immune response, lymphocytes interfere with disease by picking up specific antigens from organisms to alter their function.

Activity B *Briefly answer the following.*

1. What does cellular membrane damage result from?

_____

_____

2. Describe how effector T cells destroy foreign organisms.

_____

_____

3. Describe four ways that disorders of the immune system occur.

_____

_____

_____

4. Distinguish between natural and acquired (active and passive) immunity.

_____

_____

_____

5. What is complement, how is it formed, and how does it function?

_____

_____

_____

6. How do biologic response modifiers (BMRs) affect the immune response?

_____

_____

7. What age-related changes affect immunologic function?

_____

_____

_____

8. What effects do adrenal corticosteroids, antimetabolites, and antibiotics have on the immune system?

_____

_____

_____

Activity C **Immunoglobulins**

Match the immunoglobulin (Ig) listed in Column II with its associated Ig activity listed in Column I. An answer may be used more than once.

Column I

___ 1. Enhances phagocytosis

___ 2. Appears in intravascular serum

___ 3. Helps defend against parasites

___ 4. Activates complement system

___ 5. Protects against respiratory infections

___ 6. Possible influence on B-lymphocyte differentiation

___ 7. Prevents absorption of antigens from food

Column II

a. IgA

b. IgD

c. IgE

d. IgG

e. IgM

Medications

Match the immune system effect listed in Column II with its corresponding medication listed in Column I. An answer may be used more than once.

Column I

___ 1. Cyclosporine

___ 2. Dactinomycin

___ 3. Indomethacin

___ 4. Methotrexate

___ 5. Mustargen

___ 6. Propylthiouracil

___ 7. Vancomycin

Column II

a. Agranulocytosis, leukopenia

b. Agranulocytosis, neutropenia

c. Leukopenia, aplastic bone marrow

d. Leukopenia, T-cell inhibition

e. Transient leukopenia

SECTION II: APPLYING YOUR KNOWLEDGE

Activity D *Consider the scenario and answer the questions.*

Mrs. Bartosh, age 63, has developed an infection of the surgical site after having a colon resection. She has a fever, elevated WBC count, and a culture of the surgical wound is positive for methicillin-resistant staphylococcus aureus (MRSA).

1. What does the first line of defense, or the *phagocytic immune response,* involve?

_____

_____

2. What is the second protective response, or the *humoral immune response*?

_____

_____

3. What is the third mechanism of defense, or the *cellular immune response*?

_____

_____

SECTION III: PRACTICING FOR NCLEX

Activity E *Answer the following questions.*

1. A patient arrives at the clinic and informs the nurse that she has a very sore throat as well as a fever. A rapid strep test returns a positive result and the patient is given a prescription for an antibiotic. How did the streptococcal organism gain access to the patient to cause this infection?

   a. Through the mucous membranes of the throat

   b. Through the skin

   c. Breathing in airborne dust

   d. From being outside in the cold weather and decreasing resistance

2. A patient developed an infection while on vacation in Central America and is now taking the antibiotic chloramphenicol (Chloromycetin). What should the patient be monitored for when taking this drug?

   a. Eosinophilia

   b. Neutropenia

   c. Aplastic anemia

   d. Hypoprothrombinemia

3. An older adult patient who is postmenopausal informs the nurse that she believes she has developed another urinary tract infection (UTI). The nurse understands that postmenopausal females are at greater risk for UTIs. What risk factors do female patients in this age group have? (Select all that apply.)

   a. Residual urine

   b. Urinary incontinence

   c. Estrogen deficiency

   d. Decreased function of the thyroid gland

   e. Dry mucous membranes of the vagina

4. The nurse is caring for an older adult patient hospitalized with cellulitis of the right lower extremity. Why is it imperative that the nurse continually assess the physical and emotional status of this patient?

   a. Older patients are at risk of developing dementia.

   b. The patient will not respond to the antibiotic treatment as well as a younger patient would.

   c. Early recognition and management of factors influencing immune response may decrease morbidity and mortality.

   d. Older adult patients develop depression and suicidal tendencies when they are faced with chronic illness.

5. The nurse is caring for a patient in the hospital who is receiving a vitamin D supplement. What does the nurse understand is the importance of supplementation with this vitamin? (Select all that apply.)

   a. Vitamin D deficiency is associated with increased risk of common cancers.

   b. Vitamin D deficiency is associated with increased risk of autoimmune disease.

   c. Vitamin D deficiency is associated with increased risk of congenital anomalies.

   d. Vitamin D deficiency is associated with increased risk of inflammatory disorders.

   e. Vitamin D deficiency is associated with increased risk of celiac disease.

6. An older adult has developed a sacral pressure ulcer. What should the nurse assess in order to ensure adequate wound healing and prevent poor outcomes for this patient? (Select all that apply.)

   a. The patient's ability to perform her own wound care

   b. Nutritional status

   c. Caloric intake

   d. Quality of food ingested

   e. The amount of carbohydrates the patient ingests

7. The nurse is caring for a female patient who has an exacerbation of lupus erythematosus. What does the nurse understand is the reason that females tend to develop autoimmune disorders more frequently than men?

   a. Androgen tends to enhance immunity.

   b. Estrogen tends to enhance immunity.

   c. Testosterone tends to enhance immunity.

   d. Leukocytes are increased in females.

8. The nurse is obtaining a history from a patient with severe psoriasis. What question would be the most important to ask this patient to determine a genetic predisposition?

   a. "How did you know you developed this disease?"

   b. "Does anyone in your family have more than one autoimmune disease?"

   c. "How many children do you have?"

   d. "Does your spouse or significant other have an autoimmune disease?"

9. A patient who has developed kidney failure is discussing options with the physician for treatment. What does the nurse understand that kidney failure is associated with?

   a. A deficiency in circulating lymphocytes

   b. A deficiency in phosphorus

   c. Decreased amount of WBCs

   d. Increased amount of macrophages

10. A patient who suffered severe partial thickness burns to the face and trunk is at risk for depletion of essential proteins and immunoglobulins. The stressors associated with this patient's major injury have caused what immune process to occur?

   a. Cortisol is released from the adrenal cortex, which contributes to immunosuppression.

   b. Circulating lymphocytes will cause lymph node enlargement and altered lymph drainage.

   c. T lymphocytes are stimulated and produce antibodies.

   d. With the help of macrophages, B lymphocytes recognize the antigen of a foreign invader.

11. When obtaining a health history from a patient with possible abnormal immune function, what question would be a priority for the nurse to ask?

   a. "Have you ever been treated for a sexually transmitted infection?"

   b. "When was your last menstrual period?"

   c. "Do you have abdominal pain or discomfort?"

   d. "Have you ever received a blood transfusion?"

12. A patient tells the nurse, "I can't believe I have ineffective immune function and am getting sick again. I exercise rigorously and compete regularly." What is the best response by the nurse?

   a. "Something must be seriously wrong. You should not be getting sick since you are so healthy."

   b. "Maybe you need to stop exercising so much. It can't be good for you."

   c. "It is possible that you are immunocompromised and may have HIV."

   d. "Rigorous exercise can cause negative effects on immune response."

13. The nurse is performing a physical assessment for a patient at the clinic and palpates enlarged inguinal lymph nodes on the left. What should the nurse document? (Select all that apply.)

a. Location

b. Size

c. Consistency

d. Reports of tenderness

e. Temperature

14. The nursing instructor is discussing the development of human immunodeficiency disease (HIV) with the students. What should the instructor inform the class about helper T cells?

a. They are activated on recognition of antigens and stimulate the rest of the immune system.

b. They attack the antigen directly by altering the cell membrane and causing cell lysis.

c. They have the ability to decrease B-cell production.

d. They are responsible for recognizing antigens from previous exposure and mounting an immune response.

15. A patient is being treated in the intensive care unit for sepsis related to ventilator-associated pneumonia. The patient is on large doses of three different antibiotics. What severe outcome should the nurse monitor for in the lab studies?

a. Leukocytosis

b. Bone marrow suppression

c. Oral thrush

d. Rash

36

Management of Patients With Immunodeficiency Disorders

1. Compare the different types of primary immunodeficiency disorders and their causes, clinical manifestations, potential complications, and treatment modalities.
2. Describe the nursing management of the patient with immunodeficiency disorders.
3. Identify the essential educational needs for a patient with an immunodeficiency disorder.

SECTION I: ASSESSING YOUR UNDERSTANDING

Activity A *Fill in the blanks.*

1. Primary immunodeficiencies predispose people to three conditions: _____, _____, and _____.

2. Five disorders of common, primary immunodeficiencies are _____, _____, _____, _____, and _____.

3. The two types of inherited B-cell deficiencies result from lack of differentiation of B-cells into _____ and _____.

4. More than 50% of patients with common variable immunodeficiency (CVID) develop the disorder _____.

5. The most prevalent cause of immunodeficiency worldwide is _____.

Activity B *Briefly answer the following.*

1. What are immunodeficiency disorders caused by?

_____
_____
_____

2. Name the cardinal symptoms of immunodeficiency.

_____
_____
_____
_____

3. List some of the common different primary immunodeficiencies.

_____
_____
_____
_____

205

4. Patients that have neutropenia are at risk for what problem?

_____

5. Describe the symptoms that infants with x-linked agammaglobulinemia present with.

_____

_____

_____

_____

Activity C *Match the immune component in Column I with the disorder in Column II.*

Column I	Column II
____ **1.** B lymphocytes	**a.** Hyperimmuno-globulinemia E
____ **2.** T lymphocytes	**b.** Angioneurotic edema
____ **3.** Complement system	**c.** DiGeorge syndrome
____ **4.** Phagocytic cells	**d.** Bruton's disease

SECTION II: APPLYING YOUR UNDERSTANDING

Activity D *Consider the scenario and answer the questions.*

A patient is in the hospital being treated for DiGeorge syndrome. The physician orders an initial dose of intravenous immunoglobulin (IVIG) infusion at 200 mg/kg.

1. What type of adverse effects should the nurse be sure to monitor for?

_____

_____

_____

_____

2. What nursing implications and interventions are involved with the infusion of IVIG?

_____

_____

_____

3. What variables may affect the risk and intensity of adverse reactions with the administration of IVIG?

_____

_____

_____

SECTION III: PRACTICING FOR NCLEX

Activity E *Answer the following questions.*

1. A patient is suspected to have an immunodeficiency disorder. The physician orders a nitroblue tetrazolium reductase (NTR) test to diagnose this patient. What does the nurse suspect that this disorder is related to?

   a. Complement

   b. B lymphocytes

   c. T lymphocytes

   d. Phagocytic cells

2. The nurse is caring for a patient with an immunodeficiency disorder. What cardinal symptoms of immunodeficiency does the nurse recognize while caring for this patient? (Select all that apply.)

   a. Chronic diarrhea

   b. Nonproductive cough

   c. Chronic or recurrent severe infections

   d. Poor response to the treatment with antibiotics

   e. Vomiting

3. An infant that is 10 hours postdelivery is observed to have tetanic contractions. What symptom does the nurse recognize can indicate DiGeorge syndrome?

   a. Chronic diarrhea

   b. Hypocalcemia

   c. Neutropenia

   d. Pernicious anemia

4. The nurse is preparing to administer the recommended dose of intravenous gamma-globulin for a 60-kg male patient. How many grams will the nurse administer?

   a. 15 g

   b. 30 g

   c. 60 g

   d. 90 g

5. A patient with CVID is extremely fatigued and not feeling well. What lab test does the nurse anticipate the patient will have to detect a common development related to the disease?

   a. Aspartate aminotransferase (AST) and alanine aminotransferase (ALT)

   b. BUN and creatinine

   c. Glucose level

   d. B_{12} level

6. What severe complication does the nurse monitor for in a patient with ataxia-telangiectasia?

   a. Acute kidney injury

   b. Chronic lung disease

   c. Neurologic dysfunction

   d. Overwhelming infection

7. The nurse is preparing to infuse gamma-globulin IV. When administering this drug, the nurse knows the speed of the infusion should not exceed what rate?

   a. 1.5 mL/min

   b. 3 mL/min

   c. 6 mL/min

   d. 10 mL/min

8. The nurse is administering an infusion of gamma-globulin to a patient in the hospital. When should the nurse discontinue the infusion? (Select all that apply.)

   a. When the patient complains of flank pain

   b. When the patient begins to have shaking chills

   c. When the patient complains of tightness in the chest

   d. When the patient voids 30/mL an hour

   e. When the patient complains of nausea

9. What treatment option does the nurse anticipate for the patient with severe combined immunodeficiency disease?

   a. Bone marrow transplantation

   b. Antibiotics

   c. Radiation therapy

   d. Removal of the thymus gland

10. What does the nurse understand will result if the patient has a deficiency in the normal level of complement?

   a. Increased susceptibility to infection

   b. Decrease in vascularity to the extremities

   c. Development of congestive heart failure

   d. Risk of stroke

Management of Patients With HIV Infection and AIDS

1. Describe the modes of transmission of human immunodeficiency virus (HIV) infection and prevention strategies.
2. Describe the host viral interaction during primary infection with HIV.
3. Explain the pathophysiology associated with the clinical manifestations of HIV and acquired immunodeficiency syndrome (AIDS).
4. Describe the gerontologic considerations related to HIV/AIDS.
5. Describe the clinical management of patients with HIV/AIDS.
6. Use the nursing process as a framework for care of the patient with HIV/AIDS.

SECTION I: ASSESSING YOUR UNDERSTANDING

Activity A *Fill in the blanks.*

1. According to the Centers for Disease Control and Prevention (CDC, 2011b), _____ million people in the United States are living with HIV.

2. The two major means of HIV transmission are _____ and _____.

3. List five types of body fluids that can transmit HIV-1: _____, _____, _____, _____, and _____.

4. HIV belongs to a group of viruses known as _____.

5. The standard new HIV testing method now used when information about HIV status is needed immediately (emergency department, labor, and delivery) is _____.

6. Drug resistance can be defined as _____.

7. A fungal infection present in nearly all patients with AIDS is _____.

8. A recommended chemotherapeutic agent for Kaposi's sarcoma is _____.

9. The second most common malignancy in people with AIDS is _____.

Activity B *Briefly answer the following.*

1. Discuss the safe sexual behaviors that a nurse should incorporate into an education plan to prevent HIV/AIDS.

_____

_____

2. How can health care providers maintain "Standard Precautions" to prevent HIV transmission?

_____

_____

3. Explain the procedures that would be used for postexposure prophylaxis for health care providers.

_____

_____

4. Describe the stage of HIV disease known as *primary infection*.

_____

_____

_____

_____

5. Describe the clinical symptoms of a patient infected with acute HIV syndrome.

_____

_____

6. What are some of the adverse effects associated with HIV treatment?

_____

_____

_____

_____

7. Describe the clinical manifestations of the immune reconstitution inflammatory syndrome (IRIS).

_____

_____

8. What would the nurse document about the appearance of the cutaneous lesions seen with Kaposi's sarcoma?

_____

_____

9. When planning the care of a patient with HIV encephalopathy, what should the nurse include in the nursing interventions?

_____

_____

10. What are the differences in the etiology and clinical manifestations of cryptococcal meningitis and cytomegalovirus retinitis?

_____

_____

Activity C *Match the AIDS-indicated category listed in Column II with its associated clinical condition listed in Column I. Answers may be used more than once.*

Column I

____ **1.** Histoplasmosis

____ **2.** Hairy leukoplakia

____ **3.** Kaposi's sarcoma

____ **4.** Acute primary HIV infection

____ **5.** *Pneumocystis carinii*

____ **6.** Bacillary angiomatosis

____ **7.** Persistent generalized lymphadenopathy (PGL)

____ **8.** Extrapulmonary cryptococcosis

Column II

a. Clinical category A

b. Clinical category B

c. Clinical category C

SECTION II: APPLYING YOUR KNOWLEDGE

Activity D *Consider the scenario and answer the questions.*

CASE STUDY: Acquired Immunodeficiency Syndrome

Brendan is a 39-year-old man who has been recently diagnosed with AIDS. He is living with his wife of 7 years who is HIV positive but without any symptoms. Brendan has a previous history of IV drug use but is no longer using drugs. He is having difficulty eating, has diarrhea, and has had a 10-lb weight loss in 1 month.

1. The nurse understands that Brendan's anorexia, diarrhea, and gastrointestinal (GI) malabsorption are all factors that identify a significant problem. What problem do these symptoms contribute to?

_____

2. What assessment data would indicate to the nurse that Brendan may be dehydrated?

_____

_____

3. What medication can be effective to manage the chronic diarrhea that Brendan is having?

_____

4. What suggestions could the nurse make to improve Brendan's nutritional status?

_____

_____

_____

SECTION III: PRACTICING FOR NCLEX

Activity E *Answer the following questions.*

1. A patient is infected with HIV after sharing needles with another IV drug abuser. Upon infection with HIV, the immune system responds by making antibodies against the virus, usually within how many weeks after infection?

a. 1 to 2 weeks

b. 3 to 6 weeks

c. 3 to 12 weeks

d. 6 to 18 weeks

2. An older adult widowed woman informs the nurse that she notices vaginal dryness now that she has become sexually active again. She is not using barrier protection because it makes the dryness worse. What education should the nurse provide to the patient?

a. Use a lamb skin condom instead of latex.

b. Vaginal dryness is common in postmenopausal women, and there are creams that can be used, but she should use a latex condom.

c. Since the patient is older, it is not likely that she will acquire HIV.

d. She should abstain from sexual activity because she is at greatest risk for acquiring HIV.

3. A patient develops GI bleeding from a gastric ulcer and requires blood transfusions. The patient states to the nurse, "I am not going to have a transfusion because I don't want to get AIDS." What is the best response by the nurse?

a. "I understand what you mean, you can never be sure if the blood is tainted."

b. "I understand your concern. The blood is screened very carefully for different viruses as well as HIV."

c. "If you don't have the blood transfusions, you may not make it through this episode of bleeding."

d. "No one has gotten HIV from blood in a long time. You have to have the transfusion."

4. A new nursing graduate is working at the hospital in the medical-surgical unit. The preceptor observes the nurse emptying a patient's wound drain without gloves on. What important information should the preceptor share with the new graduate about standard precautions?

a. Standard precautions should be used with all patients to reduce the risk of transmission of bloodborne pathogens.

b. Standard precautions should only be used with patients who are HIV positive to reduce the risk of transmission of the HIV virus.

c. It is only necessary to use gloves when you are emptying reservoirs that have body fluids in them.

d. If you are careful and do not expose yourself to blood or body fluids, it is not necessary to use gloves all of the time.

5. A patient with HIV has been on antiretroviral therapy (ART) for 6 months. The patient comes to the clinic with home medications and the nurse observes that there are too many pills in the container. What does the nurse know about the factors associated with nonadherence to ART? (Select all that apply.)

a. Lives alone

b. Active substance abuse

c. Taking other medication

d. Depression

e. Lack of social support

6. A patient is on ART for the treatment of HIV. What does the nurse know would be an adequate CD4 count to determine the effectiveness of treatment for a patient per year?

   a. 1 mm^3 to 10 mm^3

   b. 10 mm^3 to 20 mm^3

   c. 20 mm^3 to 45 mm^3

   d. 50 mm^3 to 150 mm^3

7. A patient had unprotected sex with an HIV-infected person and arrives in the clinic requesting HIV testing. Results determine a negative HIV antibody test and an increased viral load. What stage does the nurse determine the patient is in?

   a. Primary infection

   b. Secondary infection

   c. Tertiary infection

   d. Latent infection

8. A patient in the clinic states, "My boyfriend told me he went to the clinic and was treated for gonorrhea." While testing for the sexually transmitted infection (STI), what else should be done for this patient?

   a. Test for HIV without informing the patient.

   b. Test for HIV, requiring the patient to sign a permit.

   c. Inform the patient that it would be beneficial to test for HIV.

   d. Administer treatment for the STI and discharge the patient.

9. A patient with HIV develops a nonproductive cough, shortness of breath, a fever of 101°F and an O$_2$ saturation of 92%. What infection caused by *Pneumocystis jiroveci* does the nurse know could occur with this patient?

   a. Mycobacterium avium complex (MAC)

   b. Pneumocystis pneumonia

   c. Tuberculosis

   d. Community-acquired pneumonia

10. A patient with AIDS informs the nurse of difficulty eating and swallowing, and shows the nurse white patches in the mouth. What problem related to AIDS does the nurse understand the patient has developed?

    a. MAC

    b. Wasting syndrome

    c. Kaposi's sarcoma

    d. Candidiasis

11. While caring for a patient with pneumocystis pneumonia, the nurse assesses flat, purplish lesions on the back and trunk. What does the nurse suspect these lesions indicate?

    a. Molluscum contagiosum

    b. Tuberculosis of the skin

    c. Kaposi's sarcoma

    d. Seborrheic dermatitis

12. The nurse receives a phone call at the clinic from the family of a patient with AIDS. They state that the patient started "acting funny" after complaining of headache, tiredness, and a stiff neck. Checking the temperature resulted in a fever of 103.2°F. What should the nurse inform the family member?

    a. "The patient probably has a case of the flu and you should give Tylenol."

    b. "The patient may have cryptococcal meningitis and will need to be evaluated by the physician."

    c. "This is one of the side effects from antiretroviral therapy and will require changing the medication."

    d. "The patient probably has pneumocystis pneumonia and will need to be evaluated by the physician."

13. A patient is diagnosed with pneumocystis pneumonia. What medication does the nurse anticipate educating the patient about for treatment?

    a. TMP-SMZ (Bactrim)

    b. Cephalexin (Keflex)

    c. Azithromycin (Zithromax)

    d. Garamycin (Gentamicin)

14. A patient with AIDS is having a recurrence of 10 to 12 loose stools a day. What medication may help this patient with controlling the chronic diarrhea?

a. Octreotide (Sandostatin)

b. Rifaximin (Xifaxan)

c. Bismuth subsalicylate (Pepto Bismol)

d. Atropine diphenoxylate (Lomotil)

15. The nurse is discussing sexual activity with a patient recently diagnosed with HIV. The patient states, "As long as I have sex with another person who is already infected, I will be okay." What is the best response by the nurse?

a. "You should avoid having unprotected sex with a person who is HIV positive because you can increase the severity of the infection in both you and your partner."

b. "Yes, since you are already infected, it won't make a difference if you have sex with a person who is HIV positive."

c. "I am not sure why you would want to have sex with another person who is HIV positive. That person may have another sexually transmitted infection."

d. "If you have sex with another person who is HIV positive, you will develop AIDS sooner."

Assessment and Management of Patients With Allergic Disorders

1. Explain the physiologic events involved with allergic reactions.
2. Describe the types of hypersensitivity.
3. Describe the management of patients with allergic disorders.
4. Describe measures to prevent and manage anaphylaxis.
5. Use the nursing process as a framework for care of the patient with allergic rhinitis.
6. Discuss the different allergic disorders according to type.

SECTION I: ASSESSING YOUR UNDERSTANDING

Activity A *Fill in the blanks.*

1. Antibodies, the most effective defense mechanisms in the body, react with antigens in three ways: _____, _____, and _____.

2. The classification of immunoglobulin (Ig) that occupies certain receptors on mast cells and produces an inflammatory response is _____.

3. Antibodies formed by lymphocytes and plasma cells in response to an immunogenic stimulus are called _____.

4. Prostaglandins are primary chemical mediators that respond to a stimulus by contracting smooth muscle and increasing capillary permeability. This response causes _____.

5. Type III hypersensitivity reactions involve the binding of antibodies to antigens. List two possible results: _____ and _____.

6. Two examples of a type IV hypersensitivity reaction (occurs 24 to 72 hours after exposure) are _____ and _____.

7. The most common cause of anaphylaxis, accounting for 75% of fatal reactions in the United States, is _____.

8. The initial medication of choice for a severe allergic reaction is _____, administered _____.

9. Patients should be advised that a "rebound" anaphylactic reaction can occur _____ hours after an initial attack, even when epinephrine has been given.

Activity B *Briefly answer the following.*

1. What happens during the physiologic response that causes an allergic reaction?

   _____

   _____

   _____

2. What is the role and function of histamine in response to an allergic threat?

   _____

   _____

3. What are the 4 types of hypersensitivity reactions (types I to IV)?

   _____

   _____

4. What are the 3 types of skin allergy tests and how are they administered?

   _____

   _____

   _____

5. What is the difference between an *atopic* and *nonatopic* IgE-mediated allergic reaction?

   _____

   _____

6. What clinical manifestations occur during an anaphylactic reaction?

   _____

   _____

   _____

7. What priority interventions are used in the treatment of an anaphylactic reaction?

   _____

   _____

8. What are the 4 types of contact dermatitis and how are they recognized?

   _____

   _____

Activity C *Match the medication in Column II with the antagonist or inhibitor in Column I.*

Column I	Column II
____ **1.** Leukotriene-receptor antagonist	**a.** Hydroxyzine (Atarax)
____ **2.** Leukotriene-receptor inhibitor	**b.** Zileuton (Zyflo CR)
____ **3.** Second-generation H_1 inhibitor	**c.** Montelukast (Singulair)
____ **4.** First-generation H_1 inhibitor	**d.** Levocetirizine (Xyzal)

SECTION II: APPLYING YOUR KNOWLEDGE

Activity D *Consider the scenarios and answer the questions.*

CASE STUDY: Allergic Rhinitis

Chris is a 26-year-old contractor who specializes in finished basements and suffers from allergies related to materials used. Because of his job, he is frequently working in environments where there are substances that stimulate an allergic reaction.

1. The nurse is educating Chris on how he can recognize symptoms that indicate an onset of an allergic reaction. An allergic reaction may be preceded by what symptoms?

   _____

   _____

2. What does the nurse inform Chris may signal a more severe form of allergic reaction?

   _____

3. What would the nurse include in the teaching plan regarding Chris's allergies?

   _____

   _____

CASE STUDY: Latex Allergy

Mindy, a new student in a nursing program, is beginning her first clinical rotation at the hospital. She and another student are giving a patient a bath wearing latex gloves when Mindy informs the other student that she is itching on both of her hands. When the gloves are removed, Mindy has erythema covering both hands.

1. What type of reaction to the latex is Mindy experiencing?

   _____

   _____

   _____

2. What can Mindy do to eliminate this type of reaction?

   _____

   _____

3. Mindy asks her instructor if it would help if she used lotion prior to donning gloves. What should the instructor inform her?

   _____

   _____

   _____

4. What types of testing can Mindy receive that will give her a definitive diagnosis of latex allergy?

   _____

   _____

   _____

SECTION III: PRACTICING FOR NCLEX

Activity E *Answer the following questions.*

1. The nurse is preparing to administer a medication that has an affinity for H1 receptors. Which medication would the nurse administer?
   a. Diphenhydramine (Benadryl)
   b. Omeprazole (Prilosec)
   c. Cimetidine (Tagamet)
   d. Ranitidine (Zantac)

2. An infant is born to a mother who had no prenatal care during her pregnancy. What type of hypersensitivity reaction does the nurse understand may have occurred?
   a. Bacterial endocarditis
   b. Rh-hemolytic disease
   c. Lupus erythematosus
   d. Rheumatoid arthritis

3. While monitoring the patient's eosinophil level, the nurse suspects a definite allergic disorder when seeing an eosinophil value of what percentage of the total leukocyte count?
   a. 1% to 3%
   b. 3% to 4%
   c. 5% to 10%
   d. 15% to 40%

4. A patient comes to the clinic with pruritus and nasal congestion after eating shrimp for lunch. The nurse is aware that the patient may be having an anaphylactic reaction to the shrimp. These symptoms typically occur within how many hours after exposure?
   a. 2 hours
   b. 6 hours
   c. 12 hours
   d. 24 hours

5. A patient is experiencing an allergic reaction to a dose of penicillin. What should the nurse look for in the patient's initial assessment?
   a. Dyspnea, bronchospasm, and/or laryngeal edema.
   b. Hypotension and tachycardia
   c. The presence and location of pruritus
   d. The severity of cutaneous warmth and flushing

6. The nurse is educating a patient with allergic rhinitis about how the condition is induced. What should the nurse include in the education on this topic?
   a. Airborne pollens or molds
   b. Ingested foods
   c. Parenteral medications
   d. Topical creams or ointments

7. A patient has a sensitivity to ragweed and tells the nurse that it comes at the same time every year. When does the patient typically notice the symptoms?

   a. Early spring

   b. Early fall

   c. Summer

   d. Midwinter

8. A patient asks the nurse if it would be all right to take an over-the-counter antihistamine for the treatment of a rash. What should the nurse educate the patient is a major side effect of antihistamines?

   a. Diarrhea

   b. Anorexia

   c. Palpitations

   d. Sedation

9. The nurse is administering a sympathomimetic drug to a patient. What areas of concern does the nurse have when administering this drug? (Select all that apply.)

   a. Causes bronchodilation

   b. Constricts integumentary smooth muscle

   c. Dilates the muscular vasculature

   d. Causes bronchoconstriction

   e. Causes laryngospasm

10. The nurse is administering injected allergens for "hyposensitization," which may produce harmful systemic reactions. Prior to administering these allergens, what medication should the nurse have at the bedside?

    a. Phenergan hydrochloride (Phenergan)

    b. Pentazocine (Talwin)

    c. Epinephrine

    d. Meclizine hydrochloride (Dramamine)

11. A patient was seen in the clinic for hypertension and received a prescription for a new antihypertensive medication. The patient arrived in the emergency department a few hours after taking the medication with severe angioedema. What medication prescribed may be responsible for the reaction?

    a. Beta blocker

    b. Angiotensin-converting enzyme (ACE) inhibitor

    c. Angiotensin receptor blocker

    d. Vasodilator

12. A patient has been diagnosed with an allergy to peanuts. What is a priority for this patient to carry at all times?

    a. A medical alert bracelet

    b. An H_1 blocker

    c. An EpiPen

    d. An oral airway

13. A patient has had a "stuffy nose" and obtained Afrin nasal spray. What education should the nurse provide to the patient in order to prevent "rebound congestion"?

    a. Be sure to use the Afrin for at least 10 days to ensure the stuffiness is gone.

    b. Use the medication every 4 hours to prevent congestion from recurring.

    c. Drink plenty of fluids.

    d. Only use the Afrin for 3 to 4 days once every 12 hours.

14. A patient was seen in the clinic 3 days previously for allergic rhinitis and was given a prescription for a corticosteroid nasal spray. The patient calls the clinic and tells the nurse that the nasal spray is not working. What is the best response by the nurse?

    a. "You need to come back to the clinic to get a different medication since this one is not working for you."

    b. "You may be immune to the effects of this medication and will need something else in its place."

    c. "The full benefit of the medication may take up to 2 weeks to be achieved."

    d. "I am sorry that you are feeling poorly but this is the only medication that will work for your problem."

15. What education should the nurse provide to the patient taking long-term corticosteroids?

    a. The patient should not stop taking the medication abruptly and should be weaned off of the medication.

    b. The patient should take the medication only as needed and not take it unnecessarily.

    c. Corticosteroids are relatively safe drugs with very few side effects.

    d. The patient should discontinue using the drug immediately if weight gain is observed.

Assessment and Management of Patients With Rheumatic Disorders

Learning Objectives

1. Explain the pathophysiology of rheumatic diseases.
2. Describe the assessment and diagnostic findings seen in patients with rheumatic diseases or disorders.
3. Use the nursing process as a framework for the care of patients with rheumatic disorders.
4. Describe the systemic effects of a connective tissue disease.
5. Devise an education plan for the patient with newly diagnosed rheumatic disease.
6. Identify modifications in interventions to accommodate changes in patients' functional ability that may occur with disease progression.

SECTION I: ASSESSING YOUR UNDERSTANDING

Activity A *Fill in the blanks.*

1. The most common symptom of rheumatic disease that causes a patient to seek medical attention is _____.

2. In the inflammatory process in rheumatic diseases, a triggering event starts the process by activating _____.

3. Synovial fluid from an inflamed joint is characteristically _____, _____, and _____.

4. The rheumatoid arthritis (RA) reaction produces enzymes that break down _____.

5. In RA, the autoimmune reaction primarily occurs in the _____.

Activity B *Briefly answer the following.*

1. What is the theory of *degradation* as it relates to the pathophysiology of rheumatic diseases?

_____

_____

2. What is the difference between *exacerbation* and *remission*?

_____

_____

_____

3. What is the difference between the patho-physiology of inflammatory rheumatic disease and that of degenerative rheumatic disease?

_____

_____

_____

4. Name three goals and corresponding manage-ment strategies for the treatment of rheumatic diseases.

_____

_____

5. What type of exercises and precautions are used to promote mobility for a patient with a rheumatic disease?

_____

_____

_____

6. What type of clinical manifestations does a patient with polymyalgia rheumatic (PMR) present with?

_____

_____

_____

7. What are the clinical manifestations of degen-erative joint disease (osteoarthritis [OA])?

_____

_____

8. What are the clinical manifestations of gout?

_____

_____

9. What nursing management options exist for fibromyalgia?

_____

_____

_____

Activity C *Match the clinical interpretation/ laboratory significance listed in Column II with its associated test listed in Column I.*

Column I

____ 1. Uric acid

____ 2. Complement

____ 3. Rheumatoid factor

____ 4. Hematocrit

____ 5. HLA-B27 antigen

____ 6. Antinuclear antibody (ANA)

____ 7. Creatinine

____ 8. C-reactive protein (CRP)

Column II

a. A decrease can be seen in chronic inflammation.

b. A positive test is associated with systemic lupus erythematosus (SLE), RA, and Raynaud's disease.

c. An increase in this substance is seen with gout.

d. This protein substance is decreased in RA and SLE.

e. This is present in 80% of those who have RA.

f. This is present in 85% of those with ankylosing spondylitis.

g. Frequently positive for RA and SLE.

h. An increase may indicate renal damage, as in scleroderma.

SECTION II: APPLYING YOUR KNOWLEDGE

Activity D *Consider the scenarios and answer the questions.*

CASE STUDY: Diffuse Connective Tissue Disease

Jane, a 33-year-old mother of two, has joint pain and stiffness, decreased mobility, and increased frequency of fatigue. She is depressed.

1. The nurse is performing an assessment when Jane comes to the clinic. What symptoms does the nurse recognize as characteristic of RA?

   _____

   _____

2. Jane has a series of laboratory studies performed and has a negative RA factor. What does the nurse understand is the significance of this result?

   _____

   _____

   _____

3. Jane has been prescribed a disease-modifying antirheumatic drug (DMARD), methotrexate (Rheumatrex), for initial treatment. When does the nurse expect she will begin to feel relief of symptoms?

   _____

   _____

4. A low-dose corticosteroid regimen is begun in conjunction with the methotrexate. Jane wants to know why she should take this medication along with the methotrexate. What explanation should the nurse provide?

   _____

   _____

   _____

CASE STUDY: Systemic Lupus Erythematosus (SLE)

Brooke is a 41-year-old mother of two teenagers who has had symptoms of joint tenderness for about 10 years. Lately, she has noticed significant morning stiffness and a slight rash over the bridge of her nose and cheeks. Her physician suspects a diagnosis of SLE.

1. When performing an assessment for Brooke, what cardiovascular symptoms should the nurse auscultate to determine if present?

   _____

   _____

2. When planning Brooke's care, the nurse anticipates that she will require education regarding her therapeutic medication regimen. What medications does the nurse provide information about?

   _____

   _____

3. Brooke has been placed on corticosteroid therapy. What should the nurse caution her about regarding the risk factors while taking corticosteroids for SLE?

   _____

   _____

   _____

SECTION III: PRACTICING FOR NCLEX

Activity E *Answer the following questions.*

1. A patient is seen in the office for complaints of joint pain, swelling, and a low-grade fever. What blood studies does the nurse know are consistent with a positive diagnosis of RA? (Select all that apply.)

   a. Positive C-reactive protein (CRP)

   b. Positive antinuclear antibody (ANA)

   c. Red blood cell (RBC) count of <4.0 million/mcL

   d. Serum complement level (C3) of >130 mg/dL

   e. Aspartate aminotransferase (AST) and alanine transaminase (ALT) levels of 7 units/L

2. A patient has a serum study that is positive for the rheumatoid factor. What does the nurse understand is the significance of this test result?

   a. Diagnostic for Sjögren's syndrome

   b. Diagnostic for SLE

   c. Specific for RA

   d. Suggestive of RA

3. The nurse knows that a patient who presents with the symptom of "blanching of fingers on exposure to cold" would be assessed for what rheumatic disease?

   a. Ankylosing spondylitis

   b. Raynaud's phenomenon

   c. Reiter's syndrome

   d. Sjögren's syndrome

4. A patient is suspected of having *myositis*. The nurse prepares the patient for what procedure that will confirm the diagnosis?

   a. Bone scan

   b. Computed tomography (CT)

   c. Magnetic resonance imaging (MRI)

   d. Muscle biopsy

5. The nurse is educating a patient about the risks of stroke related to the new prescription for a COX-2 inhibitor and what symptoms they should report. Which COX-2 inhibitor is the nurse educating the patient about?

   a. Ibuprofen (Motrin)

   b. Celecoxib (Celebrex)

   c. Piroxicam (Feldene)

   d. Tolmetin sodium (Tolectin)

6. A patient is prescribed a DMARD that is successful in the treatment of RA but has side effects, including retinal eye changes. What medication does the nurse anticipate educating the patient about?

   a. Azathioprine (Imuran)

   b. Diclofenac (Voltaren)

   c. Hydroxychloroquine (Plaquenil)

   d. Aurothioglucose (Solganal)

7. A patient is receiving gold sodium thiomalate (Myochrysine) for the treatment of RA. What does the nurse understand about the action of this compound?

   a. Inhibits DNA synthesis

   b. Inhibits lysosomal enzymes

   c. Inhibits platelet aggregation

   d. Inhibits T- and B-cell activity

8. A patient with an acute exacerbation of arthritis is temporarily confined to bed. What position can the nurse recommend to prevent flexion deformities?

   a. Prone

   b. Semi-Fowler's

   c. Side-lying with pillows supporting the shoulders and legs

   d. Supine with pillows under the knees

9. A patient comes to the clinic with an inflamed wrist. How should the nurse splint the joint to immobilize it?

   a. Slight dorsiflexion

   b. Extension

   c. Hyperextension

   d. Internal rotation

10. A patient arrives at the clinic with complaints of pain in the left great toe. The nurse assesses a swollen, warm, erythematous left great toe. What does the nurse determine that the symptoms are most likely related to?

    a. Rheumatoid arthritis

    b. Osteoarthritis

    c. Fibromyalgia

    d. Gout

11. The nurse is educating the patient with gout about ways to prevent reoccurrence of an attack. What foods should the nurse encourage the patient to avoid?

    a. Baked chicken

    b. Steak

    c. Asparagus

    d. Pineapple

12. The nurse is assessing a patient with a diagnosis of scleroderma. What clinical manifestations of scleroderma does the nurse assess? (Select all that apply.)

a. Decreased ventilation owing to lung scarring

b. Dysphagia owing to hardening of the esophagus

c. Dyspnea owing to fibrotic cardiac tissue

d. Productive cough

e. Butterfly-shaped rash on the face

13. A patient is hospitalized with a severe case of gout. The patient has gross swelling of the large toe and rates pain a 10 out of 10. With a diagnosis of gout, what should the laboratory results reveal?

a. Glucosuria

b. Hyperuricemia

c. Hyperproteinuria

d. Ketonuria

14. A patient is being placed on a purine-restricted diet. What food should be suggested by the nurse?

a. Dairy products

b. Organ meats

c. Raw vegetables

d. Shellfish

15. A patient is taking NSAIDs for the treatment of osteoarthritis. What education should the nurse give the patient about the medication?

a. Take the medication on an empty stomach in order to increase effectiveness.

b. Since the medication is able to be obtained over the counter, it has few side effects.

c. Take the medication with food to avoid stomach upset.

d. Inform the physician if there is ringing in the ears.

Musculoskeletal Function

Assessment of Musculoskeletal Function

Learning Objectives

1. Describe the basic structure and function of the musculoskeletal system.
2. Discuss the significance of the health history to the assessment of musculoskeletal health.
3. Describe the significance of physical assessment to the diagnosis of musculoskeletal dysfunction.
4. Specify diagnostic tests used for assessment of musculoskeletal function.

SECTION I: ASSESSING YOUR UNDERSTANDING

Activity A *Fill in the blanks.*

1. The leading cause of musculoskeletal-related disability in the United States is

   _____.

2. The approximate percentage of total body calcium present in the bones is

   _____.

3. In the human body, there are _____ bones.

4. Approximately _____ mg of calcium daily is essential to maintain adult bone mass.

5. Red bone marrow is located in the shaft of four long and flat bones: the

   _____, _____,

   _____, and _____.

6. The major hormonal regulators of calcium homeostasis are _____ and

   _____.

7. _____ describes the grating, crackling sound heard over irregular joint surfaces like the knee.

Activity B *Briefly answer the following.*

1. What are the general functions of the musculoskeletal system?

   _____

   _____

   _____

2. What are the differences in the function of *osteoblasts, osteocytes,* and *osteoclasts*?

   _____

   _____

   _____

3. How does vitamin D regulate the balance between bone formation and bone resorption?

   _____

   _____

4. What is the role of the sex hormones testosterone and estrogen on bone remodeling?

_____

_____

_____

_____

5. What is the process of fracture healing, including the three stages of progression?

_____

_____

6. What is the difference between isotonic and isometric contractions?

_____

_____

_____

_____

7. What are the age-related changes of the musculoskeletal system specific to bones, muscles, joints, and ligaments?

_____

_____

8. What is the difference between kyphosis, lordosis, and scoliosis?

_____

_____

Activity C *Match the test used to assess peripheral nerve function sensation in Column II with the nerve being assessed in Column I.*

Column I

_____ **1.** Peroneal

_____ **2.** Tibial

_____ **3.** Radial

_____ **4.** Ulnar

_____ **5.** Median

Column II

a. Prick the medial and lateral surface of the sole.

b. Prick the distal fat pad of the small finger.

c. Prick the skin midway between the great and second toe.

d. Prick the skin midway between the thumb and second finger.

e. Prick the top or distal surface of the index finger.

SECTION II: APPLYING YOUR KNOWLEDGE

Activity D *Consider the scenario and answer the questions.*

Kevin, a 32-year-old man, was jogging and tripped over a rock in the path. He fell on his right knee and had immediate pain but was able to get up and walk home. The next day, the knee was swollen and painful and he decided to see his physician.

1. The physician determines Kevin has an effusion. How was that detected?

_____

_____

_____

2. The physician orders a magnetic resonance imaging (MRI) study. What should the nurse educate the patient about prior to having the test?

_____

_____

_____

_____

3. What procedure will the physician perform to remove the fluid from Kevin's knee?

_____

_____

SECTION III: PRACTICING FOR NCLEX

Activity E *Answer the following questions.*

1. A patient has a fracture of the right femur sustained in an automobile accident. What process of fracture healing does the nurse understand will occur with this patient?

   a. Reactive phase, reparative phase, remodeling phase

   b. Primary phase, secondary phase, third phase

   c. First intention, secondary intention, third intention

   d. Active phase, dormant phase, restructure phase

2. A patient has a fracture that is being treated with open rigid compression plate fixation devices. How will the progress of bone healing be monitored?

   a. Remove the plate and determine if the bone is growing back.

   b. Serial x-rays

   c. Arthroscopy

   d. The bone will heal on its own without intervention.

3. A patient tells the physician about shoulder pain that is present even without any strenuous movement. The physician identifies a sac filled with synovial fluid. What condition should the nurse educate the patient about?

   a. A fracture of the clavicle

   b. Osteoarthritis of the shoulder

   c. Bursitis

   d. Ankylosing spondylitis

4. A patient has had a stroke and is unable to move the right upper and lower extremity. During assessment the nurse picks up the arm and it is limp and without tone. How would the nurse document this finding?

   a. Rigidity

   b. Flaccidity

   c. Atonic

   d. Tetanic

5. A patient tells the nurse, "I was working out and lifting weights and now that I have stopped, I am flabby and my muscles have gone!" What is the best response by the nurse?

   a. "While you are lifting weights, endorphins are released, creating increase in muscle mass, but if the muscles are not used they will atrophy."

   b. "The muscle mass has decreased from the lack of calcium in the cells."

   c. "Your muscles were in a state of hypertrophy from the weight lifting but it will persist only if the exercise is continued."

   d. "Once you stop exercising, the contraction of the muscle does not regain its strength."

6. After a bone density test, an older adult female patient tells the nurse, "I don't understand why I have osteoporosis because I eat well and take my calcium." What does the nurse understand is the reason that the patient may have osteoporosis?

   a. Everyone gets osteoporosis and there is nothing you can do to prevent it.

   b. Men lose more bone mass than women but women still lose some.

   c. In order to prevent bone loss, women have to take hormones.

   d. The loss is from withdrawal of estrogen and a decrease in activity levels.

7. A patient comes to the clinic and informs the nurse of numbness, tingling, and a burning sensation in the arm from the elbow down to the fingers. What type of symptom would this be documented as?

   a. Paresthesia

   b. Flaccidity

   c. Atonia

   d. Effusion

8. The nurse is performing an assessment on an older adult patient and observes the patient has an increased forward curvature of the thoracic spine. What does the nurse understand this common finding is known as?

   a. Lordosis

   b. Scoliosis

   c. Osteoporosis

   d. Kyphosis

9. The nurse assesses soft subcutaneous nodules along the line of the tendons in a patient's hand and wrist. What does this finding indicate to the nurse?

   a. The patient has osteoarthritis.

   b. The patient has lupus erythematosus.

   c. The patient has rheumatoid arthritis.

   d. The patient has neurofibromatosis.

10. The nurse is caring for a pregnant patient with pregnancy-induced hypertension. When assessing the reflexes in the ankle, the nurse observes rhythmic contractions of the muscle when dorsiflexing the foot. What would the nurse document this finding as?

    a. Positive Babinski reflex

    b. Clonus

    c. Hypertrophy

    d. Ankle reflex

11. The nurse is performing an assessment for a patient who may have peripheral neurovascular dysfunction. What signs does the patient present with that indicate circulation is impaired? (Select all that apply.)

    a. Pale, cyanotic, or mottled color

    b. Cool temperature of the extremity

    c. More than 3-second capillary refill

    d. Tenting skin turgor

    e. Limited range of motion

12. A patient is scheduled for a procedure that will allow the physician to visualize the knee joint in order to diagnose the patient's pain. What procedure will the nurse prepare the patient for?

    a. Arthrocentesis

    b. Bone scan

    c. Electromyography

    d. Arthroscopy

13. A patient is having repeated tears of the joint capsule in the shoulder, and the physician orders an arthrogram. What intervention should the nurse provide after the procedure is completed? (Select all that apply.)

    a. Apply a compression bandage to the area.

    b. Apply heat to the area for 48 hours.

    c. Administer a mild analgesic.

    d. Inform the patient that a clicking or crackling noise in the joint may persist for a couple of days.

    e. Actively exercise the area immediately after the procedure.

CHAPTER 41

Musculoskeletal Care Modalities

Learning Objectives

1. Identify the preventive and health education needs of the patient with a cast, splint, or brace.
2. Describe the nursing management of the patient with a cast, splint, or brace.
3. Describe the various types of traction and the principles of effective traction.
4. Identify the preventive nursing care needs of the patient with an external fixator or in traction.
5. Describe the nursing management of the patient with an external fixator or in traction.
6. Compare the nursing needs of the patient undergoing total hip arthroplasty with those of the patient undergoing total knee arthroplasty.
7. Use the nursing process as a framework for care of the patient undergoing orthopedic surgery.

SECTION I: ASSESSING YOUR UNDERSTANDING

Activity A *Fill in the blanks.*

1. The most effective cleansing solution for care of a pin site is _____.

2. A nursing goal for a patient with skeletal traction is to avoid infection and the development of _____ at the site of pin insertion.

3. The nurse knows to assess a patient for deep vein thrombosis (DVT) by assessing the lower extremities for:

   _____, _____, _____, and _____.

4. The nurse assesses for perineal nerve injury by checking the patient's casted leg for the primary symptoms of _____, _____, and _____.

5. The nurse expects that _____ of weight can be used for a patient in skeletal traction.

6. An artificial joint for total hip replacement involves an implant that consists of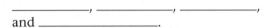
   _____, _____, and _____.

7. The nurse caring for a postoperative hip replacement patient knows that the patient should not cross his or her legs at any time for _____ after surgery.

8. After a total hip replacement, stair climbing is kept to a minimum for _____ to _____ months.

9. After a total hip replacement, the patient is usually able to resume daily activities after _____.

10. Unrelieved pain for a patient in a cast must be *immediately reported* to avoid _____, _____, _____, and _____.

Activity B *Briefly answer the following.*

1. Name four purposes for having a cast application.

_____

_____

2. Compare the advantages of a fiberglass cast to those of a plaster cast.

_____

_____

3. The nurse completes a neurovascular assessment of either the fingers or toes of a casted extremity to determine circulatory status. What expected outcomes does the nurse anticipate will occur?

_____

_____

4. What are the five "Ps" that should be assessed as part of the neurovascular check?

_____

5. List the danger signs of possible circulatory constriction that the nurse should assess for in a casted extremity.

_____

_____

_____

6. Name three major complications of an extremity that is casted, braced, or splinted.

_____

7. List four reasons for a patient to have traction application.

_____

_____

8. What potential immobility-related complications may develop when a patient is in skeletal traction?

_____

_____

9. Describe compartment syndrome.

_____

_____

10. What is a Volkmann's contracture?

_____

_____

_____

11. What methods for preventing hip prosthesis dislocation would the nurse teach a patient?

_____

_____

_____

_____

Activity C *Match the description in Column II with the common orthopedic surgical procedure in Column I.*

Column I

____ 1. Open reduction

____ 2. Internal fixation

____ 3. Arthroplasty

____ 4. Hemiarthroplasty

____ 5. Meniscectomy

____ 6. Amputation

____ 7. Bone graft

____ 8. Tendon transfer

____ 9. Fasciotomy

Column II

a. The placement of bone tissue (autologous or homologous grafts) to promote healing, to stabilize, or to replace diseased bone

b. The removal of a body part

c. The excision of damaged joint fibrocartilage

d. The insertion of a tendon to improve function

e. The incision and diversion of the muscle fascia to relieve muscle constriction, as in compartment syndrome, or to reduce fascia contracture

f. The correction and alignment of the fracture after surgical dissection and exposure of the fracture

g. The repair of joint problems through the operating arthroscope (an instrument that allows the surgeon to operate within a joint without a large incision) or through open joint surgery

h. The replacement of one of the articular surfaces

i. The stabilization of the reduced fracture by the use of metal screws, plates, wires, nails, and pins

SECTION II: APPLYING YOUR KNOWLEDGE

Activity D *Consider the scenarios and answer the questions.*

CASE STUDY: External Fixator

Felicia is a 36-year-old on a ski trip with her friends. While skiing, she fell and sustained an open fracture to the left forearm with soft tissue swelling. She was rescued by the ski patrol and taken to the nearest hospital, where the orthopedic surgeon applied an external fixator.

1. What is the benefit of applying an external fixator versus an open reduction and internal fixation for this type of fracture?

   _____

   _____

   _____

2. Felicia is concerned about the bulk of the fixator and how she will look. She tells the nurse, "I am going to look like Frankenstein with this thing on!" What interventions can the nurse provide to promote acceptance of the fixator?

   _____

   _____

   _____

3. How often should the nurse monitor the neurovascular status of the arm?

   _____

4. The nurse is monitoring the pin site every 8 hours. What should be documented with every assessment to ensure that pin site infection is not developing?

   _____

   _____

CASE STUDY: Total Hip Replacement

Tom is a 62-year-old athletic coach at a high school. Sports activities, especially baseball, have been the focus of his energies since he was in high school and college. Because of prior hip joint injuries and degenerative joint disease, he is scheduled for a total hip replacement.

1. Tom informs the nurse that he is hoping for a drastic change in his life after hip replacement. What improvements can Tom expect to see after hip replacement?

   _____

   _____

2. Tom has been taking a nonsteroidal anti-inflammatory drug (NSAID) for the discomfort he has had in his hip. Why is it important for him to discontinue the use of this medication 1 week prior to his surgery?

   _____

   _____

3. The nurse is discussing how Tom will be positioned after his procedure to avoid dislocating the hip prosthesis. What information is Tom given?

   _____

   _____

   _____

4. Tom should be informed about the signs and symptoms of prosthetic dislocation. What signs and symptoms is he instructed about verbally and in writing?

   _____

   _____

   _____

SECTION III: PRACTICING FOR NCLEX

Activity E *Answer the following questions.*

1. A patient with an arm cast complains of pain. What nursing interventions should the nurse provide in order to reduce the incidence of complications? (Select all that apply.)
   a. Assess the fingers for color and temperature.
   b. Administer a prescribed analgesic to promote comfort and allay anxiety.
   c. Assess for a pressure sore
   d. Determine the exact site of the pain.
   e. Cut the cast with a cast saw

2. A patient arrives in the emergency department with a suspected bone fracture of the right arm. How does the nurse expect the patient to describe the pain?
   a. A dull, deep, boring ache
   b. Sharp and piercing
   c. Similar to "muscle cramps"
   d. Sore and aching

3. The nurse suspects "compartment syndrome" for a casted extremity. What characteristic symptoms would the nurse assess that would confirm these suspicions? (Select all that apply.)
   a. Decreased sensory function
   b. Excruciating pain
   c. Loss of motion
   d. Capillary refill less than 3 seconds
   e. 2+ peripheral pulses in the affected distal pulse

4. The nurse suspects that a patient with an arm cast has developed a pressure ulcer. Where should the nurse assess for the presence of the ulcer?
   a. Lateral malleolus
   b. Olecranon
   c. Radial styloid
   d. Ulna styloid

5. A patient has a cast removed after bone healing takes place. What should the nurse instruct the patient to do after removal? (Select all that apply.)
   a. Apply an emollient lotion to soften the skin.
   b. Control swelling with elastic bandages, as directed.
   c. Gradually resume activities and exercise.
   d. Use friction to remove dead surface skin by rubbing the area with a towel.
   e. Use a razor to shave the dead skin off.

6. A patient has a long leg cast applied. Where does the nurse understand a common pressure problem may occur?
   a. Dorsalis pedis
   b. Peroneal nerve
   c. Popliteal artery
   d. Posterior tibialis

7. The nurse is very concerned about the potential debilitating complication of peroneal nerve injury. What symptom does the nurse recognize as a result of that complication?
   a. Permanent paresthesias
   b. Footdrop
   c. Deep vein thrombosis (DVT)
   d. Infection

8. A patient in pelvic traction needs circulatory status assessed. How should the nurse assess for a positive Homans' sign?
   a. Have the patient extend both hands while the nurse compares the volume of both radial pulses.
   b. Have the patient extend each leg and dorsiflex each foot to determine if pain or tenderness is present in the lower leg.
   c. Have the patient plantar flex both feet while the nurse performs the blanch test on all of the patient's toes.
   d. Have the patient squeeze the nurse's hands with his or her hands to evaluate any difference in strength.

9. An older adult patient had a hip replacement. When should the patient begin with assisted ambulation with a walker?

 a. 24 hours

 b. 72 hours

 c. 1 week

 d. 2 to 3 weeks

10. A patient had a total hip replacement. What recommended leg position should the nurse ensure is maintained to prevent prosthesis dislocation?

 a. Abduction

 b. Adduction

 c. Flexion

 d. Internal rotation

11. The nurse is caring for a patient with a total hip replacement. How should the nurse allow the patient to turn?

 a. 45 degrees onto the unoperated side if the affected hip is kept abducted

 b. From the prone to the supine position only, and the patient must keep the affected hip extended and abducted

 c. To any comfortable position as long as the affected leg is extended

 d. To the operative side if the affected hip remains extended

12. The nurse is caring for a patient who had a total hip replacement. What lethal postoperative complication should the nurse closely monitor for?

 a. Atelectasis

 b. Hypovolemia

 c. Pulmonary embolism

 d. Urinary tract infection

13. A patient had a total left hip arthroplasty. What clinical manifestation would indicate to the nurse that the prosthesis is dislocated?

 a. The left leg is internally rotated.

 b. The leg length is the same as the right leg.

 c. The patient has discomfort when moving in the bed.

 d. Diminished peripheral pulses on the affected extremity

14. The nurse assesses a patient after total right hip arthroplasty and observes a shortening of the extremity, and the patient complains of severe pain in the right side of the groin. What is the priority action of the nurse?

 a. Apply Buck's traction.

 b. Notify the physician.

 c. Externally rotate the extremity.

 d. Bend the knee and rotate the knee internally.

15. The nurse is caring for a patient postoperatively following orthopedic surgery. The nurse assesses an oxygen saturation of 89%, confusion, and a rash on the upper torso. What does the nurse suspect is occurring with this patient?

 a. Polyethylene-induced infection

 b. Pneumonia

 c. Fat emboli syndrome

 d. Disseminated intravascular coagulation

Management of Patients With Musculoskeletal Disorders

Learning Objectives

1. Describe the nursing management, rehabilitation, and health education needs of the patient with low back pain.
2. Describe common musculoskeletal disorders of the hand, wrist, shoulder, and foot and nursing care of the patient undergoing surgery to correct these disorders.
3. Explain the pathogenesis, prevention, and management of osteoporosis.
4. Use the nursing process as a framework for care of the patient with osteoporotic vertebral fracture.
5. Identify the causes and related management of patients with osteomalacia, Paget's disease, and septic arthritis.
6. Use the nursing process as a framework for care of the patient with osteomyelitis.
7. Describe the causes and related management of the patient with a primary or metastatic bone tumor.

SECTION I: ASSESSING YOUR UNDERSTANDING

Activity A *Fill in the blanks.*

1. The major consequence of osteoporosis is

   _____.

2. Primary osteoporosis in women usually begins between the ages of _____ and

   _____.

3. The primary deficit in osteomalacia is
   _____, which promotes calcium absorption from the gastrointestinal tract.

4. Three medications used to treat Paget's disease are _____, _____, and _____.

5. The intervertebral disks that are subject to the greatest mechanical stress and greatest degenerative changes are _____, _____, and _____.

6. The layman's term for onychocryptosis, a common foot condition, is _____.

7. Osteomyelitis with vascular insufficiency, which most commonly affects the feet, is seen most often among patients with _____ and _____.

8. The recommended adequate intake (RAI) level of calcium for all individuals is _____ to _____ mg daily.

9. Bone formation is enhanced by _____, _____, and _____.

10. The most common benign bone tumor is _____.

Activity B *Briefly answer the following.*

1. Identify at least five musculoskeletal problems that can cause acute low back pain.

   _____

   _____

2. Explain the difference between bursitis and tendinitis.

   _____

   _____

3. What is *impingement syndrome* and what measures are necessary to promote shoulder healing?

   _____

   _____

   _____

4. Describe the assessment technique used for Tinel's sign.

   _____

   _____

   _____

5. Name the risk factors (modifiable and non-modifiable) associated with osteoporosis.

   _____

   _____

6. Describe the clinical manifestations associated with septic arthritis.

   _____

   _____

   _____

Activity C *Match the diagnostic procedures for low back pain in Column I with their definitions in Column II.*

Column I

____ 1. Bone scan

____ 2. Computed tomography (CT) scan

____ 3. Magnetic resonance imaging (MRI) scan

____ 4. Electromyogram (EMG)

____ 5. Myelogram

____ 6. Ultrasound

Column II

a. Used to evaluate spinal nerve root disorders (radiculopathies)

b. Useful in identifying underlying problems, such as obscure soft tissue lesions adjacent to the vertebral column and problems of vertebral disks

c. May disclose infections, tumors, and bone marrow abnormalities

d. Permits visualization of the nature and location of spinal pathology

e. Permits visualization of segments of the spinal cord that may have herniated or may be compressed (infrequently performed; indicated when MRI scan is contraindicated)

f. Useful in detecting tears in ligaments, muscles, tendons, and soft tissues in the back

SECTION II: APPLYING YOUR KNOWLEDGE

Activity D *Consider the scenario and answer the questions.*

CASE STUDY: Osteoporosis

Emily is a 49-year-old administrative assistant at a community college who has just been diagnosed with osteoporosis. The physician has asked you to answer some of Emily's questions and explain the physician's directions for her level of activity and her nutritional needs.

1. What would the nurse tell Emily about why she is losing bone mass?

   _____

   _____

   _____

2. What two reasons could the nurse share to explain why women develop osteoporosis more frequently than men?

   _____

   _____

3. The nurse advises Emily that the development of osteoporosis is significantly dependent on what factors?

   _____

   _____

4. How much calcium should the nurse advise Emily that she needs daily?

   _____

SECTION III: PRACTICING FOR NCLEX

Activity E *Answer the following questions.*

1. A patient comes back to the clinic with a continued complaint of back pain. What time frame does the nurse understand constitutes "chronic pain"?
   a. 4 weeks
   b. 3 months
   c. 6 months
   d. 1 year

2. A patient is having low back pain. What position can the nurse suggest to relieve this discomfort?
   a. High-Fowler's to allow for maximum hip flexion
   b. Supine, with the knees slightly flexed and the head of the bed elevated 30 degrees
   c. Prone, with a pillow under the shoulders
   d. Supine, with the bed flat and a firm mattress in place

3. The nurse is educating the patient with low back pain about the proper way to lift objects. What muscle should the nurse encourage the patient to maximize?
   a. Gastrocnemius
   b. Latissimus dorsi
   c. Quadriceps
   d. Rectus abdominis

4. The nurse has educated a patient with low back pain about techniques to relieve the back pain and prevent further complications. What statement by the patient shows understanding of the education the nurse provided?
   a. "I will lie prone with my legs slightly elevated."
   b. "I will bend at the waist when I am lifting objects from the floor."
   c. "I will avoid prolonged sitting or walking."
   d. "Instead of turning around to grasp an object, I will twist at the waist."

5. A patient diagnosed with carpal tunnel syndrome (CTS) asks the nurse about numbness in the fingers and pain in the wrist. In responding to the patient, how would the nurse best describe CTS?
   a. "CTS is a neuropathy that is characterized by bursitis and tendinitis."
   b. "CTS is a neuropathy that is characterized by flexion contracture of the fourth and fifth fingers."
   c. "CTS is a neuropathy that is characterized by compression of the median nerve at the wrist."
   d. "CTS is a neuropathy that is characterized by pannus formation in the shoulder."

6. The nurse is assessing the feet of a patient and observes an overgrowth of the horny layer of the epidermis. What does the nurse recognize this condition as?

   a. Bunion

   b. Clawfoot

   c. Corn

   d. Hammer toe

7. A patient has been diagnosed with osteomalacia. What common symptoms does the nurse recognize that correlate with the diagnosis?

   a. Bone fractures and kyphosis

   b. Bone pain and tenderness

   c. Muscle weakness and spasms

   d. Softened and compressed vertebrae

8. A patient stepped on an acorn while walking barefoot in the backyard and developed an infection progressing to osteomyelitis. What microorganism does the nurse understand is most often the cause of the development of osteomyelitis?

   a. *Proteus*

   b. *Pseudomonas*

   c. *Salmonella*

   d. *Staphylococcus aureus*

9. A patient is diagnosed with osteomyelitis of the right leg. What signs and symptoms does the nurse recognize that are associated with this diagnosis? (Select all that apply.)

   a. Pain

   b. Erythema

   c. Fever

   d. Leukopenia

   e. Purulent drainage

10. A patient comes to the clinic complaining of low back pain radiating down the left leg. After diagnostic studies rule out any pathology, the physician orders a serotonin-norepinephrine reuptake inhibitor (SNRI). Which medication does the nurse anticipate educating the patient about?

    a. Amitriptyline (Elavil)

    b. Duloxetine (Cymbalta)

    c. Gabapentin (Neurontin)

    d. Cyclobenzaprine (Flexeril)

11. A patient shows the nurse a round, firm nodule on the wrist. The pain is described as aching, with some weakness of the fingers. What treatment does the nurse anticipate assisting with? (Select all that apply.)

    a. Educating the patient on the use of gabapentin

    b. Active range-of-motion exercises

    c. Corticosteroid injections

    d. Surgical excision

    e. Aspiration of the cyst

12. A patient had hand surgery to correct a Dupuytren's contracture. What nursing intervention is a priority postoperatively?

    a. Changing the dressing

    b. Applying a cock-up splint and immobilization

    c. Having the patient exercise the fingers to avoid future contractures

    d. Performing hourly neurovascular assessments for the first 24 hours

13. A patient is diagnosed with osteogenic sarcoma. What laboratory studies should the nurse monitor for the presence of elevation?

    a. Magnesium level

    b. Potassium level

    c. Alkaline phosphatase

    d. Troponin levels

14. The nurse is caring for a patient with bone metastasis from a primary breast cancer. The patient complains of muscle weakness and nausea and is voiding large amounts frequently. Cardiac dysrhythmias are observed on the telemetry monitor. What should the nurse suspect based on these clinical manifestations?

a. Hypercalcemia

b. Hypocalcemia

c. Hypokalemia

d. Hyperkalemia

15. The hospice nurse is assigned to care for a patient with metastatic bone cancer who wants to remain at home. What is the therapeutic goal in the care of this patient?

a. Prevent the patient from having to go to the hospital for care.

b. Relieve pain and discomfort while promoting quality of life.

c. Increase the activity level of the patient to prevent complications related to immobility.

d. Ensure that the family accepts the patient's imminent death.

Management of Patients With Musculoskeletal Trauma

1. Differentiate between contusions, strains, sprains, dislocations, and subluxations.
2. Identify the signs and symptoms of an acute fracture.
3. Describe the treatment procedures of fracture reduction, fracture immobilization, and management of open and intra-articular fractures.
4. Describe the prevention and management of immediate and delayed complications of fractures.
5. Describe the rehabilitation needs of patients with fractures of the upper and lower extremities, pelvis, and hips.
6. Use the nursing process as a framework for care of the older adult patient with a fracture of the hip.
7. Identify sports- and occupation-related musculoskeletal disorders and their signs, symptoms, and treatments.
8. Describe the rehabilitation and health education needs of the patient who has had an amputation.
9. Use the nursing process as a framework for care of the patient with an amputation.

SECTION I: ASSESSING YOUR UNDERSTANDING

Activity A *Fill in the blanks.*

1. A muscle tear that is microscopic and due to overuse is called a _____.

2. The femur fracture that commonly leads to avascular necrosis or nonunion due to an abundant supply of blood vessels in the area is a fracture of the _____.

3. Patients with open fractures risk three major complications: _____, _____, and _____.

4. _____ is the most common fracture of the distal radius is.

5. The most common complication of hip fractures in the elderly is _____.

6. Common pulmonary complications for the elderly following a hip fracture include _____ and _____.

7. Three range-of-motion activities are avoided for a patient with a lower extremity amputation: _____, _____, and _____.

8. The residual limb should never be placed on a pillow to avoid

   _____.

9. Patients who experience a fracture of the humeral neck are advised that healing will take an average of _____ weeks, with restricted vigorous activity for an additional _____ weeks.

10. The longest immobilization time necessary for fracture union occurs with a fracture of the _____.

Activity B *Briefly answer the following.*

1. Joint dislocation can lead to avascular necrosis if it is not treated. What is avascular necrosis?

   _____

   _____

2. The nurse feels a grating sensation in a patient's extremity. What is this sensation caused by? How would the nurse document this sensation?

   _____

   _____

   _____

3. Name three early and three delayed complications of fractures.

   _____

   _____

   _____

   _____

4. A patient is in early shock from a fracture. What five activities are involved in the treatment?

   _____

   _____

   _____

   _____

5. List three early and serious complications associated with bed rest and reduced skeletal muscle contractions for a patient with an open fracture.

   _____

   _____

6. What immediate nursing and medical management techniques are used for an open fracture?

   _____

   _____

   _____

   _____

7. Describe the difference between open and closed reduction as management techniques for fractures.

   _____

   _____

   _____

   _____

8. List five factors that can enhance fracture healing and five factors that can inhibit it.

   _____

   _____

Activity C *Match the type of fracture in Column II with its descriptive terminology listed in Column I.*

PART I

Column I	Column II
____ **1.** A break occurs across the entire section of the bone.	**a.** Avulsion
	b. Comminuted
____ **2.** A fragment of the bone is pulled off by a ligament or tendon.	**c.** Complete
	d. Epiphyseal
____ **3.** Bone is splintered into several fragments.	**e.** Greenstick
____ **4.** One side of a bone is broken and the other side is bent.	
____ **5.** A fracture that occurs through the epiphysis.	

PART II

Column I	Column II
___ **1.** A fracture occurs at an angle across the bone.	**a.** Compressed
___ **2.** Fragments are driven inward.	**b.** Depressed
	c. Oblique
___ **3.** The fractured bone is compressed by another bone.	**d.** Open
	e. Pathologic
___ **4.** The fracture extends through the skin.	
___ **5.** A fracture occuring through an area of diseased bone.	

SECTION II: APPLYING YOUR KNOWLEDGE

Activity D *Consider the scenario and answer the questions.*

CASE STUDY: Above-the-Knee Amputation

William, a 70-year-old priest, lives in a center city rectory. He is scheduled to have an above-the-knee amputation of his left leg because of peripheral vascular disease.

1. The nurse is assessing William prior to the surgical procedure. What should the nurse look for to assess the circulatory status of the affected limb?

_____

_____

2. What factors should be accounted for in determining the level of William's amputation?

_____

_____

_____

3. The nurse needs to assist William in exercising the muscles needed for crutch walking. What major muscle would the nurse assist with strengthening?

_____

_____

4. William experiences phantom limb sensations postoperatively. What is the most appropriate nursing response?

_____

_____

5. William's amputation is treated with a soft compression dressing. What nursing interventions should the nurse perform?

_____

_____

_____

_____

6. The nurse should be aware of what problems that can delay prosthetic fittings?

_____

_____

7. The nurse is preparing to apply a bandage to William's residual limb. What technique should the nurse use to apply the bandage?

_____

_____

SECTION III: PRACTICING FOR NCLEX

Activity E *Answer the following questions.*

1. A patient has stepped in a hole in the yard, causing an ankle injury. The ankle is edematous and painful to palpation. How long should the nurse inform the patient that the acute inflammatory stage will last?

a. Less than 24 hours

b. Between 24 and 48 hours

c. About 72 hours

d. At least 1 week

2. The nurse is caring for a patient after arthroscopic surgery for a rotator cuff tear. The nurse informs the patient that full activity can usually resume after what period of time?

a. 3 to 4 weeks

b. 8 weeks

c. 3 to 4 months

d. 6 to 12 months

3. A patient had an above-the-knee amputation of the left leg related to complications from PVD. The nurse enters the patient's room and observes the dressing and bed covers saturated with blood. What is the first action by the nurse?

   a. Notify the physician.

   b. Apply a tourniquet.

   c. Use skin clips to close the wound.

   d. Reinforce the dressing.

4. A patient sustains an open fracture with extensive soft tissue damage. The nurse determines that this fracture would be classified as what grade?

   a. I

   b. II

   c. III

   d. IV

5. A patient sustains an open fracture of the left arm after an accident at the roller skating rink. What does emergency management of this fracture involve? (Select all that apply.)

   a. Covering the area with a clean dressing if the fracture is open

   b. Immobilizing the affected site

   c. Splinting the injured limb

   d. Asking the patient if he or she is able to move the arm

   e. Wrapping the arm in an ace bandage

6. The nurse is caring for a patient who sustained an open fracture of the right femur in an automobile accident. What does the nurse understand is the most serious complication of an open fracture?

   a. Infection

   b. Muscle atrophy caused by loss of supporting bone structure

   c. Necrosis of adjacent soft tissue caused by blood loss

   d. Nerve damage

7. The nurse is monitoring a patient who sustained an open fracture of the left hip. What type of shock should the nurse be aware can occur with this type of injury?

   a. Cardiogenic

   b. Hypovolemic

   c. Neurogenic

   d. Septicemic

8. A patient sustained an open fracture of the femur 24 hours ago. While assessing the patient, the nurse observes the patient is having difficulty breathing, and oxygen saturation decreases to 88% from a previous 99%. What does the nurse understand is likely occurring with this patient?

   a. Spontaneous pneumothorax

   b. Cardiac tamponade

   c. Pneumonia

   d. Fat emboli

9. A patient sustains a fracture of the arm. When does the nurse anticipate pendulum exercise should begin?

   a. As soon as tolerated, after a reasonable period of immobilization

   b. In 2 to 3 weeks, when callus ossification prevents easy movements of bony fragments

   c. In about 4 to 5 weeks, after new bone is well established

   d. In 2 to 3 months, after normal activities are resumed

10. A patient falls while skiing and sustains a supracondylar fracture. What does the nurse know is the most serious complication of a supracondylar fracture of the humerus?

    a. Hemarthrosis

    b. Paresthesia

    c. Malunion

    d. Volkmann's ischemic contracture

11. While riding a bicycle on a narrow road, the patient was hit from behind and thrown into a ditch, sustaining a pelvic fracture. What complications does the nurse know to monitor for that are common to pelvic fractures?

    a. Paresthesia and ischemia

    b. Hemorrhage and shock

    c. Paralytic ileus and a lacerated urethra

    d. Thrombophlebitis and infection

12. The nurse is caring for a patient with a pelvic fracture. What nursing assessment for a pelvic fracture should be included? (Select all that apply.)

    a. Checking the urine for hematuria

    b. Palpating peripheral pulses in both lower extremities

    c. Testing the stool for occult blood

    d. Assessing level of consciousness

    e. Assessing pupillary response

13. A patient has suffered a femoral shaft fracture in an industrial accident. What is an immediate nursing concern for this patient?

    a. Hypovolemic shock

    b. Infection

    c. Knee and hip dislocation

    d. Pain resulting from muscle spasm

14. A nurse is caring for a patient who has had an amputation. What interventions can the nurse provide to foster a positive self-image? (Select all that apply.)

    a. Encouraging the patient to care for the residual limb

    b. Allowing the expression of grief

    c. Encourage the patient to have family and friends view the residual limb to decrease self-consciousness.

    d. Encouraging family and friends to refrain from visiting temporarily because this may increase the patient's embarrassment.

    e. Introducing the patient to local amputee support groups.

15. A patient was climbing a ladder, slipped on a rung, and fell on the right side of the chest. X-ray studies reveal three rib fractures, and the patient is complaining of pain with inspiration. What is the anticipated treatment for this patient?

    a. Chest strapping

    b. Mechanical ventilation

    c. Coughing and deep breathing with pillow splinting

    d. Thoracentesis

Digestive and Gastrointestinal Function

Assessment of Digestive and Gastrointestinal Function

1. Describe the structure and function of the organs of the gastrointestinal (GI) tract.
2. Describe the mechanical and chemical processes involved in digesting and absorbing nutrients and eliminating waste products.
3. Use assessment parameters appropriate for determining the status of GI function.
4. Discriminate between normal and abnormal GI function.
5. Identify the appropriate preparation, patient education, and follow-up care for patients who are undergoing diagnostic evaluation of the GI tract.

SECTION I: ASSESSING YOUR UNDERSTANDING

Activity A *Fill in the blanks.*

1. Three pancreatic secretions that contain digestive enzymes are _____, _____, and _____.

2. Chyme, partially digested food that is mixed with gastric contents, stimulates segmented contractions, which are _____, and intestinal peristalsis, which is _____.

3. It takes _____ hours after eating for food to pass into the terminal ileum. It takes _____ hours for food to reach and distend the rectum.

4. Structural changes in the esophagus that occur as the result of aging include _____, _____, and _____.

5. Reflux of food into the esophagus from the stomach is prevented by contraction of the _____.

6. The digestion of starches begins in the mouth with the secretion of the enzyme _____.

7. The stomach, which derives its acidity from hydrochloric acid, has a pH of approximately _____.

8. Intrinsic factor is a gastric secretion necessary for the intestinal absorption of vitamin _____, which prevents pernicious anemia.

9. A hormonal regulatory substance that inhibits stomach contraction and gastric secretions is _____.

10. _____, which is secreted by the gallbladder, is responsible for fat emulsification.

11. The stomach has four anatomic regions: the _____, _____, _____, and _____.

12. The major carbohydrate that tissues use for fuel is _____.

Activity B   *Briefly answer the following.*

1. What role do the sympathetic and parasympathetic portions of the autonomic nervous system play in GI function?

_____

_____

_____

_____

2. Describe what results from obstruction of the GI tract.

_____

_____

_____

3. A flexible sigmoidoscope permits how much of the lower bowel to be viewed?

_____

4. When the patient is to perform a Hemoccult II test, what should the nurse inform the patient to avoid in order to prevent a false-positive result?

_____

_____

_____

_____

5. When is a magnetic resonance imaging (MRI) test contraindicated?

_____

_____

_____

6. What will occur if there is a lack of intrinsic factor secreted by the gastric mucosa?

_____

_____

_____

_____

Activity C   *Match the major digestive enzyme in Column II with its associated digestive action listed in Column I.*

Column I

_____ **1.** Helps convert protein into amino acids.

_____ **2.** Facilitates the production of dextrins and maltose.

_____ **3.** Digests protein and helps form polypeptides.

_____ **4.** Digests carbohydrates and helps form fructose.

_____ **5.** Glucose is a product of this enzyme's action.

_____ **6.** Helps form galactose.

Column II

a. Amylase

b. Maltase

c. Sucrase

d. Lactase

e. Pepsin

f. Trypsin

SECTION II: APPLYING YOUR KNOWLEDGE

Activity D   *Consider the scenario and answer the questions.*

Carl is a 54-year-old patient who comes to the clinic and informs the nurse that he has been having blood in his stools for the past 2 weeks. He states that he has no pain or discomfort and has never had any trouble with his bowel movements. The physician schedules Carl for a colonoscopy with moderate sedation.

1. The nurse is giving Carl instructions about preparation of the bowel prior to the procedure. What is the importance of the bowel preparation for a colonoscopy?

_____

_____

2. What information should the nurse provide with regard to the position Carl will be placed in during the procedure?

_____

_____

_____

3. The nurse informs Carl that he will be monitored during the entire procedure. What monitoring will occur during the procedure?

_____

_____

4. During the colonoscopy, for what complications should Carl be continuously monitored?

_____

_____

_____

SECTION III: PRACTICING FOR NCLEX

Activity E *Answer the following questions.*

1. The nurse is performing an initial assessment of a patient complaining of increased stomach acid related to stress. The nurse knows that the physician will want to consider the influence of what neuroregulator?

   a. Gastrin

   b. Cholecystokinin

   c. Norepinephrine

   d. Secretin

2. The nurse is performing an assessment of a patient. During the assessment the patient informs the nurse of some recent "stomach trouble." What does the nurse know is the most common symptom of patients with GI dysfunction?

   a. Diffuse pain

   b. Dyspepsia

   c. Constipation

   d. Abdominal bloating

3. The nurse is investigating a patient's complaint of pain in the duodenal area. Where should the nurse perform the assessment?

   a. Epigastric area and consider possible radiation of pain to the right subscapular region

   b. Hypogastrium in the right or left lower quadrant

   c. Left lower quadrant

   d. Periumbilical area, followed by the right lower quadrant

4. A patient is complaining of abdominal pain associated with indigestion. What is characteristic of this type of pain?

   a. Described as crampy or burning

   b. In the left lower quadrant

   c. Less severe after an intake of fatty foods

   d. Relieved by the intake of coarse vegetables, which stimulate peristalsis

5. The nurse is collecting a stool specimen from a patient. What characteristic of the stool indicates to the nurse that the patient may have an upper GI bleed?

   a. Clay-colored

   b. Greasy and foamy

   c. Tarry and black

   d. Threaded with mucus

6. The nurse is performing an abdominal assessment for a patient in the hospital with complaints of abdominal pain. What part of the assessment should the nurse perform first?

   a. Percussion

   b. Palpation

   c. Auscultation

   d. Inspection

7. The nurse has been directed to position a patient for an examination of the abdomen. What position should the nurse place the patient in for the examination?

   a. Prone position with pillows positioned to alleviate pressure on the abdomen

   b. Semi-Fowler's position with the left leg bent to minimize pressure on the abdomen

   c. Supine position with the knees flexed to relax the abdominal muscles

   d. Reverse Trendelenburg position to facilitate the natural propulsion of intestinal contents

8. The nurse auscultates the abdomen to assess bowel sounds. She documents five to six sounds heard in less than 30 seconds. How does the nurse document the bowel sounds?

   a. Normal

   b. Hypoactive

   c. Hyperactive

   d. Borborygmi

9. The nurse is providing instructions to a patient scheduled for a gastroscopy. What should the nurse be sure to include in the instructions? (Select all that apply.)

   a. The patient must fast for 8 hours before the examination.

   b. The throat will be sprayed with a local anesthetic.

   c. After gastroscopy, the patient cannot eat or drink until the gag reflex returns (1 to 2 hours).

   d. The physician will be able to determine if there is a presence of bowel disease.

   e. The patient must have bowel cleansing prior to the procedure.

10. A patient is scheduled for a fiberoptic colonoscopy. What does the nurse know that fiberoptic colonoscopy is most frequently used to diagnose?

    a. Bowel disease of unknown origin

    b. Cancer screening

    c. Inflammatory bowel disease

    d. Occult bleeding

11. A patient is being prepared for esophageal manometry. The nurse should inform the patient to withhold what medication for 48 hours prior to the procedure?

    a. Amiodarone (Cordarone)

    b. Calan (Verapamil)

    c. Aspirin

    d. Metoprolol (Lopressor)

12. The nurse is assisting the physician with a gastric acid stimulation test for a patient. What medication should the nurse prepare to administer subcutaneously to stimulate gastric secretions?

    a. Pentagastrin

    b. Atropine

    c. Robinul (glycopyrrolate)

    d. Mucomyst

13. The nurse is assisting the physician with a colonoscopy for a patient with rectal bleeding. The physician requests the nurse to administer glucagon during the procedure. Why is the nurse administering this medication during the procedure?

    a. The patient is probably hypoglycemic and requires the glucagon.

    b. To relieve anxiety during the procedure for moderate sedation.

    c. To reduce air accumulation in the colon.

    d. To relax colonic musculature and reduce spasm.

14. A patient is in the outpatient recovery area after having a colonoscopy and informs the nurse of abdominal cramping. What is the best response by the nurse?

    a. "We may need to go back in and see what is wrong. You shouldn't have discomfort."

    b. "I will call the physician and let him know. He may have put too much air in your colon."

    c. "I will call the physician and see if I can give you pain medication. Sometimes the pain can be caused by having a biopsy."

    d. "The cramping is caused by the air insufflated in the colon during the procedure."

15. During a colonoscopy with moderate sedation, the patient groans with obvious discomfort and begins bleeding from the rectum. The patient is diaphoretic and has an increase in abdominal girth from distention. What complication of this procedure is the nurse aware may be occurring?

    a. Infection

    b. Bowel perforation

    c. Colonic polyp

    d. Rectal fissure

Digestive and Gastrointestinal Treatment Modalities

Learning Objectives

1. Describe the purposes and types of enteral and parenteral nutrition access devices.
2. Identify the purposes, indications for, and administration techniques of enteral and parenteral nutrition formulas.
3. Discuss nursing management of the patient who has a nasally placed feeding tube, stomal tube, or intravenous catheter.
4. Use the nursing process as a framework for care of the patient receiving enteral or parenteral nutrition support.
5. Describe the nursing measures used to prevent complications from enteral and parenteral nutrition support.

SECTION I: ASSESSING YOUR UNDERSTANDING

Activity A *Fill in the blanks.*

1. A nasally placed feeding tube is for short-term use and should stay in place for no more than ____ weeks before being replaced with a new tube.

2. Nasogastric feeding tubes are used for patients who have the ability to _____ and _____ nutrition, fluids, and medications adequately by the gastric route.

3. Prokinetic agents can be administered to facilitate _____ movement of the feeding tube into the duodenum.

4. Feeding patients through tubes placed beyond the _____ or using _____ agents can decrease the frequency of feeding regurgitation and aspiration.

5. _____ or _____ feeding is indicated when the esophagus and stomach need to be bypassed or when the patient is at risk for aspiration.

6. When giving an initial tube feeding, the nurse would be looking for _____ around the tube site on the abdomen.

7. A dressing over the tube outlet and the gastrostomy tube protects the skin around the incision from _____ and _____.

Activity B *Briefly answer the following.*

1. Describe the purpose of gastric intubation.

_____

_____

_____

_____

2. What is the visual difference between the color of gastric aspirate and the color of intestinal aspirate?

_____

_____

_____

3. Name three common causes of constipation for a patient who is receiving enteral feedings.

_____

_____

_____

4. What is the Sengstaken-Blakemore tube used for?

_____

_____

5. Why must extra caution be taken when inserting a feeding tube with a stylet?

_____

_____

Activity C *Match the description of the type of nasogastric, nasoenteric, and regular feeding tube in Column II with its appropriate name listed in Column I.*

Column I

____ **1.** Sengstaken–Blakemore

____ **2.** Levin

____ **3.** Gastric-Sump Salem

____ **4.** Moss

____ **5.** Dobbhoff or EnteraFlo

Column II

a. Triple-lumen nasogastric tube that also has a duodenal lumen for postoperative feedings

b. Nasoenteric feeding tube about 6 ft in length

c. Single-lumen, plastic, or rubber nasogastric tube about 4 ft in length

d. Double-lumen, plastic nasogastric tube about 20 cm in length

e. Triple-lumen, rubber nasogastric tube (two lumens are used to inflate the gastric and esophageal balloons)

SECTION II: APPLYING YOUR KNOWLEDGE

Activity D *Consider the scenarios and answer the questions.*

CASE STUDY: Dumping Syndrome

Nancy is 37 years old, 5 ft 7 in tall, and weighs 140 lb. She receives 250 mL of a feeding over a 15-minute period every 4 hours through a nasogastric tube. Nancy has had esophageal surgery for carcinoma.

1. Nancy tells the nurse that she has diarrhea. The nurse suspects Nancy is experiencing the dumping syndrome. What other possible causes should the nurse eliminate?

_____

_____

_____

2. The nurse notes a residual gastric content of 50 mL. What is the priority action by the nurse?

_____

3. What intervention can the nurse provide to Nancy to decrease peristalsis during feedings?

_____

4. What complications may occur with dumping syndrome that the nurse should monitor for?

_____

CASE STUDY: Total Parenteral Nutrition

Penny is 30 years old and single. She is 5 ft 7 in tall, weighs 150 lb, and is receiving parenteral nutrition solution at the rate of 3 L/day. Her postoperative condition warrants receiving nutrients by the intravenous route.

1. The nurse knows that, to spare body protein, Penny's daily caloric intake should be at what level?

_____

2. The nurse estimates Penny's caloric intake for each 1,000 mL of total parenteral nutrition to yield a glucose concentration of how many calories?

_____

3. The nurse should observe Penny for signs of rapid fluid intake. What signs does the nurse determine would indicate rapid fluid intake?

SECTION III: PRACTICING FOR NCLEX

Activity E *Answer the following questions.*

1. The physician ordered a nasoenteric feeding tube with a tungsten-weighted tip. The nurse knows to obtain what kind of tube?
   a. Dobbhoff
   b. Levin
   c. Salem
   d. Sengstaken–Blakemore

2. A nurse prepares a patient for insertion of a nasoenteric tube. What position should the nurse place the patient in?
   a. In high-Fowler's position
   b. Flat in bed
   c. On his or her right side
   d. In semi-Fowler's position with his or her head turned to the left

3. The nurse is inserting a Levin tube for a patient for gastric decompression. The tube should be inserted to 6 to10 cm beyond what length?
   a. A length of 50 cm (20 in)
   b. A point that equals the distance from the nose to the xiphoid process
   c. The distance measured from the tip of the nose to the earlobe and from the earlobe to the xiphoid process
   d. The distance determined by measuring from the tragus of the ear to the xiphoid process

4. The nurse inserts a nasogastric tube into the right nares of a patient. When testing the tube aspirate for pH to confirm placement, what does the nurse anticipate the pH will be if placement is in the lungs?
   a. 1
   b. 2
   c. 4
   d. 6

5. The nurse is managing a gastric (Salem) sump tube for a patient who has an intestinal obstruction and will be going to surgery. What interventions should the nurse perform to make sure the tube is functioning properly?
   a. Maintain intermittent or continuous suction at a rate greater than 120 mm Hg.
   b. Keep the vent lumen above the patient's waist to prevent gastric content reflux.
   c. Irrigate only through the vent lumen.
   d. Tape the tube to the head of the bed to avoid dislodgement.

6. The nurse is inserting a nasoenteric tube for a patient with a paralytic ileus. How long does the nurse anticipate the tube will be required? (Select all that apply.)
   a. Until bowel sound is present
   b. Until flatus is passed
   c. Until peristalsis is resumed
   d. Until the patient stops vomiting
   e. Until the tube comes out on its own

7. The nurse assesses a patient who recently had a nasoenteric intubation. Symptoms of oliguria, lethargy, and tachycardia in the patient would indicate to the nurse what common complication?
   a. A cardiac dysrhythmia
   b. Fluid volume deficit
   c. Mucous membrane irritation
   d. Pulmonary complications

8. The nurse checks residual content before each intermittent tube feeding. When should the patient be reassessed?
   a. When the residual is about 50 mL
   b. When the residual is between 50 and 80 mL
   c. When the residual is about 100 mL
   d. When the residual is greater than 200 mL

9. The nurse is caring for a patient who has dumping syndrome from high-carbohydrate foods being administered over a period of less than 20 minutes. What is a nursing measure to prevent or minimize the dumping syndrome?

   a. Administer the feeding at a warm temperature to decrease peristalsis.

   b. Administer the feeding by bolus to prevent continuous intestinal distention.

   c. Administer the feeding with about 100 mL of fluid to dilute the high-carbohydrate concentration.

   d. Administer the feeding with the patient in semi-Fowler's position to decrease transit time influenced by gravity.

10. The nurse is caring for a comatose patient and administering gastrostomy feedings. What does the nurse understand is the reason that gastrostomy feedings are preferred to nasogastric feedings in the comatose patient?

   a. Gastroesophageal sphincter is intact, lessening the possibility of regurgitation.

   b. Digestive process occurs more rapidly because the feedings do not have to pass through the esophagus.

   c. Feedings can be administered with the patient in the recumbent position.

   d. The patient cannot experience the deprivational stress of not swallowing.

11. A patient has had a gastrostomy tube inserted. What does the nurse anticipate the initial fluid nourishment will be after the insertion of the gastrostomy tube?

   a. Distilled water

   b. 10% glucose and tap water

   c. Milk

   d. High-calorie liquids

12. The nurse is caring for a patient who has a gastrostomy tube feeding. Upon initiating her care, the nurse aspirates the gastrotomy tube for gastric residual volume (GRV) and obtains 200 mL of gastric contents. What is the priority action by the nurse?

   a. Discontinue the infusion.

   b. Place the patient in a Fowler's position with the head of the bed at 45 degrees.

   c. Remove the aspirated fluid and do not reinstill.

   d. Dilute the gastric tube feeding solution with water and continue the feeding.

13. The nurse is inserting a sump tube in a patient with Crohn's disease who is suspected of having a bowel obstruction. What does the nurse understand is the benefit of the gastric (Salem) sump tube in comparison to some of the other tubes?

   a. The tube is radiopaque.

   b. The tube is shorter.

   c. The tube is less expensive.

   d. The tube can be connected to suction and others cannot.

14. The nurse is inserting a nasogastric tube for a patient with pancreatitis. What intervention can the nurse provide to allow facilitation of the tube insertion?

   a. Spray the oropharynx with an anesthetic spray.

   b. Have the patient maintain a backward tilt head position.

   c. Allow the patient to sip water as the tube is being inserted.

   d. Have the patient eat a cracker as the tube is being inserted.

15. The nurse is inserting a nasogastric tube and the patient begins coughing and is unable to speak. What does the nurse suspect has occurred?

   a. The nurse has inserted a tube that is too large for the patient.

   b. The nurse has inadvertently inserted the tube into the trachea.

   c. This is a normal occurrence and the tube should be left in place.

   d. The tube is most likely defective and should be immediately removed.

CHAPTER 46

Management of Patients With Oral and Esophageal Disorders

Learning Objectives

1. Describe the nursing management of patients with conditions of the oral cavity.
2. Describe the relationship of dental hygiene and dental problems to nutrition and to disease.
3. Describe the nursing management of patients with abnormalities of the oral cavity, jaw, and salivary glands.
4. Describe the nursing management of patients with cancer of the oral cavity.
5. Use the nursing process as a framework for care of patients undergoing neck dissection.
6. Use the nursing process as a framework for care of patients with various conditions of the esophagus.
7. Describe the various conditions of the esophagus and their clinical manifestations and management.

SECTION I: ASSESSING YOUR UNDERSTANDING

Activity A *Fill in the blanks.*

1. Digestion normally begins in the _____.

2. _____ percent of adults 45 to 64 years of age have severe periodontal disease.

3. A common lesion of the mouth that is also referred to as a "canker sore" is _____.

4. The incidence of most dental caries is directly related to an increase in the dietary intake of _____.

5. Preventive orthodontics for malocclusion can start as early as age _____.

6. Mumps, a viral infection affecting children, is usually an inflammation of the _____ gland.

7. If detected early, prior to lymph node involvement, the 5-year survival rate for oral cancer is about _____ percent.

8. The most common site for cancer of the oral cavity is the _____.

Activity B *Briefly answer the following.*

1. How does tooth decay begin?

_____

_____

2. What measures can the nurse encourage patients to take to prevent and control dental caries?

_____

_____

_____

_____

3. What intervention can be provided to relieve the discomfort of a patient with a tooth abscess in the early stage?

_____

_____

_____

4. What is the difference between sialadenitis and sialolithiasis?

_____

_____

5. What potential postoperative complications may be involved with the patient who has had a radical neck dissection?

_____

_____

Activity C *Match the abnormality of the lips, mouth, or gums listed in Column II with its associated symptomatology of the lip, mouth, or gums listed in Column I.*

Column I

_____ 1. Ulcerated and painful, white papules

_____ 2. Reddened area or rash associated with itching

_____ 3. Painful, inflamed, swollen gums

_____ 4. White overgrowth of horny layer of epidermis

_____ 5. Shallow ulcer with a red border and white or yellow center

_____ 6. Hyperkeratotic white patches usually in buccal mucosa

_____ 7. Reddened circum-scribed lesion that ulcerates and becomes encrusted

_____ 8. White patches with rough, hairlike projec-tions usually found on the tongue

Column II

a. Actinic cheilitis

b. Leukoplakia

c. Chancre

d. Canker sore

e. Gingivitis

f. Lichen planus

g. Contact dermatitis

h. Hairy leukoplakia

SECTION II: APPLYING YOUR KNOWLEDGE

Activity D *Consider the scenarios and answer the questions.*

CASE STUDY: Radical Neck Dissection

J.R., a 64-year-old patient with a 40-year history of using oral tobacco products, has been diagnosed with a malignancy of the neck and is scheduled for a radical neck dissection. J.R. will be accompanied to the hospital by his wife, who will be assisting with his care when he is discharged.

1. The nurse is preparing J.R. for surgery. What two common morbidities does the nurse know are associated with a radical neck dissection?

_____

2. What postoperative complications should the nurse observe for after J.R.'s surgery?

_____

3. J.R. has returned to the postanesthesia care unit after surgery. What position should the nurse maintain the patient in postoperatively?

_____

4. Postoperatively, what finding should be immediately reported because it may indicate airway obstruction?

_____

5. The nurse observes excessive drooling during a postoperative assessment. What nerve should the nurse assess for damage?

_____

6. What can be done prior to J.R.'s discharge to assist the wife with his care?

_____

_____

CASE STUDY: Mandibular Fracture

William, a 17-year-old student, suffered a mandibular fracture while playing football. He is presently having jaw repositioning surgery under general anesthesia. His parents are in the waiting area.

1. How should the nurse position William in the immediate postoperative period?

_____

2. What should the nurse tell William and his family to explain why nasogastric suctioning is needed?

_____

_____

3. For emergency use, which of the following should the nurse be sure is available at the head of the bed?

_____

4. What initial postoperative diet would be recommended for William?

_____

CASE STUDY: Cancer of the Mouth

Edith, a 64-year-old mother of two, has been a chain smoker for 20 years. During the past month, she noticed a dryness in her mouth and a roughened area that is irritating. She mentioned her symptoms to her dentist, who referred her to a medical internist.

1. On the basis of the patient's health history, the nurse suspects oral cancer. What would the nurse expect the lesion to look like?

_____

2. During the health history, the nurse noted that Edith did not mention a late-occurring symptom of mouth cancer. What does the nurse know is a symptom of late mouth cancer?

_____

3. On physical examination, Edith evidenced changes associated with cancer of the mouth. What changes would the nurse know are characteristic of cancer of the mouth?

_____

_____

SECTION III: PRACTICING FOR NCLEX

Activity E _Answer the following questions._

1. The nurse is performing an assessment for a patient who presents to the clinic with a lip lesion. The lesion is erythemic, is fissuring, and has white hyperkeratosis. What does the nurse suspect that these findings are characteristic of?

a. Actinic cheilitis

b. Human papillomavirus lesion

c. Frey syndrome

d. Sialadenitis

2. A patient is experiencing painful, inflamed, and swollen gums, and when brushing the teeth, the gums bleed. What common disease of the oral tissue does the nurse understand these symptoms indicate?

a. Candidiasis

b. Gingivitis

c. Herpes simplex

d. Cancer of the oral mucosa

3. The nurse is caring for a patient after drainage of a dentoalveolar or periapical abscess. What should the care of the patient include in the postoperative phase? (Select all that apply.)

a. Soft diet after 24 hours

b. Fluid restriction for the first 48 hours because the gums are swollen and painful

c. External heat by pad or compress to hasten the resolution of the inflammatory swelling

d. Warm saline mouthwashes every 2 hours while awake

e. Gargle with peroxide and saline every 4 hours

4. A patient complains about an inflamed salivary gland below his right ear. The nurse documents probable inflammation of which gland?

a. Buccal

b. Parotid

c. Sublingual

d. Submandibular

5. An older adult patient who has been living at home alone is diagnosed with parotitis. What causative bacteria does the nurse suspect is the cause of the parotitis?

   a. Methicillin-resistant *Streptococcus aureus* (MRSA)

   b. *Pneumococcus*

   c. *Staphylococcus aureus*

   d. *Streptococcus viridans*

6. A nurse inspects the Stensen duct of the parotid gland to determine inflammation and possible obstruction. What area in the oral cavity would the nurse examine?

   a. Buccal mucosa next to the upper molars

   b. Dorsum of the tongue

   c. Roof of the mouth next to the incisors

   d. Posterior segment of the tongue near the uvula

7. The nurse is obtaining a history on a patient who comes to the clinic. What symptom described by the patient is one of the first symptoms associated with esophageal disease?

   a. Dysphagia

   b. Malnutrition

   c. Pain

   d. Regurgitation of food

8. A patient tells the nurse that it feels like food is "sticking" in the lower portion of the esophagus. What motility disorder does the nurse suspect these symptoms indicate?

   a. Achalasia

   b. Diffuse spasm

   c. Gastroesophageal reflex disease

   d. Hiatal hernia

9. A patient is brought to the emergency department by a family member, who states that the patient "drank drain cleaner." What intervention does the nurse anticipate providing to treat this patient? (Select all that apply.)

   a. Administering an irritant that will stimulate vomiting

   b. Aspirating secretions from the pharynx if respirations are affected

   c. Neutralizing the chemical

   d. Washing the esophagus with large volumes of water

   e. Administering activated charcoal

10. While caring for a patient who has had radical neck surgery, the nurse notices an abnormal amount of serosanguineous secretions in the wound suction unit during the first postoperative day. What does the nurse know is an expected amount of drainage in the wound unit?

    a. Between 40 and 80 mL

    b. Approximately 80 to 120 mL

    c. Between 120 and 160 mL

    d. Greater than 160 mL

11. A patient describes a burning sensation in the esophagus, pain when swallowing, and frequent indigestion. What does the nurse suspect that these clinical manifestations indicate?

    a. Peptic ulcer disease

    b. Esophageal cancer

    c. Gastroesophageal reflux disease

    d. Diverticulitis

12. A patient has been diagnosed with Zenker's diverticulum. What treatment does the nurse anticipate educating the patient about?

    a. A low-residue diet

    b. Chemotherapeutic agents

    c. Radiation therapy

    d. Surgical removal of the diverticulum

13. A patient who is HIV positive comes to the clinic and is experiencing white patches with rough hairlike projections. The nurse observes the lesions on the lateral border of the tongue. What abnormality of the mouth does the nurse determine these lesions are?

    a. Aphthous stomatitis

    b. Nicotine stomatitis

    c. Erythroplakia

    d. Hairy leukoplakia

14. A patient comes to the clinic complaining of a sore throat. When assessing the patient, the nurse observes a reddened ulcerated lesion on the lip. The patient tells the nurse that it has been there for a couple of weeks but it does not hurt. What should the nurse consult with the physician about testing for?

a. HIV

b. Syphilis

c. Gonorrhea

d. Herpes simplex

15. A patient has been taking a 10-day course of antibiotics for pneumonia. The patient has been having white patches that look like milk curds in the mouth. What treatment will the nurse educate the patient about?

a. Nystatin (Mycostatin)

b. Cephalexin (Rocephin)

c. Fluocinolone acetonide oral base gel

d. Acyclovir (Zovirax)

47

Management of Patients With Gastric and Duodenal Disorders

Learning Objectives

1. Compare the etiology, clinical manifestations, and management of acute gastritis, chronic gastritis, and peptic ulcer.
2. Use the nursing process as a framework for care of patients with peptic ulcer.
3. Describe the pharmacologic, dietary, and surgical treatment of peptic ulcer.
4. Describe the causes, classifications, and morbid complications associated with obesity and management strategies for treating obesity.
5. Use the nursing process as a framework of care of patients who undergo bariatric surgical procedures.
6. Use the nursing process as a framework for care of patients with gastric cancer.
7. Identify the complications of bariatric or other gastric surgical procedures and their prevention and management.
8. Describe the home health care needs of the patient who has had bariatric or other gastric surgical procedures.
9. Discuss the etiology, clinical manifestations, and management of tumors of the small intestine.

SECTION I: ASSESSING YOUR UNDERSTANDING

Activity A *Fill in the blanks.*

1. The most common site for peptic ulcer formation is the _____.

2. Peptic ulcers occur with the most frequency in those between the ages of _____ and _____ years.

3. A frequently prescribed proton pump inhibitor of gastric acid is _____.

4. The most common complication of peptic ulcer disease that occurs in 10% to 20% of patients is _____.

5. The average weight loss after bariatric surgery is about _____% of previous body weight.

6. _____ is the bacillus commonly associated with the formation of gastric, and possibly duodenal, ulcers.

7. _____, _____, _____, and _____ are some of the major potential complications of a peptic ulcer.

8. The stomach pouch created by gastric bypass or bonding surgery can hold up to _____ mL of food and fluids.

Activity B *Briefly answer the following.*

1. Describe the priority intervention that should be used to treat the ingestion of a corrosive acid or alkali.

_____

_____

_____

2. Explain why patients who have gastritis due to a vitamin deficiency usually have malabsorption of vitamin B_{12}.

_____

_____

3. Name two conditions that are specifically related to peptic ulcer development.

_____

_____

4. List several findings characteristic of Zollinger–Ellison syndrome.

_____

_____

5. What does the term "stress ulcer" mean?

_____

_____

6. What is the difference between Cushing and Curling's ulcer in terms of cause and location?

_____

_____

_____

7. Explain the current theory about diet modification for peptic ulcer disease.

_____

_____

_____

_____

8. Describe the clinical manifestations associated with a peptic ulcer perforation.

_____

_____

_____

9. How does bariatric surgery work?

_____

_____

Activity C **Pharmacologic Therapy for Peptic Ulcer Disease and Gastritis**

Match the specific drug in Column II with the drug type in Column I.

Column I

____ **1.** Antibiotics

____ **2.** Antidiarrheal

____ **3.** Histamine-2 receptor antagonist

____ **4.** Proton pump inhibitors

____ **5.** Prostaglandin E1 analogue

Column II

a. Bismuth subsalicylate (Pepto Bismol)

b. Clarithromycin (Biaxin)

c. Misoprostol (Cytotec)

d. Famotidine (Pepcid)

e. Pantoprazole (Protonix)

SECTION II: APPLYING YOUR KNOWLEDGE

Activity D *Consider the scenario and answer the questions.*

CASE STUDY: Gastric Cancer

Mr. Jackson, a 66-year-old African American, has recently been seen by a physician to confirm a diagnosis of gastric cancer. He has a history of tobacco use and was diagnosed 10 years ago with pernicious anemia. He and his family are shocked about the possibility of this diagnosis because he has been asymptomatic prior to recent complaints of pain and multiple gastrointestinal symptoms.

1. The nurse is assessing Mr. Jackson and has progressed to palpation of the abdomen. What indication does the nurse have that metastasis to the liver may have occurred?

_____

2. What type of diagnostic procedures will the nurse educate Mr. Jackson about that will most likely be performed?

_____

_____

3. The surgical team has decided that a Billroth II would be the best approach to treatment. What does the nurse explain to the family that this procedure involves?

_____

_____

4. The nurse explains that combination chemotherapy, more effective than single-agent chemotherapy, frequently follows surgery. What primary agent does the nurse anticipate will be used?

_____

SECTION III: PRACTICING FOR NCLEX

Activity E *Answer the following questions.*

1. A patient has been diagnosed with acute gastritis and asks the nurse what could have caused it. What is the best response by the nurse? (Select all that apply.)

a. "It can be caused by ingestion of strong acids."

b. "You may have ingested some irritating foods."

c. "Is it possible that you are overusing aspirin."

d. "It is a hereditary disease."

e. "It is probably your nerves."

2. The nurse is caring for a patient who has been diagnosed with gastritis. To promote fluid balance when treating gastritis, the nurse knows that what minimal daily intake of fluids is required?

a. 1.0 L

b. 1.5 L

c. 2.0 L

d. 2.5 L

3. A patient who had a Roux-en-Y bypass procedure for morbid obesity ate a chocolate chip cookie after a meal. After ingestion of the cookie, the patient complained of cramping pains, dizziness, and palpitation. After having a bowel movement, the symptoms resolved. What should the patient be educated about regarding this event?

a. Gastric outlet obstruction

b. Dumping syndrome

c. Bile reflux

d. Celiac disease

4. A patient comes to the clinic with the complaint, "I think I have an ulcer." What is a characteristic associated with peptic ulcer pain that the nurse should inquire about? (Select all that apply.)

a. Burning sensation localized in the back or mid-epigastrium

b. Feeling of emptiness that precedes meals from 1 to 3 hours

c. Severe gnawing pain that increases in severity as the day progresses

d. Pain that radiates to the shoulder or jaw

e. Vomiting without associated nausea

5. The nurse is educating a patient about the discharge medication. When should the nurse instruct the patient to take the antacid medication?

a. With the meal

b. 30 minutes before the meal

c. 1 to 3 hours after the meal

d. Immediately after the meal

6. A patient is scheduled for a Billroth I procedure for ulcer management. What does the nurse understand will occur when this procedure is performed?

a. A partial gastrectomy is performed with anastomosis of the stomach segment to the duodenum.

b. A sectioned portion of the stomach is joined to the jejunum.

c. The antral portion of the stomach is removed and a vagotomy is performed.

d. The vagus nerve is cut and gastric drainage is established.

7. The nurse is developing a plan of care for a patient with peptic ulcer disease. What nursing interventions should be included in the care plan? (Select all that apply.)

   a. Making neurovascular checks every 4 hours

   b. Frequently monitoring hemoglobin and hematocrit levels

   c. Observing stools and vomitus for color, consistency, and volume

   d. Checking the blood pressure and pulse rate every 15 to 20 minutes

   e. Inserting an indwelling catheter for incontinence

8. The nurse is caring for a patient who is suspected to have developed a peptic ulcer hemorrhage. Which action would the nurse perform first?

   a. Place the patient in a recumbent position with the legs elevated.

   b. Prepare a peripheral and central line for intravenous infusion.

   c. Assess vital signs.

   d. Call the physician.

9. A patient sustained second- and third-degree burns over 30% of the body surface area approximately 72 hours ago. What type of ulcer should the nurse be alert for while caring for this patient?

   a. Curling's ulcer

   b. Peptic ulcer

   c. Esophageal ulcer

   d. Meckel's ulcer

10. A patient is in the hospital for the treatment of peptic ulcer disease. The nurse finds the patient vomiting and complaining of a sudden severe pain in the abdomen. The nurse then assesses a board-like abdomen. What does the nurse suspect these symptoms indicate?

   a. The treatment for the peptic ulcer is ineffective.

   b. A reaction to the medication given for the ulcer

   c. Gastric penetration

   d. Perforation of the peptic ulcer

11. A patient taking metronidazole (Flagyl) for the treatment of *H. pylori* states that the medication is causing nausea. What suggestion can the nurse provide to the patient to alleviate this problem?

   a. Discontinue the use of the medication.

   b. Tell the patient to ask the physician to prescribe another type of antibiotic.

   c. Take the medication with meals to decrease the nausea.

   d. Crush the medication and put it in applesauce.

12. The nurse is educating a patient with peptic ulcer disease about the disease process. What decreases the secretion of bicarbonate from the pancreas into the duodenum, resulting in increased acidity of the duodenum?

   a. Smoking

   b. Eating spicy foods

   c. Drinking carbonated beverages

   d. Taking antacids

13. A patient is complaining of diarrhea after having bariatric surgery. What nonpharmacologic treatment can the nurse suggest to decrease the incidence of diarrhea?

   a. Decrease the fat content in the diet.

   b. Increase the fiber content in the diet.

   c. Decrease the amount of fluid the patient is drinking.

   d. Increase the protein content in the diet.

14. A patient has a Class II classification of obesity. What level of health risk does this pose for the patient?

   a. Mild risk

   b. Moderate risk

   c. Severe risk

   d. Very severe risk

15. A patient has a BMI ranger greater than 40 kg/m². What would this patient's obesity classification be?

   a. Overweight

   b. Class I

   c. Class II

   d. Class III

Management of Patients With Intestinal and Rectal Disorders

Learning Objectives

1. Identify the health care learning needs of patients with constipation or diarrhea.
2. Compare the conditions of malabsorption with regard to their pathophysiology, clinical manifestations, and management.
3. Use the nursing process as a framework for care of patients with diverticular disease.
4. Compare Crohn's disease (regional enteritis) and ulcerative colitis with regard to their pathophysiology; clinical manifestations; diagnostic evaluation; and medical, surgical, and nursing management.
5. Use the nursing process as a framework for care of the patient with inflammatory bowel disease.
6. Describe the responsibilities of the nurse in meeting the needs of the patient with an intestinal diversion.
7. Describe the various types of intestinal obstructions and their management.
8. Use the nursing process as a framework for care of the patient with colorectal cancer.
9. Describe the nursing management of the patient with an anorectal condition.

SECTION I: ASSESSING YOUR UNDERSTANDING

Activity A *Fill in the blanks.*

1. The two diseases of the colon that are commonly associated with constipation are _____ and _____.

2. The recommended dietary intake of fiber is _____ grams per day. This intake, along with 1.5 to 2 L of fluids daily, should prevent constipation that occurs with fewer than _____ bowel movements per week.

3. The most common bacteria found in antibiotic-associated diarrhea is _____ _____.

4. The three most common causes of small bowel obstruction are _____, _____, and _____.

5. The majority of large bowel obstructions are caused by _____.

6. A disorder of malabsorption that inactivates pancreatic enzymes is _____ _____.

7. Malabsorption diseases may affect the ability of the digestive system to absorb the major water-soluble _____.

8. The most common site for the presence of diverticulitis is the _____.

9. Common clinical manifestations of Crohn's disease are _____ and _____.

10. The nurse is irrigating a colostomy. The catheter should be advanced into the stoma _____ to _____ inches.

Activity B *Briefly answer the following.*

1. Name four complications associated with diverticulitis.

   _____

   _____

2. List the common bacteria found in a patient who has developed peritonitis.

   _____

   _____

3. List six risk factors for colorectal cancer that the nurse can educate the public about.

   _____

   _____

   _____

   _____

   _____

   _____

4. Describe the physiologic response that occurs when a patient has a Valsalva maneuver while straining during defecation.

   _____

   _____

   _____

   _____

5. What medications may be prescribed for the patient with constipation that will enhance colonic transit by increasing propulsive motor activity?

   _____

   _____

   _____

   _____

   _____

   _____

6. Name at least four factors that may be associated with the development of irritable bowel syndrome.

   _____

   _____

   _____

   _____

7. Name the hallmark signs of malabsorption syndrome.

   _____

   _____

   _____

   _____

Activity C

PART 1: Key Terms

Match the term in Column II with its associated definition in Column I.

Column I	Column II
____ **1.** A tubular fibrous tract that extends from an opening beside the anus into the anal canal	**a.** Valsalva maneuver
	b. Tenesmus
____ **2.** Dilated and atonic colon caused by a fecal mass	**c.** Stoma
	d. Corn
____ **3.** A chemotherapeutic agent used to treat colon cancer	**e.** Fistula
	f. Peritonitis
____ **4.** A food to avoid for a patient with an ileostomy	**g.** Crohn's disease
	h. TPN
____ **5.** Straining at stool	**i.** 5-FU
____ **6.** Another name for regional enteritis	**j.** Effluent
	k. CEA
____ **7.** A highly reliable blood study used to diagnose appendicitis	**l.** Laxatives
	m. Megacolon
____ **8.** Painful straining at stool	**n.** Borborygmus
____ **9.** The most common bacteria associated with peritonitis	**o.** Celery
	p. *E. coli*
____ **10.** Another term for fecal matter	
____ **11.** An ileal outlet on the abdomen	
____ **12.** Intestinal rumbling	
____ **13.** Another food to avoid for a patient with an ileostomy	
____ **14.** The most popular over-the-counter medication purchased in the United States	
____ **15.** Intravenous nutrition used for inflammatory bowel disease	
____ **16.** The most common complication of colon cancer	

PART 2: Laxative Classification and Action

Match the type of laxative listed in Column III with its classification in Column II. Then match the classification in Column II with its action listed in Column I.

Column I	Column II	Column III
____ **1.** Magnesium ions alter stool consistency.	**a.** Bulk forming	**1.** Mineral oil
	b. Stimulant	**2.** Metamucil
____ **2.** Surfactant action hydrates stool.	**c.** Fecal softener	**3.** Milk of magnesia
	d. Lubricant	**4.** Dulcolax
____ **3.** Electrolytes induce diarrhea.	**e.** Saline agent	**5.** Colace
	f. Osmotic agent	**6.** Colyte
____ **4.** Polysaccharides and cellulose mix with intestinal contents.		
____ **5.** Colon is irritated and sensory nerve endings stimulated.		
____ **6.** Hydrocarbons soften fecal matter.		

SECTION II: APPLYING YOUR KNOWLEDGE

Activity D *Consider the scenario and answer the questions.*

CASE STUDY: Appendicitis

Rory, an 18-year-old girl, is admitted to the hospital with a possible diagnosis of appendicitis. She became symptomatic approximately 24 hours prior to her hospital admission.

1. Since Rory has been symptomatic for 24 hours, what symptoms does the nurse expect to find when obtaining subjective and objective data that correlates with a diagnosis of appendicitis?

   _____

   _____

   _____

   _____

2. Before the nurse sends Rory to have any diagnostic x-rays, what procedure should be performed?

   _____

   _____

3. Two hours after admission, the nurse observes Rory lying motionless and supine in the bed and she tells the nurse that she feels worse. What does the nurse suspect may have occurred during this time frame?

   _____

SECTION III: PRACTICING FOR NCLEX

Activity E *Answer the following questions.*

1. The nurse is assessing a patient with appendicitis. The nurse is attempting to elicit a Rovsing's sign. Where should the nurse palpate for this indicator of acute appendicitis?

   a. Right lower quadrant
   b. Left lower quadrant
   c. Right upper quadrant
   d. Left upper quadrant

2. A patient is not having daily bowel movements and has begun taking a laxative for this problem. What should the nurse educate the patient about regarding laxative use?

   a. When taking the laxatives, plenty of fluid should be taken as well.
   b. The laxatives should be taken no more than 3 times a week or laxative addiction will result.
   c. Laxatives should not be routinely taken due to destruction of nerve endings in the colon.
   d. Laxatives should never be the first response for the treatment of constipation; natural methods should be employed first.

3. A patient is admitted to the hospital after not having had a bowel movement in several days. The nurse observes the patient is having small liquid stools, a grossly distended abdomen, and abdominal cramping. What complication can this patient develop related to this problem?

   a. Appendicitis
   b. Rectal fissures
   c. Bowel perforation
   d. Diverticulitis

4. The nurse is performing an abdominal assessment for a patient with diarrhea and auscultates a loud rumbling sound in the left lower quadrant. What will the nurse document this sound as on the nurse's notes?

   a. Loud bowel sounds
   b. Borborygmus
   c. Tenesmus
   d. Peristalsis

5. The nurse is caring for an older adult patient experiencing fecal incontinence. When planning the care of this patient, what should the nurse designate as a priority goal?

   a. Maintaining skin integrity
   b. Beginning a bowel program to establish continence
   c. Instituting a diet high in fiber and increase fluid intake
   d. Determining the need for surgical intervention to correct the problem

6. A patient with irritable bowel syndrome has been having more frequent symptoms lately and is not sure what lifestyle changes may have occurred. What suggestion can the nurse provide to identify a trigger for the symptoms?

   a. Document how much fluid is being taken to determine if the patient is overhydrating.

   b. Discontinue the use of any medication presently being taken to determine if medication is a trigger.

   c. Begin an exercise regimen and biofeedback to determine if external stress is a trigger.

   d. Keep a 1- to 2-week symptom and food diary to identify food triggers.

7. The nurse is caring for a patient who has malabsorption syndrome with an undetermined cause. What procedure will the nurse assist with that is the best diagnostic test for this illness?

   a. Ultrasound

   b. Endoscopy with mucosal biopsy

   c. Stool specimen for ova and parasites

   d. Pancreatic function tests

8. A patient arrives in the emergency department with complaints of right lower abdominal pain that began 4 hours ago and is getting worse. The nurse assesses rebound tenderness at McBurney's point. What does this assessment data indicate to the nurse?

   a. Crohn's disease

   b. Ulcerative colitis

   c. Appendicitis

   d. Diverticulitis

9. The nurse is caring for a patient who has had an appendectomy. What is the best position for the nurse to maintain the patient in after the surgery?

   a. Prone

   b. Sims' left lateral

   c. High Fowler's

   d. Supine with head of bed elevated 15 degrees

10. A patient is suspected to have diverticulosis without symptoms of diverticulitis. What diagnostic test does the nurse anticipate educating the patient about prior to scheduling?

    a. Colonoscopy

    b. Barium enema

    c. Flexible sigmoidoscopy

    d. CT scan

11. The nurse is admitting a patient with a diagnosis of diverticulitis and assesses that the patient has a boardlike abdomen, no bowel sounds, and complains of severe abdominal pain. What is the nurse's first action?

    a. Start an IV with lactated Ringer's solution.

    b. Notify the physician.

    c. Administer a retention enema.

    d. Administer an opioid analgesic.

12. The nurse is assigned to care for a patient 2 days after an appendectomy due to a ruptured appendix with resultant peritonitis. The nurse has just assisted the patient with ambulation to the bedside commode when the patient points to the surgical site and informs the nurse that "something gave way." What does the nurse suspect may have occurred?

    a. A drain may have become dislodged.

    b. Wound dehiscence has occurred.

    c. Infection has developed.

    d. The surgical wound has begun to bleed.

13. A patient is having a diagnostic workup for complaints of frequent diarrhea, right lower abdominal pain, and weight loss. The nurse is reviewing the results of the barium study and notes the presence of "string sign." What does the nurse understand that this is significant of?

    a. Crohn's disease

    b. Ulcerative colitis

    c. Irritable bowel syndrome

    d. Diverticulitis

14. A patient is being seen in the clinic for complaints of painful hemorrhoids. The nurse assesses the patient and observes the hemorrhoids are prolapsed but able to be placed back in the rectum manually. The nurse documents the hemorrhoids as what degree?

a. First degree

b. Second degree

c. Third degree

d. Fourth degree

15. The nurse is irrigating a colostomy when the patient says, "You will have to stop, I am cramping so badly." What is the priority action by the nurse?

a. Inform the patient that it will only last a minute and continue with the procedure.

b. Clamp the tubing and give the patient a rest period.

c. Stop the irrigation and remove the tube.

d. Replace the fluid with cooler water since it is probably too warm.

Metabolic and Endocrine Function

Assessment and Management of Patients With Hepatic Disorders

Learning Objectives

1. Identify the metabolic functions of the liver and the alterations that occur with hepatic disorders.
2. Explain liver function tests and the clinical manifestations of liver dysfunction in relation to pathophysiologic alterations of the liver.
3. Relate jaundice, portal hypertension, ascites, varices, nutritional deficiencies, and hepatic coma to pathophysiologic alterations of the liver.
4. Describe the medical, surgical, and nursing management of patients with esophageal varices.
5. Compare the various types of hepatitis and their causes, prevention, clinical manifestations, management, prognosis, and home health care needs.
6. Use the nursing process as a framework for care of the patient with cirrhosis of the liver.
7. Compare the nonsurgical and surgical management of patients with cancer of the liver.
8. Describe the postoperative nursing care of the patient undergoing liver transplantation.

SECTION I: ASSESSING YOUR UNDERSTANDING

Activity A *Fill in the blanks.*

1. Liver function tests are not abnormal until _____ % of the liver is revealed to be damaged.

2. The two major complications of a liver biopsy are _____ and _____.

3. The mortality rate for hepatitis B can be as high as _____%.

4. The most common reason for liver transplantation is exposure to _____.

5. Hepatocellular carcinoma is caused by _____, _____, _____, and _____.

6. The leading cause of death after liver transplantation is _____.

7. The majority of blood supply to the liver, which is rich in nutrients from the gastrointestinal tract, comes from the _____.

8. The liver synthesizes prothrombin only if there is enough _____.

9. The substance necessary for the manufacture of bile salts by hepatocytes is _____.

10. Hepatic lobectomy for cancer can be successful when the primary site is localized. Because of the regenerative capacity of the liver, a surgeon can remove up to _____ % of liver tissue.

11. _____, caused by contaminated needles shared by drug users, is also the most common reason for liver transplantation.

12. _____ is the most common single cause of death in patients with cirrhosis.

Activity B *Briefly answer the following.*

1. What age-related changes are significant in the hepatobiliary system?

   _____

   _____

2. What role does the liver play in glucose metabolism?

   _____

   _____

3. Describe the differences between hemolytic, hepatocellular, and obstructive jaundice in regard to etiology.

   _____

   _____

   _____

   _____

4. What is the main function of bile salts?

   _____

5. What are the indications for postexposure vaccination with hepatitis B immunoglobulin?

   _____

   _____

6. Name the chemicals most commonly implicated in toxic hepatitis.

   _____

7. Cirrhosis results in shunting of portal system blood into collateral blood vessels in the gastrointestinal tract. What are the most common sites of engorged collateral blood vessels?

   _____

   _____

8. Name three signs of advanced liver disease.

   _____

Activity C *Match the vitamin listed in Column II with the signs of deficiency due to severe chronic liver disease listed in Column I.*

Column I

____ 1. Hypoprothrombinemia

____ 2. Beriberi and polyneuritis

____ 3. Hemorrhagic lesions of scurvy

____ 4. Night blindness

____ 5. Macrocytic anemia

____ 6. Skin and neurologic changes

____ 7. Mucous membrane lesions

Column II

a. Vitamin A

b. Vitamin C

c. Vitamin K

d. Folic acid

e. Thiamine

f. Riboflavin

g. Pyridoxine

SECTION II: APPLYING YOUR KNOWLEDGE

Activity D *Consider the scenarios and answer the questions.*

CASE STUDY: Liver Biopsy

Veronica, age 46, is scheduled for a liver biopsy to determine if she has cirrhosis of the liver. The nurse assigned to care for Veronica is to accompany her to the treatment room.

1. What preparation is required by the nurse prior to beginning the procedure?

   _____

   _____

2. The nurse is positioning Veronica for the biopsy. What position will the nurse place her in to ensure adequate access to the biopsy site?

   _____

3. What should the nurse instruct Veronica to do immediately before needle insertion?

   _____

   _____

   _____

4. What position should the nurse assist Veronica to maintain immediately after the biopsy is performed?

_____

_____

CASE STUDY: Paracentesis

Wendy, a 62-year-old patient, is scheduled for a paracentesis because of ascites formation subsequent to cirrhosis of the liver.

1. Before the procedure, the nurse obtains several drainage bottles. What is the maximum amount of fluid that should be aspirated during the procedure?

_____

2. What position will the nurse assist Wendy to maintain during the paracentesis?

_____

_____

3. The nurse is monitoring Wendy for signs of vascular collapse. What signs and symptoms would indicate to the nurse that this is occurring?

_____

CASE STUDY: Alcoholic or Nutritional Cirrhosis

Nathan, a 50-year-old physically disabled veteran, has lived alone for 30 years. He has maintained his independence despite chronic back pain resulting from a war injury. He has a long history of depression and limited food intake. He drinks 6 to 10 bottles of beer daily. He was recently admitted to a veteran's hospital with a diagnosis of alcoholic or nutritional cirrhosis. He was asymptomatic for ascites.

1. What early clinical manifestations indicative of alcoholic or nutritional cirrhosis does the nurse assess in Nathan?

_____

2. Nathan is 5 ft 8 in tall and weighs 154 lb. The physician recommends 50 cal/kg for weight gain. What should Nathan's daily caloric intake be?

_____

_____

3. The physician recommends a sodium-restricted diet. What does the nurse expect the suggested sodium intake to be?

_____

CASE STUDY: Liver Transplantation

Denise, a 54-year-old mother of three, is scheduled for a liver transplantation subsequent to an extensive hepatic malignancy with multifocal tumors greater than 8 cm in diameter.

1. What postoperative complication that is common after liver transplant should the nurse monitor Denise for?

_____

2. Denise will be receiving cyclosporine to prevent rejection of the transplanted liver. What potential side effects of the medication may Denise experience?

_____

3. What interventions can the nurse provide for Denise prior to the liver transplant to assist her psychologically to prepare for the procedure?

_____

_____

_____

SECTION III: PRACTICING FROM NCLEX

Activity E *Answer the following questions.*

1. The nurse is educating a patient with cirrhosis about the importance of maintaining a low-sodium diet. What food item would be permitted on a low sodium diet?
   a. Peanut butter
   b. A pear
   c. Hot dog
   d. Sliced ham

2. The nurse is caring for a patient who has ascites as a result of hepatic dysfunction. What intervention can the nurse provide to determine if the ascites is increasing? (Select all that apply.)

   a. Measure urine output every 8 hours.

   b. Assess and document vital signs every 4 hours.

   c. Measure abdominal girth daily.

   d. Perform daily weights.

   e. Monitor number of bowel movements per day.

3. The nurse is concerned about potassium loss when a diuretic is prescribed for a patient with ascites and edema. What diuretic may be ordered that spares potassium and prevents hypokalemia?

   a. Furosemide (Lasix)

   b. Spironolactone (Aldactone)

   c. Acetazolamide (Diamox)

   d. Bumetanide (Bumex)

4. The nurse is caring for a patient with ascites due to cirrhosis of the liver. What position does the nurse understand will activate the renin-angiotensin-aldosterone and sympathetic nervous system and decrease responsiveness to diuretic therapy?

   a. Prone

   b. Supine

   c. Left-lateral Sims'

   d. Upright

5. A patient is scheduled for a diagnostic paracentesis, but when coagulation studies were reviewed, the nurse observed they were abnormal. How does the nurse anticipate the physician will proceed with the paracentesis?

   a. The physician will use an ultrasound-guided paracentesis

   b. The physician will not perform the procedure

   c. The physician will proceed with the paracentesis at the bedside

   d. The physician will have the nurse administer packed RBCs prior to the paracentesis.

6. What intervention does the nurse anticipate providing for the patient with ascites that will help correct the decrease in effective arterial blood volume that leads to sodium retention?

   a. Diuretic therapy

   b. Therapeutic paracentesis

   c. Platelet infusions

   d. Albumin infusion

7. The nurse is providing care to a patient with gross ascites who is maintaining a position of comfort in the high semi-Fowler's position. What is the nurse's priority assessment of this patient?

   a. Respiratory assessment related to increased thoracic pressure

   b. Urinary output related to increased sodium retention

   c. Peripheral vascular assessment related to immobility

   d. Skin assessment related to increase in bile salts

8. A patient with suspected esophageal varices is scheduled for an upper endoscopy with moderate sedation. After the procedure is performed, how long should the nurse withhold food and fluids?

   a. For 2 hours after the last dose of medication is given

   b. Until the gag reflex returns

   c. Until the patient expresses thirst

   d. For 6 hours after the procedure

9. A patient who had a recent myocardial infarction was brought to the emergency department with bleeding esophageal varices and is presently receiving fluid resuscitation. What first-line pharmacologic therapy does the nurse anticipate administering to control the bleeding from the varices?

   a. Vasopressin (Pitressin)

   b. Epinephrine

   c. Octreotide (Sandostatin)

   d. Glucagon

10. A patient with bleeding esophageal varices has had pharmacologic therapy with Octreotide (Sandostatin) and endoscopic therapy with esophageal varices banding, but the patient has continued to have bleeding. What procedure that will lower portal pressure does the nurse prepare the patient for?

    a. Transjugular intrahepatic portosystemic shunting (TIPS)

    b. Vasopressin (Pitressin)

    c. Sclerotherapy

    d. Balloon tamponade

11. The nurse is educating a patient who has been treated for hepatic encephalopathy about dietary restrictions to prevent ammonia accumulation. What should the nurse include in the teaching?

    a. Decrease the amount of fats in the diet.

    b. Increase the amount of potassium in the diet.

    c. Decrease the amount of protein in the diet.

    d. Increase the amount of magnesium in the diet.

12. The nurse is caring for a patient with cirrhosis of the liver and observes that the patient is having hand-flapping tremors. What does the nurse document this finding as?

    a. Constructional apraxia

    b. Fetor hepaticus

    c. Ataxia

    d. Asterixis

13. The nurse is administering Cephulac (lactulose) to decrease the ammonia level in a patient who has hepatic encephalopathy. What should the nurse carefully monitor for that may indicate a medication overdose?

    a. Watery diarrhea

    b. Vomiting

    c. Ringing in the ears

    d. Asterixis

14. A patient with severe chronic liver dysfunction comes to the clinic with bleeding of the gums and blood in the stool. What vitamin deficiency does the nurse suspect the patient may be experiencing?

    a. Riboflavin deficiency

    b. Folic acid deficiency

    c. Vitamin A deficiency

    d. Vitamin K deficiency

15. A student accepted into a nursing program must begin receiving the hepatitis B series of injections. The student asks when the next two injections should be administered. What is the best response by the instructor?

    a. "You must have the second one in 2 weeks and the third in 1 month."

    b. "You must have the second one in 1 month and the third in 6 months."

    c. "You must have the second one in 6 months and the third in 1 year."

    d. "You must have the second one in 1 year and the third the following year."

50

Assessment and Management of Patients With Biliary Disorders

Learning Objectives

1. Identify the structure and function of the biliary tract and pancreas.
2. Compare approaches to management of cholelithiasis.
3. Use the nursing process as a framework for care of patients with cholelithiasis and those undergoing laparoscopic or open cholecystectomy.
4. Differentiate between acute and chronic pancreatitis.
5. Use the nursing process as a framework for care of patients with acute pancreatitis.
6. Describe the nutritional and metabolic effects of surgical treatment of tumors of the pancreas.

SECTION I: ASSESSING YOUR UNDERSTANDING

Activity A *Fill in the blanks.*

1. The capacity of the gallbladder for bile storage is _____ mL.

2. The endocrine secretions of the pancreas are
_____, _____, and _____.

3. Digestive enzymes are secreted by the pancreas: _____ aids in the digestion of carbohydrates, _____ aids in protein digestion, and _____ aids in the digestion of fats.

4. _____ is the cause of more than 90% of cases of acute cholecystitis.

5. The most serious complication after a laparoscopic cholecystectomy is _____ _____.

6. A major cause of morbidity and mortality in patients with acute pancreatitis is _____.

7. Bile is stored in the _____.

8. The major stimulus for increased bicarbonate secretion from the pancreas is _____ _____.

9. Statistics show that there is a greater incidence of gallbladder disease for women who are
_____, _____, and _____.

Activity B *Briefly answer the following.*

1. Describe what occurs when a gallstone obstructs the cystic duct.

2. Why does jaundice occur in patients with gallbladder disease?

_____

_____

3. A patient is scheduled for an outpatient laparoscopic cholecystectomy. Because the patient will only be at the hospital for less than a day, intensive education is necessary. What should the nurse include in the education?

_____

_____

_____

_____

4. Percutaneous cholecystostomy has been used in the treatment and diagnosis of acute cholecystitis in patients who are poor risks for any surgical procedure or for general anesthesia. What type of patients fit these conditions?

_____

_____

5. Name four clinical signs for predicting the severity of pancreatitis and associated mortality.

_____

Activity C *Match the diagnostic study in Column I with the description/purpose of the study in Column II.*

Column I

_____ **1.** Cholecystogram, cholangiogram

_____ **2.** Celiac axis arteriography

_____ **3.** Laparoscopy

_____ **4.** Endoscopic retrograde cholangiopancreatography

_____ **5.** Endoscopic ultrasound (EUS)

Column II

a. Identifies small tumors and facilitates fine needle aspiration biopsy.

b. Visualizes the gallbladder and bile duct.

c. Visualizes the liver and pancreas.

d. Visualizes the biliary structure.

e. Visualizes the pancreas via endoscopy.

SECTION II: APPLYING YOUR KNOWLEDGE

Activity D *Consider the scenario and answer the questions.*

CASE STUDY: Cholecystectomy

Brenda, a 33-year-old obese mother of four, is diagnosed as having acute gallbladder inflammation. She is 5 ft 4 in tall and weighs 190 lb. The physician decides to delay surgical intervention until Brenda's acute symptoms subside.

1. What does the nurse anticipate that Brenda's initial course of treatment will probably consist of?

_____

2. As foods are added to Brenda's diet, she needs to know that she should avoid what type of foods?

_____

3. Brenda is being medicated with chenodeoxycholic acid. What education should the nurse provide to Brenda about the decreased effectiveness of the drug when taken in conjunction with certain items?

_____

CASE STUDY: Cholecystectomy: Postoperative Situation

Because Brenda's symptoms continue to recur, she is scheduled for gallbladder surgery.

1. Brenda is scheduled for a laparoscopic cholecystectomy under general anesthesia. The physician determines that the common bile duct may be obstructed by a gallstone. What should be performed prior to the surgery?

_____

_____

2. What should the nurse assess for postoperatively in order to prevent complications?

_____

_____

3. Brenda needs to know that dietary fat restriction is usually lifted after the biliary ducts dilate to accommodate bile once held by the gallbladder. How long will this take?

_____

SECTION III: PRACTICING FOR NCLEX

Activity E *Answer the following questions.*

1. A patient is diagnosed with gallstones in the bile ducts. What laboratory results should the nurse review?
   a. Serum ammonia concentration of 90 mg/dL
   b. Serum albumin concentration of 4.0 g/dL
   c. Serum bilirubin level greater than 1.0 mg/dL
   d. Serum globulin concentration of 2.0 g/dL

2. A patient is admitted to the hospital with a possible common bile duct obstruction. What clinical manifestations does the nurse understand are indicators of this problem? (Select all that apply.)
   a. Amber-colored urine
   b. Clay-colored feces
   c. Pruritus
   d. Jaundice
   e. Pain in the left upper abdominal quadrant

3. A patient is admitted to the hospital with possible cholelithiasis. What diagnostic test of choice will the nurse prepare the patient for?
   a. X-ray
   b. Oral cholecystography
   c. Cholecystography
   d. Ultrasonography

4. A patient is receiving pharmacologic therapy with ursodeoxycholic acid or chenodeoxycholic acid for treatment of small gallstones. The patient asks the nurse how long the therapy will take to dissolve the stones. What is the best answer the nurse can give?
   a. 1 to 2 months
   b. 3 to 5 months
   c. 6 to 8 months
   d. 6 to 12 months

5. A patient is diagnosed with mild acute pancreatitis. What does the nurse understand is characteristic of this disorder?
   a. Edema and inflammation
   b. Pleural effusion
   c. Sepsis
   d. Disseminated intravascular coagulopathy

6. The nurse is admitting a patient to the intensive care unit with a diagnosis of acute pancreatitis. What does the nurse expect was the reason the patient came to the hospital?
   a. Severe abdominal pain
   b. Fever
   c. Jaundice
   d. Mental agitation

7. The nurse should assess for an important early indicator of acute pancreatitis. What prolonged and elevated level would the nurse determine is an early indicator?
   a. Serum calcium
   b. Serum lipase
   c. Serum bilirubin
   d. Serum amylase

8. When caring for the patient with acute pancreatitis, the nurse must consider pain relief measures. What nursing interventions could the nurse provide? (Select all that apply.)
   a. Encouraging bed rest to decrease the metabolic rate
   b. Assisting the patient into the prone position
   c. Withholding oral feedings to limit the release of secretin
   d. Administering parenteral opioid analgesics as ordered
   e. Administering prophylactic antibiotics

9. A patient is suspected to have pancreatic carcinoma and is having diagnostic testing to determine insulin deficiency. What would the nurse determine is an indicator for insulin deficiency in this patient? (Select all that apply.)
   a. An abnormal glucose tolerance
   b. Glucosuria
   c. Hyperglycemia
   d. Elevated lipase level
   e. Hypoglycemia

10. A nurse should monitor blood glucose levels for a patient diagnosed with hyperinsulinism. What blood value does the nurse recognize as inadequate to sustain normal brain function?
    a. 30 mg/dL
    b. 50 mg/dL
    c. 70 mg/dL
    d. 90 mg/dL

11. The nurse is caring for a patient with acute pancreatitis. The patient has an order for an anticholinergic medication. The nurse explains that the patient will be receiving that medication for what reason?
    a. To decrease metabolism
    b. To depress the central nervous system and increase the pain threshold
    c. To reduce gastric and pancreatic secretions
    d. To relieve nausea and vomiting

12. The patient admitted with acute pancreatitis has passed the acute stage and is now able to tolerate solid foods. What type of diet will increase caloric intake without stimulating pancreatic enzymes beyond the ability of the pancreas to respond?
    a. Low-sodium, high-potassium, low-fat diet
    b. High-carbohydrate, high-protein, low-fat diet
    c. Low-carbohydrate, high-potassium diet
    d. High-carbohydrate, low-protein, low-fat diet

13. When the nurse is caring for a patient with acute pancreatitis, what intervention can be provided in order to prevent atelectasis and prevent pooling of respiratory secretions?
    a. Frequent changes of positions
    b. Placing the patient in the prone position
    c. Perform chest physiotherapy
    d. Suction the patient every 4 hours

14. A patient with acute pancreatitis puts the call bell on to tell the nurse about an increase in pain. The nurse observes the patient guarding; the abdomen is boardlike and no bowel sounds are detected. What is the major concern for this patient?
    a. The patient requires more pain medication.
    b. The patient is developing a paralytic ileus.
    c. The patient has developed peritonitis.
    d. The patient has developed renal failure.

15. What is a major concern for the nurse when caring for a patient with chronic pancreatitis?
    a. Pain
    b. Weight loss
    c. Nausea
    d. Mental status changes

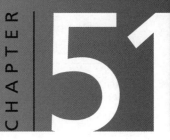
Assessment and Management of Patients With Diabetes

Learning Objectives

1. Differentiate between type 1 and type 2 diabetes.
2. Describe etiologic factors associated with diabetes.
3. Relate the clinical manifestations of diabetes to the associated pathophysiologic alterations.
4. Identify the diagnostic and clinical significance of blood glucose test results.
5. Explain the dietary modifications used for management of people with diabetes.
6. Describe the relationships among diet, exercise, and medication (i.e., insulin or oral antidiabetic agents) for people with diabetes.
7. Develop an education plan for insulin self-management.
8. Identify the role of oral antidiabetic agents in therapy for patients with diabetes.
9. Use the nursing process as a framework for care of patients who have hyperglycemia with diabetic ketoacidosis or hyperglycemic hyperosmolar syndrome.
10. Describe management strategies for a person with diabetes to use during "sick days."
11. Describe the major macrovascular, microvascular, and neuropathic complications of diabetes and the self-care behaviors that are important in their prevention.
12. Identify the programs and community support groups available for people with diabetes.

SECTION I: ASSESSING YOUR UNDERSTANDING

Activity A *Fill in the blanks.*

1. It is estimated that more than _____ million people in the United States have diabetes, although almost one third of these cases are undiagnosed.

2. In the United States, diabetes is the leading cause of _____, _____, and _____.

3. The major classifications of diabetes are: _____, _____, _____, and diabetes associated with other conditions or syndromes.

4. Because insulin normally inhibits _____ and _____, these processes occur in an unrestrained fashion in people with insulin deficiency and contribute further to hyperglycemia.

5. When excess glucose is excreted in the urine, it is accompanied by excessive loss of fluids and electrolytes, which is called _____.

6. Insulin resistance refers to a _____ tissue sensitivity to insulin.

7. Uncontrolled type 2 diabetes may lead to an acute problem—_____ _____.

8. Gestational diabetes occurs in as many as ____% of pregnant women and increases their risk for hypertensive disorders during pregnancy.

9. Goals for blood glucose levels during pregnancy are _____ or less before meals and _____ or less 2 hours after meals.

10. Classic clinical manifestations of diabetes include the "three Ps": _____, _____, and _____.

11. A finding of _____ is the basic criterion for the diagnosis of diabetes.

12. Type 2 diabetes is the _____ leading cause of death and affects approximately ____% of older adults.

13. A woman at average risk for the development of hyperglycemia during pregnancy should be tested at _____ weeks of gestation.

14. _____ is the most common risk of insulin pump therapy.

15. _____, _____, and _____ are the three metabolic derangements that occur in diabetic ketoacidosis.

Activity B *Briefly answer the following.*

1. Why does the economic cost of diabetes continue to increase?

_____

_____

2. Why does hyperglycemia develop during pregnancy?

_____

_____

3. What are two main problems related to insulin in type 2 diabetes?

_____

_____

4. When educating a patient with diabetes about increasing fiber intake, what risks should be discussed?

_____

_____

_____

5. Describe how insulin regulation is altered in the diabetic state.

_____

_____

_____

_____

6. List the clinical manifestations characteristic of hyperglycemic hyperosmolar syndrome.

_____

_____

7. How do sulfonylureas act for patients with type II diabetes?

_____

_____

Activity C *Match the physiologic change listed in Column II with its associated term listed in Column I.*

Column I

____ **1.** Gluconeogenesis

____ **2.** Glucosuria

____ **3.** Glycogenolysis

____ **4.** Nephropathy

____ **5.** Retinopathy

Column II

a. Filtered glucose that the kidney cannot absorb spills over into urine.

b. Glycogen breaks down in the liver through the action of glucagon.

c. New glucose is produced from amino acids.

d. Microvascular changes develop in the eyes.

e. Small vessel disease affects the kidneys.

SECTION II: APPLYING YOUR KNOWLEDGE

Activity D *Consider the scenarios and answer the questions.*

CASE STUDY: Type 1 Diabetes

Albert, a 35-year-old, insulin-dependent diabetic patient, is admitted to the hospital with a diagnosis of pneumonia. He has been febrile since admission. His daily insulin requirement is 24 units of NPH.

1. Every morning Albert is given NPH (neutral protamine Hagedorn) insulin at 7:30 AM. Meals are served at 8:30 AM, 12:30 PM, and 6:30 PM. Between what hours does the nurse expect that the NPH insulin will reach its maximum effect (peak)?

   _____

2. A bedtime snack is provided for Albert. This is based on the knowledge that intermediate-acting insulins are effective for what duration of time?

   _____

3. Albert refuses his bedtime snack. What is a priority for the nurse to assess due to his refusal of a snack?

   _____

   _____

CASE STUDY: Hypoglycemia

Betty, an 18-year-old type 1 diabetic patient, is unconscious when admitted to the hospital. Her daily dose of insulin has been 32 units of NPH each morning. Her mother informs the nurse that Betty and her boyfriend just broke up prior to both going away to college and she hasn't been eating well since the breakup.

1. What factors may have contributed to the development of Betty's hypoglycemia?

   _____

2. Betty is given 1 mg of glucagon hydrochloride, subcutaneously, in the emergency department. What latent symptoms should the nurse monitor for related to the action of the glucagon?

   _____

   _____

3. After Betty is medically stabilized, she is admitted to the clinical area for observation and health teaching. What warning symptoms should the nurse educate Betty about associated with hypoglycemia?

   _____

   _____

4. What information can the nurse provide to Betty to help prevent future events of hypoglycemia?

   _____

   _____

   _____

CASE STUDY: Diabetic Ketoacidosis

Christine, a 64-year-old woman, is admitted to the clinical area with a diagnosis of diabetic ketoacidosis. Christine lives alone and is frequently noncompliant with her dietary and medication regimen. She has had several admissions prior to this one. On admission, she is drowsy yet responsive.

1. What priority actions should the nurse take in caring for Christine?

   _____

   _____

   _____

2. What rehydrating intravenous solution does the nurse expect to infuse?

   _____

3. What laboratory results would the nurse expect to find that may be associated with Christine's condition?

   _____

4. The physician orders an insulin drip to be started at 5 units/hr. When hanging the drip, what should the nurse do prior to connecting the drip to the patient?

   _____

   _____

   _____

5. As blood glucose levels approach normal, what electrolyte imbalance should the nurse assess for?

   _____

SECTION III: PRACTICING FOR NCLEX

Activity E *Answer the following questions.*

1. A patient is diagnosed with type 1 diabetes. What clinical characteristics does the nurse expect to see in this patient? (Select all that apply.)
   a. Ketosis-prone
   b. Little endogenous insulin
   c. Obesity at diagnoses
   d. Younger than 30 years of age
   e. Older than 65 years of age

2. When the nurse is caring for a patient with type 1 diabetes, what clinical manifestation would be a priority to closely monitor?
   a. Hypoglycemia
   b. Hyponatremia
   c. Ketonuria
   d. Polyphagia

3. A female diabetic patient who weighs 130 lb has an ideal body weight of 116 lb. For weight reduction of 2 lb/week, approximately what should her daily caloric intake be?
   a. 1000 calories
   b. 1200 calories
   c. 1500 calories
   d. 1,800 calories

4. The nurse is preparing to administer intermediate-acting insulin to a patient with diabetes. Which insulin will the nurse administer?
   a. NPH
   b. Iletin II
   c. Humalog (Lispro)
   d. Glargine (Lantus)

5. An older adult patient that has diabetes type 2 comes to the emergency department with second-degree burns to the bottom of both feet and states, "I didn't feel too hot but my feet must have been too close to the heater." What does the nurse understand is most likely the reason for the decrease in temperature sensation?
   a. A faulty heater
   b. Autonomic neuropathy
   c. Peripheral neuropathy
   d. Sudomotor neuropathy

6. The nurse is caring for a patient with an abnormally low blood glucose concentration. What glucose level will the nurse observe when assessing laboratory results?
   a. Lower than 50–60 mg/dL
   b. Between 60 and 80 mg/dL
   c. Between 75 and 90 mg/dL
   d. 95 mg/dL

7. A patient with diabetic ketoacidosis has had a large volume of fluid infused for rehydration. What potential complication from rehydration should the nurse monitor for?
   a. Hypokalemia
   b. Hyperkalemia
   c. Hyperglycemia
   d. Hyponatremia

8. The nurse is assessing a patient with nonproliferative (background) retinopathy. When examining the retina, what would the nurse expect to assess? (Select all that apply.)
   a. Leakage of fluid or serum (exudates)
   b. Microaneurysms
   c. Focal capillary single closure
   d. Detachment
   e. Blurred optic discs

9. A nurse is caring for a diabetic patient with a diagnosis of nephropathy. What would the nurse expect the urinalysis report to indicate?
   a. Albumin
   b. Bacteria
   c. Red blood cells
   d. White blood cells

10. The nurse expects that a type 1 diabetic patient may receive what percentage of his or her usual morning dose of insulin preoperatively?
    a. 10% to 20%
    b. 25% to 40%
    c. 50% to 60%
    d. 85% to 90%

11. An older adult patient is in the hospital being treated for sepsis related to a urinary tract infection. The patient has started to have an altered sense of awareness, profound dehydration, and hypotension. What does the nurse suspect the patient is experiencing?

   a. Systemic inflammatory response syndrome

   b. Hyperglycemic hyperosmolar syndrome

   c. Multiple-organ dysfunction syndrome

   d. Diabetic ketoacidosis

12. The nurse is preparing to administer IV fluids for a patient with ketoacidosis who has a history of hypertension and congestive heart failure. What order for fluids would the nurse anticipate infusing for this patient?

   a. D5W

   b. 0.9% normal saline

   c. 0.45 normal saline

   d. D5 normal saline

13. A patient has been newly diagnosed with type 2 diabetes, and the nurse is assisting with the development of a meal plan. What step should be taken into consideration prior to making the meal plan?

   a. Making sure that the patient is aware that quantity of foods will be limited

   b. Ensuring that the patient understands that some favorite foods may not be allowed on the meal plan and substitutes will need to be found

   c. Determining whether the patient is on insulin or taking oral antidiabetic medication

   d. Reviewing the patient's diet history to identify eating habits and lifestyle and cultural eating patterns

14. The nurse is educating the patient with diabetes about the importance of increasing dietary fiber. What should the nurse explain is the rationale for the increase? (Select all that apply.)

   a. May improve blood glucose levels

   b. Decrease the need for exogenous insulin

   c. Help reduce cholesterol levels

   d. May reduce postprandial glucose levels

   e. Increase potassium levels

15. The nurse is educating a patient about the benefits of fruit versus fruit juice in the diabetic diet. The patient states, "What difference does it make if you drink the juice or eat the fruit? It is all the same." What is the best response by the nurse?

   a. "Eating the fruit is more satisfying than drinking the juice. You will get full faster."

   b. "Eating the fruit will give you more vitamins and minerals than the juice will."

   c. "The fruit has less sugar than the juice."

   d. "Eating the fruit instead of drinking juice decreases the glycemic index by slowing absorption."

16. The nurse is administering an insulin drip to a patient in ketoacidosis. What insulin does the nurse know is the only one that can be used intravenously?

   a. NPH

   b. Regular

   c. Lispro

   d. Lantus

CHAPTER 52

Assessment and Management of Patients With Endocrine Disorders

Learning Objectives

1. Describe the functions of each of the endocrine glands and their hormones.
2. Identify the diagnostic tests used to determine alterations in function of each of the endocrine glands.
3. Use the nursing process as a framework for care of patients with hyperthyroidism.
4. Develop a plan of nursing care for the patient undergoing thyroidectomy.
5. Compare hyperparathyroidism and hypoparathyroidism: their causes, clinical manifestations, management, and nursing interventions.
6. Compare Addison's disease with Cushing syndrome: their causes, clinical manifestations, management, and nursing interventions.
7. Describe nursing management of patients with adrenal insufficiency.
8. Use the nursing process as a framework for care of patients with Cushing syndrome.
9. Identify the education needs of patients requiring corticosteroid therapy.

SECTION I: ASSESSING YOUR UNDERSTANDING

Activity A *Fill in the blanks.*

1. The term used to describe the regulation of hormone concentration in the bloodstream is
_____.

2. The _____ is the major structure that balances the rapid action of the nervous system with slower hormonal action.

3. The two major hormones secreted by the posterior lobe of the pituitary gland are
_____, which controls
_____, and
_____, which facilitates
_____.

4. Oversecretion of adrenocorticotropic hormone (ACTH), or the growth hormone, results in
_____ or _____.

5. A deficiency of ADH or vasopressin can result in the disorder known as _____,
which is characterized by
_____ and
_____.

6. The thyroid gland produces three hormones: _____, _____, and _____.

7. The most common cause of hypothyroidism is _____.

8. Primary hyperthyroidism occurs two to four times more often in _____ than in _____.

9. The most common type of hyperthyroidism is _____.

10. The two most common medications used to treat hyperthyroidism are _____ and _____.

11. Tetany is evidenced when either of these signs are positive: _____ or _____.

12. The three types of steroid hormones produced by the adrenal cortex are _____, _____, and _____.

13. One of the most important and frequently occurring complications of hyperparathyroidism is _____.

14. _____ is the most common cause of thyrotoxicosis in the older adult patient.

Activity B *Briefly answer the following.*

1. Name the hormones that the anterior pituitary gland is responsible for secreting.

   _____

   _____

2. List four ways that hormones are classified.

   _____

   _____

3. What does the nurse understand are the objectives in the management of hypothyroidism?

   _____

   _____

   _____

4. Describe how radioactive iodine would be administered to a patient with cancer of the thyroid gland.

   _____

   _____

   _____

Activity C *Match the hormonal function listed in Column II with its corresponding hormone listed in Column I.*

Column I

_____ 1. Glucagon

_____ 2. Aldosterone

_____ 3. Oxytocin

_____ 4. Somatotropin

_____ 5. Vasopressin

_____ 6. Calcitonin

_____ 7. Prolactin

_____ 8. Melatonin

_____ 9. Parathormone

_____ 10. Insulin

Column II

a. Controls excretion of water by the kidneys.

b. Lowers blood sugar.

c. Inhibits bone resorption.

d. Influences metabolism that is essential for normal growth.

e. Supports sexual maturation.

f. Promotes the secretion of milk.

g. Stimulates the reabsorption of sodium and the elimination of potassium.

h. Promotes glycogenolysis.

i. Increases the force of uterine contractions during parturition.

j. Regulates serum calcium.

SECTION II: APPLYING YOUR KNOWLEDGE

Activity D *Consider the scenarios and answer the questions.*

CASE STUDY: Primary Hypothyroidism

Connie, age 28, has been hospitalized for 2 days for symptoms leading to the diagnosis of primary hypothyroidism.

1. What tests does the nurse know will assist with the confirmation of diagnosis of primary hypothyroidism for Connie?

   _____

   _____

2. What clinical manifestations that are consistent with Connie's diagnosis should be monitored?

_____

_____

_____

3. What comfort measures can the nurse include in Connie's care?

_____

_____

4. Connie is ordered Synthroid 0.125 mg orally daily. What education should the nurse provide?

_____

_____

_____

_____

CASE STUDY: Hyperparathyroidism

Emily is a 65-year-old woman who has been complaining of continued emotional irritability. Her family describes her as always being "on edge" and neurotic. After several months of exacerbated symptoms, Emily underwent a complete physical examination and was diagnosed with hyperparathyroidism.

1. Emily is having difficulty closing her eyes and has to use artificial tears because her eyes are so dry. What condition does the nurse observe that Emily has that causes this problem?

_____

_____

2. Emily also complains of "feeling like my heart is beating out of my chest." What does the nurse explain to Emily is causing this feeling?

_____

_____

3. Emily is started on methimazole (Tapazole) for treatment of the hyperthyroidism. What education does the nurse provide about the medication?

_____

_____

_____

CASE STUDY: Subtotal Thyroidectomy

Darrell, a 37-year-old father of two, has just returned to the clinical area from the recovery room. Darrell has had a subtotal thyroidectomy.

1. Postoperatively, Darrell is assisted from the stretcher to the bed. What position of comfort should the nurse help Darrell to maintain?

_____

2. The nurse should assess for the common manifestation of recurrent laryngeal nerve damage. What is an indicator for this type of nerve damage?

_____

3. What should the nurse be sure to have available to administer if tetany occurs?

_____

SECTION III: PRACTICING FOR NCLEX

Activity E *Answer the following questions.*

1. When thyroid hormone is administered for prolonged hypothyroidism for a patient, what should the nurse monitor for?
   a. Angina
   b. Depression
   c. Mental confusion
   d. Hypoglycemia

2. A patient comes to the clinic with complaints of severe thirst. The patient has been drinking up to 10 L of cold water a day, and the patient's urine looks like water. What diagnostic test does the nurse anticipate the physician will order for diagnosis?
   a. Complete blood count (CBC)
   b. Fluid deprivation test
   c. Urine specific gravity
   d. TSH test

3. What clinical manifestations does the nurse recognize would be associated with a diagnosis of hyperthyroidism? (Select all that apply.)
   a. A pulse rate slower than 90 bpm
   b. An elevated systolic blood pressure
   c. Muscular fatigability
   d. Weight loss.
   e. Intolerance to cold

4. The nurse is caring for a patient with hyperthyroidism who suddenly develops symptoms related to thyroid storm. What symptoms does the nurse recognize that are indicative of this emergency?

a. Heart rate of 62

b. Blood pressure 90/58 mm Hg

c. Oxygen saturation of 96%

d. Temperature of 102°F

5. What pharmacologic therapy does the nurse anticipate administering when the patient is experiencing thyroid storm? (Select all that apply.)

a. Acetaminophen

b. Iodine

c. Propylthiouracil

d. Synthetic levothyroxine

e. Dexamethasone (Decadron)

6. The nurse assesses a patient who has an obvious goiter. What type of deficiency does the nurse recognize is most likely the cause of this?

a. Thyrotropin

b. Iodine

c. Thyroxine

d. Calcitonin

7. What breakfast items would the nurse recommend when assisting with the breakfast menu for a patient with hyperthyroidism?

a. Cereal with milk and bananas

b. Fried eggs and bacon

c. Orange juice and toast

d. Pork sausage and cranberry juice

8. A patient is suspected of having a pheochromocytoma and is having diagnostic tests done in the hospital. What symptoms does the nurse recognize as most significant for a patient with this disorder?

a. Blood pressure varying between 120/86 and 240/130 mm Hg

b. Heart rate of 56–64 bpm

c. Shivering

d. Complaints of nausea

9. A patient is diagnosed with overactivity of the adrenal medulla. What epinephrine value does the nurse recognize is a positive diagnostic indicator for overactivity of the adrenal medulla?

a. 50 pg/mL

b. 100 pg/mL

c. 100 to 300 pg/mL

d. 450 pg/mL

10. The nurse is caring for a patient with hyperparathyroidism and observes a calcium level of 16.2 mg/dL. What interventions does the nurse prepare to provide to reduce the calcium level? (Select all that apply.)

a. Administration of calcitonin

b. Administration of calcium carbonate

c. Intravenous isotonic saline solution in large quantities

d. Monitoring the patient for fluid overload

e. Administration of a bronchodilator

11. A patient is ordered desmopressin (DDAVP) for the treatment of diabetes insipidus. What therapeutic response does the nurse anticipate the patient will experience?

a. A decrease in blood pressure

b. A decrease in blood glucose levels

c. A decrease in urine output

d. A decrease in appetite

12. The nurse auscultates a bruit over the thyroid glands. What does the nurse understand is the significance of this finding?

a. The patient may have hypothyroidism.

b. The patient may have thyroiditis.

c. The patient may have hyperthyroidism.

d. The patient may have Cushing disease.

13. A patient with a history of hypothyroidism is admitted to the intensive care unit unconscious and with a temperature of 95.2°F. A family member informs the nurse that the patient has not taken thyroid medication in over 2 months. What does the nurse suspect that these findings indicate?

a. Thyroid storm

b. Myxedema coma

c. Diabetes insipidus

d. Syndrome of inappropriate antidiuretic hormone (SIADH)

14. The nurse on the telemetry floor is caring for a patient with long-standing hypothyroidism who has been taking synthetic thyroid hormone replacement sporadically. What is a priority that the nurse monitors for in this patient?

   a. Symptoms of acute coronary syndrome

   b. Dietary intake of foods with saturated fats

   c. Symptoms of pneumonia

   d. Heat intolerance

15. A patient taking corticosteroids for exacerbation of Crohn's disease comes to the clinic and informs the nurse that he wants to stop taking them because of the increase in acne and moon face. What can the nurse educate the patient regarding these symptoms?

   a. The symptoms are permanent side effects of the corticosteroid therapy.

   b. The moon face and acne will resolve when the medication is tapered off.

   c. Those symptoms are not related to the corticosteroid therapy.

   d. The dose of the medication must be too high and should be lowered.

16. A patient has been taking tricyclic antidepressants for many years for the treatment of depression. The patient has developed SIADH and has been admitted to the acute care facility. What should the nurse carefully monitor when caring for this patient? (Select all that apply.)

   a. Strict intake and output

   b. Neurologic function

   c. Urine and blood chemistry

   d. Liver function tests

   e. Signs of dehydration

Kidney and Urinary Function

Assessment of Kidney and Urinary Function

Learning Objectives

1. Describe the anatomy and physiology of the renal and urinary systems.
2. Discuss the role of the kidneys in regulating fluid and electrolyte balance, acid–base balance, and blood pressure.
3. Describe the gerontologic considerations related to upper and lower urinary tract function.
4. Describe the diagnostic studies used to determine upper and lower urinary tract function.
5. Identify the assessment parameters used for determining the status of upper and lower urinary tract function.
6. Initiate education and preparation for patients undergoing assessment of the urinary system.

SECTION I: ASSESSING YOUR UNDERSTANDING

Activity A *Fill in the blanks.*

1. The functional unit of each kidney is the _____, located in the _____ of the kidney.

2. Normal adult bladder capacity is _____ mL of urine.

3. The urine osmolality level that indicates an early sign of kidney disease is _____.

4. The regulation of the amount of sodium excreted depends on the hormone _____.

5. When a person is dehydrated, the urine osmolality is _____.

6. Water is reabsorbed, rather than excreted, under the control of the _____ _____.

7. The normal serum pH is _____; urine pH is ____.

8. The major waste product of protein metabolism is _____, with approximately _____ g produced and excreted daily.

9. The test that most accurately reflects glomerular filtration and renal excretory function is the _____ test.

Activity B *Briefly answer the following.*

1. At what point will a patient receive renal replacement therapy?

_____

_____

2. Name the three areas of the ureters that have a propensity for obstruction by renal calculi.

_____

_____

3. Where are amino acids and glucose usually filtered?

_____

_____

4. Where is the antidiuretic hormone (ADH), or vasopressin, secreted?

_____

_____

5. What does the regulation of sodium volume excreted depend on?

_____

_____

Activity C *Match the description of pain in Column II with the pain location in Column I.*

Column I

____ **1.** Kidney

____ **2.** Bladder

____ **3.** Ureteral

____ **4.** Prostatic

____ **5.** Urethral

Column II

a. Severe, sharp, stabbing, colicky

b. Dull, constant ache

c. Vague discomfort

d. Dull continuous pain, intense when voiding

e. Pain variable, most severe during and immediately after voiding

SECTION II: APPLYING YOUR KNOWLEDGE

Activity D *Consider the scenario and answer the questions.*

Carol, age 55, is having a kidney biopsy to determine the cause of her frequent episodes of hematuria. Carol has had several other diagnostic tests performed with inconclusive results and is experiencing blood in her urine.

1. Before the biopsy is carried out, what laboratory studies should be conducted for Carol in order to identify any risk of postbiopsy bleeding?

_____

_____

2. What position will the nurse assist Carol in maintaining during the procedure?

_____

_____

3. What intervention does the nurse anticipate providing to clear any blood from the urine after the procedure?

_____

_____

SECTION III: PRACTICING FOR NCLEX

Activity E *Answer the following questions.*

1. A patient has an increase in blood osmolality when the nurse reviews the laboratory work. What can this increase indicate for the patient?

   a. ADH stimulation

   b. An increase in urine volume

   c. Diuresis

   d. Less reabsorption of water

2. A patient is being seen in the clinic for possible kidney disease. What major sensitive indicator of kidney disease does the nurse anticipate the patient will be tested for?

   a. Blood urea nitrogen level

   b. Creatinine clearance level

   c. Serum potassium level

   d. Uric acid level

3. The nurse is caring for a patient with end-stage kidney disease in the hospital and smells a fetid odor from the patient's breath. What major manifestation of uremia will be present?

   a. A decreased serum phosphorus level

   b. Hyperparathyroidism

   c. Hypocalcemia with bone changes

   d. Increased secretion of parathormone

4. The nurse is assessing a patient upon admission to the hospital. What significant nursing assessment data is relevant to renal function? (Select all that apply.)

   a. Any voiding disorders

   b. The patient's occupation

   c. The presence of hypertension or diabetes

   d. The patient's financial status

   e. The ability of the patient to manage activities of daily living

5. The nurse is assigned to care for a patient in the oliguric phase of kidney failure. When does the nurse understand that oliguria is said to be present?

   a. When the urine output is less than 30 mL/h

   b. When the urine output is about 100 mL/h

   c. When the urine output is between 300 and 500 mL/h

   d. When the urine output is between 500 and 1,000 mL/h

6. A 24-hour urine collection is scheduled to begin at 8:00 AM. When should the nurse initiate the procedure?

   a. After discarding the 8:00 AM specimen

   b. At 8:00 AM, with or without a specimen

   c. 6 hours after the urine is discarded

   d. With the first specimen voided after 8:00 AM

7. The nurse is educating a patient about preparation for an IV urography. What should the nurse be sure to include in the preparation instructions?

   a. A liquid restriction for 8 to 10 hours before the test is required

   b. The patient may have liquids before the test.

   c. The patient will have enemas until the urine is clear.

   d. The patient is restricted from eating or drinking from midnight until after the test.

8. A patient had a renal angiography and is being brought back to the hospital room. What nursing interventions should the nurse carry out after the procedure to detect complications? (Select all that apply.)

   a. Assess peripheral pulses.

   b. Compare color and temperature between the involved and uninvolved extremities.

   c. Examine the puncture site for swelling and hematoma formation.

   d. Apply warm compresses to the insertion site to decrease swelling.

   e. Increase the amount of IV fluids to prevent clot formation.

9. A patient is having an MAG3 renogram and is informed that radioactive material will be injected to determine kidney function. What should the nurse instruct the patient to do during the procedure?

   a. Lie still on the table for approximately 35 minutes.

   b. Drink contrast material at various intervals during the procedure.

   c. Turn from side to side to get a variety of views during the procedure.

   d. Take deep breaths and hold them at various times throughout the procedure.

10. A patient is scheduled for a test with contrast to determine kidney function. What statement made by the patient should the nurse inform the physician about prior to testing?

    a. "I don't like needles."

    b. "I am allergic to shrimp."

    c. "I take medication to help me sleep at night."

    d. "I have had a test similar to this one in the past."

CHAPTER 54

Management of Patients With Kidney Disorders

Learning Objectives

1. Describe the key factors associated with the development of kidney disorders.
2. Differentiate between the causes of chronic kidney disease and acute kidney injury.
3. Compare and contrast the pathophysiology, clinical manifestations, medical management, and nursing management for patients with kidney disorders.
4. Describe the nursing management of patients with chronic kidney disease and acute kidney injury.
5. Compare and contrast the renal replacement therapies including hemodialysis, peritoneal dialysis, continuous renal replacement therapies, and kidney transplantation.
6. Describe the nursing management of the patient on dialysis who is hospitalized.
7. Develop a postoperative plan of nursing care for the patient undergoing kidney surgery and transplantation.

SECTION I: ASSESSING YOUR UNDERSTANDING

Activity A *Fill in the blanks.*

1. The primary cause of chronic kidney disease is _____.

2. Nephrosclerosis is primarily caused by _____ and _____.

3. Two blood levels that are significantly increased in acute kidney injury (AKI) are _____ and _____.

4. _____ is the leading cause of death for patients undergoing chronic hemodialysis.

5. The most common and serious complication of continuous ambulatory peritoneal dialysis (CAPD) is _____.

6. Two complications of renal surgery that are believed to be caused by reflex paralysis of intestinal peristalsis and manipulation of the colon or duodenum during surgery are _____ and _____.

7. The most accurate indicator of fluid loss or gain in an acutely ill patient is _____.

8. The major manifestation of nephrotic syndrome is _____.

9. The most common type of renal carcinoma arises from the renal epithelium and accounts for more than ____% of all kidney tumors.

10. The four phases of acute kidney injury are _____, _____, _____, and _____.

11. _____ is the type of renal failure characterized by increased glomerular permeability and manifested by massive proteinuria.

Activity B *Briefly answer the following.*

1. List some of the signs that a patient with chronic glomerulonephritis may be developing heart failure:

   _____

   _____

   _____

2. Name the clinical findings that the nurse would expect to find in a patient who has nephrotic syndrome:

   _____

   _____

   _____

3. What is the difference between autosomal-dominant and autosomal-recessive polycystic kidney disease?

   _____

   _____

   _____

   _____

4. How can the nurse assist the patient with all of the testing required to detect a possible renal tumor?

   _____

   _____

   _____

5. List the factors that influence mortality rate in patients with acute kidney injury:

   _____

   _____

Activity C *Match the symptom listed in Column II with its associated fluid or electrolyte imbalance listed in Column I.*

Column I

____ 1. Calcium deficit

____ 2. Calcium excess

____ 3. Fluid volume deficit

____ 4. Fluid volume excess

____ 5. Magnesium deficit

____ 6. Potassium deficit

____ 7. Potassium excess

____ 8. Protein deficit

____ 9. Sodium deficit

____ 10. Sodium excess

Column II

a. Carpopedal spasm and tetany

b. Muscle hypotonicity and flank pain

c. Oliguria and weight loss

d. Positive Chvostek's sign

e. Crackles and dyspnea

f. Chronic weight loss and fatigability

g. Fingerprinting on the sternum

h. Irritability and intestinal colic

i. Rough, dry tongue and thirst

j. Soft, flabby muscles and weakness

SECTION II: APPLYING YOUR KNOWLEDGE

Activity D *Consider the scenarios and answer the questions.*

CASE STUDY: Continuous Ambulatory Peritoneal Dialysis (CAPD)

Edward is a 29-year-old diabetic patient with end-stage kidney disease (ESKD). He had had a kidney transplant that was rejected and chose CAPD as a way of managing his ESKD. The nurse has been educating Edward about the use of CAPD and will have a home health nurse come in to the home and ensure that he will be able to manage the regimen.

1. Why does the nurse believe that Edward chose to manage his ESKD with CAPD?

   _____

   _____

2. Using CAPD, how often would Edward need to dialyze himself?

   _____

3. Edward needs to be aware that toxic wastes are exchanged during the equilibration or dwell time. How long is he instructed to allow the fluid to dwell?

_____

4. The nurse is educating Edward about the dietary modifications that are necessary to decrease the amount of accumulated waste products. What should the nurse be sure to include in the education?

_____

CASE STUDY: Acute Kidney Injury

Fran, a 42-year-old patient, is hospitalized with a diagnosis of AKI resulting from the administration of gentamicin sulfate for a pseudomonal infection. Fran is acutely ill upon admission and experiencing an altered level of consciousness.

1. The nurse is concerned that Fran may experience reduced kidney blood flow. What symptoms would the nurse assess for?

_____

2. During the oliguric phase of AKI, what should Fran's protein intake for her 156-lb body weight be?

_____

3. When Fran has passed the diuretic phase, what diet should the nurse recommend for her?

_____

4. After the oliguric phase, Fran will experience a period of recovery. How long would the nurse expect the recovery period to last?

_____

SECTION III: PRACTICING FOR NCLEX

Activity E *Answer the following questions.*

1. The nurse notes that a patient who is retaining fluid had a 1-kg weight gain. The nurse knows that this is equivalent to about how many mL?
   a. 250 mL
   b. 500 mL
   c. 750 mL
   d. 1,000 mL

2. A patient admitted with electrolyte imbalance has carpopedal spasm, ECG changes, and a positive Chvostek's sign. What deficit does the nurse suspect the patient has?
   a. Calcium
   b. Magnesium
   c. Phosphorus
   d. Sodium

3. The nurse is reviewing a patient's laboratory results. What findings does the nurse assess that are consistent with acute glomerulonephritis? (Select all that apply.)
   a. Red blood cells in the urine
   b. Polyuria.
   c. Proteinuria
   d. White cell casts in the urine
   e. Hemoglobin of 12.8 g/dL

4. The nurse is caring for a patient in the oliguric phase of AKI. What does the nurse know would be the daily urine output?
   a. 1.5 L
   b. 1.0 L
   c. Less than 400 mL
   d. Less than 50 mL

5. The nurse is educating a patient who is required to restrict potassium intake. What foods would the nurse suggest the patient eliminate that are rich in potassium?
   a. Butter
   b. Citrus fruits
   c. Cooked white rice
   d. Salad oils

6. A patient has AKI with a negative nitrogen balance. How much weight does the nurse expect the patient to lose?
   a. 0.5 kg/day
   b. 1.0 kg/day
   c. 1.5 kg/day
   d. 2.0 kg/day

7. A patient has stage 3 chronic kidney failure. What would the nurse expect the patient's glomerular filtration rate (GFR) to be?
   a. A GFR of 90 mL/min/1.73 m²
   b. A GFR of 30–59 mL/min/1.73 m²
   c. A GFR of 120 mL/min/1.73 m²
   d. A GFR of 85 mL/min/1.73 m²

8. A patient with chronic kidney failure experiences decreased levels of erythropoietin. What serious complication related to those levels should the nurse assess for when caring for this patient?

   a. Anemia

   b. Acidosis

   c. Hyperkalemia

   d. Pericarditis

9. At the end of five peritoneal exchanges, a patient's fluid loss was 500 mL. How much is this loss equal to?

   a. 0.5 lb

   b. 1.0 lb

   c. 1.5 lb

   d. 2 lb

10. The nurse is caring for a patient after kidney surgery. What major danger should the nurse closely monitor for?

    a. Abdominal distention owing to reflex cessation of intestinal peristalsis

    b. Hypovolemic shock caused by hemorrhage

    c. Paralytic ileus caused by manipulation of the colon during surgery

    d. Pneumonia caused by shallow breathing because of severe incisional pain

11. A patient undergoing a CT scan with contrast has a baseline creatinine level of 3 mg/dL, identifying this patient as at a high risk for developing kidney failure. What is the most effective intervention to reduce the risk of developing radiocontrast-induced nephropathy (CIN)?

    a. Performing the test without contrast

    b. Administering Garamycin (gentamicin) prophylactically

    c. Hydrating with saline intravenously before the test

    d. Administering sodium bicarbonate after the procedure

12. The nurse is reviewing the potassium level of a patient with kidney disease. The results of the test are 6.5 mEq/L, and the nurse observes peaked T waves on the ECG. What priority intervention does the nurse anticipate the physician will order to reduce the potassium level?

    a. Administration of an insulin drip

    b. Administration of a loop diuretic

    c. Administration of sodium bicarbonate

    d. Administration of sodium polystyrene sulfonate [Kayexalate])

13. The nurse is administering calcium acetate (PhosLo) to a patient with ESKD. When is the best time for the nurse to administer this medication?

    a. With food

    b. 2 hours before meals

    c. 2 hours after meals

    d. At bedtime with 8 ounces of fluid

14. A patient with ESKD is scheduled to have an arteriovenous fistula created. The nurse explains that the patient will have a temporary dialysis catheter because the fistula has to "mature." The nurse will explain that the patient will have to wait how long before using the fistula?

    a. 1 to 2 weeks

    b. 2 to 3 weeks

    c. 1 month

    d. 2 to 3 months

15. A patient is placed on hemodialysis for the first time. The patient complains of a headache with nausea and begins to vomit, and the nurse observes a decreased level of consciousness. What does the nurse determine has happened?

    a. The dialysis was performed too rapidly.

    b. The patient is having an allergic reaction to the dialysate.

    c. The patient is experiencing a cerebral fluid shift.

    d. Too much fluid was pulled off during dialysis.

CHAPTER 55

Management of Patients With Urinary Disorders

Learning Objectives

1. Identify factors contributing to upper and lower urinary tract infections (UTIs).
2. Use the nursing process as a framework for care of the patient with a lower UTI.
3. Differentiate between the various adult dysfunctional voiding patterns.
4. Develop a patient education plan for a patient who has mixed (stress and urge) urinary incontinence.
5. Identify potential causes of an obstruction of the urinary tract along with the medical and surgical management of the patient with this condition.
6. Use the nursing process as a framework for care of the patient with kidney stones.
7. Describe the pathophysiology, clinical manifestations, medical management, and nursing management for patients with genitourinary trauma and urinary tract cancers.
8. Use the nursing process as a framework for care of the patient undergoing urinary diversion surgery.

SECTION I: ASSESSING YOUR UNDERSTANDING

Activity A *Fill in the blanks.*

1. The three natural defenses to bacterial invasion of the urinary tract are _____ (protein), _____ (immunoglobulin), and _____ _____, which interfere with the adherence of *Escherichia coli.*

2. Three organisms most frequently found in UTIs are _____, _____, and _____.

3. The most common cause of recurrent UTIs in elderly males is _____.

4. The most common site of a lower UTI is the _____.

5. The type of incontinence that results from a sudden increase in intra-abdominal pressure is _____.

6. Fluid management as a method of behavioral therapy for incontinence requires a daily liquid intake of _____ mL.

7. The major complication of neurogenic bladder is _____.

8. The major cause of death for patients with neurologic impairment of the bladder is _____.

9. A woman is taught to catheterize herself by inserting the catheter _____ inches into the urethra.

10. A major clinical manifestation of renal stones is _____.

Activity B *Briefly answer the following.*

1. Name six categories of risk factors for UTIs.

   _____

   _____

2. Name seven factors that contribute to UTIs in older adult patients.

   _____

   _____

   _____

   _____

3. Name ten common risk factors for urinary incontinence.

   _____

   _____

   _____

   _____

4. List the various causes of transient incontinence.

   _____

   _____

   _____

5. Explain the general principles/guidelines that the nurse should follow to prevent infection in a patient with an indwelling urinary catheter.

   _____

   _____

6. Name the eight risks factors for bladder cancer:

   _____

   _____

   _____

   _____

Activity C *Match the type of medication in Column II with the specific medication used to treat UTIs and pyelonephritis in Column I.*

Column I

_____ 1. Nitrofurantoin (Macrodantin)

_____ 2. Cephalexin (Keflex)

_____ 3. Ciprofloxacin (Cipro)

_____ 4. Ampicillin (Omnipen)

_____ 5. Co-trimoxazole (Bactrim, Septra)

_____ 6. Phenazopyridine (Pyridium)

Column II

a. Trimethoprim-sulfamethoxazole

b. Urinary analgesic agent

c. Penicillin antibiotic

d. Anti-infective, urinary tract

e. Fluoroquinolone antibiotic

f. Bactericidal antibiotic

SECTION II: APPLYING YOUR KNOWLEDGE

Activity D *Consider the scenario and answer the questions.*

CASE STUDY: Acute Pyelonephritis

Janice, age 24, arrives in the emergency department with complaints of chills, low back pain, nausea, and vomiting. She informs the nurse that it is painful to urinate. The symptoms began approximately 8 hours ago and she has been taking acetaminophen (Tylenol) for a fever of 102°F. The physician suspects that she has acute pyelonephritis.

1. The nurse is aware that a test must be performed to isolate the causative organism in order that the appropriate antibiotic be given. What type of specimen should the nurse collect?

   _____

2. The nurse is performing a physical assessment of the patient and knows that what findings are consistent with the diagnosis of acute pyelonephritis?

   _____

   _____

3. The patient is suspected to have an obstruction in the urinary tract. What type of testing may be performed in order to locate the obstruction?

   _____

SECTION III: PRACTICING FOR NCLEX

Activity E *Answer the following questions.*

1. A patient comes to the clinic suspecting a possible UTI. What symptoms of a UTI would the nurse recognize from the assessment data gathered?

   a. Rebound tenderness at McBurney's point

   b. An output of 200mL with each voiding

   c. Cloudy urine

   d. Urine with a specific gravity of 1.005–1.022

2. A patient has been diagnosed with a UTI and is prescribed an antibiotic. What first-line fluoroquinolone antibacterial agent for UTIs has been found to be significantly effective?

   a. Bactrim

   b. Cipro

   c. Macrodantin

   d. Septra

3. A patient with a UTI is having burning and pain when urinating. What urinary analgesic is prescribed for relief of these symptoms?

   a. Bactrim

   b. Levaquin

   c. Pyridium

   d. Septra

4. The nurse is educating a patient with urolithiasis about preventative measures to avoid another occurrence. What should the patient be encouraged to do?

   a. Increase fluid intake so that the patient can excrete 2,500 to 4,000 mL every day, which will help prevent additional stone formation.

   b. Participate in strenuous exercises so that the tone of smooth muscle in the urinary tract can be strengthened to help propel calculi.

   c. Add calcium supplements to the diet to replace losses to renal calculi.

   d. Limit voiding to every 6 to 8 hours so that increased volume can increase hydrostatic pressure, which will help push stones along the urinary system.

5. The nurse is providing an education program for the nursing assistants in a long-term care facility in order to decrease the number of UTIs in the female population. What interventions should the nurse introduce in the program? (Select all that apply.)

   a. For those patients who are incontinent, insert indwelling catheters.

   b. Perform hand hygiene prior to patient care.

   c. Assist the patients with frequent toileting.

   d. Provide careful perineal care.

   e. Encourage patients to wear briefs.

6. The nurse is caring for a patient with dementia in the long-term care facility when the patient has a change in cognitive function. What should the nurse suspect this patient may be experiencing?

   a. A UTI

   b. A stroke

   c. An aneurysm

   d. Fecal impaction

7. The nurse is educating a female patient with a UTI on the pharmacologic regimen for treatment. What is important for the nurse to instruct the patient to do?

   a. Take the antibiotic as well as an antifungal for the yeast infection she will probably have.

   b. Take the antibiotic for 3 days as prescribed.

   c. Understand that if the infection reoccurs, the dose will be higher next time.

   d. Be sure to take the medication with grapefruit juice.

8. A patient informs the nurse that every time she sneezes or coughs, she urinates in her pants. What type of incontinence does the nurse recognize the patient is experiencing?

   a. Urge incontinence

   b. Functional incontinence

   c. Stress incontinence

   d. Iatrogenic incontinence

9. A patient taking an alpha-adrenergic medication for the treatment of hypertension is having a problem with incontinence. What does the nurse tell the patient?

   a. The medication has caused permanent damage to the bladder sphincter and will require surgical correction.

   b. Relaxation of the supporting ligaments has occurred and the patient will need to perform pelvic floor exercises to strengthen them.

   c. The patient will require a medication regimen to decrease the overactivity of the bladder.

   d. When the medication is discontinued or changed, the incontinence will resolve.

10. The patient has been diagnosed with urge incontinence. What classification of medication does the nurse expect the patient will be placed on to help alleviate the symptoms?

    a. Antispasmodic agents

    b. Urinary analgesics

    c. Antibiotics

    d. Anticholinergic agents

11. A patient has a suprapubic catheter inserted postoperatively. What would be the advantages of the suprapubic catheter versus a urethral catheter? (Select all that apply.)

    a. The suprapubic catheter can be kept in longer than a urethral catheter.

    b. The patient can void sooner than with a urethral catheter.

    c. The suprapubic catheter allows for more mobility.

    d. The patient is not at risk for a UTI with a suprapubic catheter.

    e. The suprapubic catheter permits measurement of residual urine without urethral instrumentation.

12. The nurse is educating a patient who will be performing self-catheterization at home. What information provided by the nurse will help reduce the incidence of infection?

    a. Clean the catheter with antibacterial soap, thoroughly rinse and dry before reinsertion.

    b. Sterilize the catheter by boiling it in water for 20 minutes.

    c. Insert the catheter for urine drainage three times per day.

    d. A new catheter must be used each time catheterization is required.

13. The nurse is caring for a patient with severe pain related to ureteral colic. What medication can the nurse administer with a physician's order that will inhibit the synthesis of prostaglandin E, reducing swelling and facilitating passage of the stone?

    a. Morphine sulfate

    b. Aspirin

    c. Ketoralac (Toradol)

    d. Meperidine (Demerol)

14. A patient who has been treated with uric acid for stones is being discharged from the hospital. What type of diet does the nurse discuss with the patient?

    a. Low-calcium diet

    b. High-protein diet

    c. Low-phosphorus diet

    d. Low-purine diet

15. A patient has had surgery to create an ileal conduit for urinary diversion. What is a priority intervention by the nurse in the postoperative phase of care?

    a. Turn the patient every 2 hours around the clock.

    b. Administer pain medication every 2 hours.

    c. Monitor urine output hourly and report output greater than 30 mL/hr.

    d. Clean the stoma with soap and water after the patient voids.

Reproductive Function

Chapter header

CHAPTER **56**

Assessment and Management of Female Physiologic Processes

Learning Objectives

1. Describe the anatomy and physiology of the female reproductive system.
2. Describe approaches to effective assessment of female physiologic processes.
3. Identify the diagnostic examinations and tests used to determine alterations in female reproductive function and describe the nurse's role before, during, and after these examinations and procedures.
4. Identify common female physiologic processes and related nursing implications.
5. Describe methods of contraception and implications for health care and education.
6. Describe the causes and management of infertility.
7. Use the nursing process to plan for care of the patient with an ectopic pregnancy.
8. Develop an education plan for women who are approaching or have completed menopause.

SECTION I: ASSESSING YOUR UNDERSTANDING

Activity A *Fill in the blanks.*

1. Puberty usually begins at ages _____ to _____ but may occur as early as age _____.

2. The pituitary gland releases two essential hormones: _____ hormone causes the ovaries to secrete estrogen and _____ hormone stimulates the production of progesterone.

3. Menopause usually begins at age _____ to _____ years with a median age of _____ years. Perimenopause can begin as early as age _____ years.

4. The menstrual cycle is dependent on hormone production. The hormone responsible for stimulating progesterone is

   _____.

5. Approximately _____ to _____ of intimate partner violence is committed by men against women; this violence can be emotional, physical, sexual, or economic in nature.

6. More than _____ in _____ women are victims of childhood sexual abuse.

7. The most accurate outpatient procedure for evaluating a woman for endometrial cancer is

   _____.

8. _____ is probably the most significant form of menstrual dysfunction because it may signal cancer, benign tumors of the uterus, or other gynecologic problems.

9. Many women currently use oral contraceptive preparations of synthetic _____ and _____ .

10. The _____ is an effective contraceptive device that consists of a round, flexible spring (50 to 90 mm wide) covered with a domelike latex rubber cup.

Activity B *Briefly answer the following.*

1. A woman comes to the clinic frequently with complaints of chronic pelvic pain. What does the nurse understand can be associated with this complaint?

_____

_____

2. Why is Pap smear follow-up important if a woman has atypical cells from the first test?

_____

3. Describe the instructions the nurse should give to a patient who has had a surgical cone biopsy.

_____

_____

_____

4. Why would a hysteroscopy be indicated for a patient experiencing abnormal uterine bleeding?

_____

_____

5. What is the premenstrual syndrome?

_____

_____

6. Describe four possible options for the treatment of an ectopic pregnancy.

_____

_____

7. Name six possible causes of ectopic implantation.

_____

_____

_____

Activity C *Match the term in Column II with its corresponding definition in Column I.*

Column I

____ **1.** Painful sexual intercourse

____ **2.** Bladder protruding into the vagina

____ **3.** Beginning of menstruation

____ **4.** Description of ovaries and fallopian tubes

____ **5.** Painful menstruation

____ **6.** Implantation of endometrial tissue in other areas of the pelvis

____ **7.** Pain on movement of the cervix

____ **8.** Absence of menstrual flow

Column II

a. Adnexa

b. Amenorrhea

c. Chandelier sign

d. Cystocele

e. Dysmenorrhea

f. Dyspareunia

g. Endometriosis

h. Menarche

SECTION II: APPLYING YOUR KNOWLEDGE

Activity D *Consider the scenario and answer the questions.*

Elaine, a 50-year-old patient, informs the nurse that she is experiencing some of the symptoms of menopause. She has not had a menstrual period in 8 months and states that she is having hot flashes.

1. What does the nurse explain to Elaine is the cause of the hot flashes?

_____

_____

2. Elaine asks the nurse about the benefits of hormone therapy. What does the nurse explain are the benefits as well as the disadvantages of hormone therapy?

_____

_____

_____

_____

3. What other methods can the nurse inform Elaine are available to treat the hot flashes?

_____

_____

_____

_____

SECTION III: PRACTICING FOR NCLEX

Activity E *Answer the following questions.*

1. A woman at an employee health fair informs the nurse that she has had vaginal bleeding for the past several days. She is postmenopausal and has not had a menstrual period for the past 4 years. What should the nurse instruct the woman to do?

   a. She should see her gynecologist or physician as soon as possible.

   b. She should mention the bleeding episode to her physician at her next appointment.

   c. She should disregard this bleeding episode, because it is probably normal.

   d. She should use a birth control method, because she may be fertile with her next ovulation.

2. During an internal vaginal examination, the nurse practitioner notes a frothy and malodorous discharge. What bacteria does the practitioner suspect is causing this disorder?

   a. *Candida*

   b. *Eschar*

   c. *Trichomonas*

   d. *Escherichia coli*

3. A postmenopausal patient is experiencing dyspareunia. What methods can the nurse recommend she use to diminish the discomfort?

   a. Ibuprofen

   b. Petroleum jelly

   c. Water-based lubricant

   d. Aspirin

4. The nurse is discussing nutritional needs for a postmenopausal patient. What dietary increase should the nurse recommend to the patient?

   a. Calcium

   b. Iron

   c. Salt

   d. Vitamin K

5. In educating a patient with PMS about changing her dietary practices, what would the nurse recommend that she increase her intake of?

   a. Magnesium

   b. Vitamin D

   c. Iron

   d. Zinc

6. An adolescent patient comes to the clinic with complaints of "terrible pain" during menstruation. What should the nurse document this subjective data as?

   a. Dysmenorrhea

   b. Amenorrhea

   c. Menorrhagia

   d. Metrorrhagia

7. The nurse is discussing contraception with a patient interested in transdermal contraceptives. What should the nurse inform the client is the most common side effect of transdermal contraceptives?

   a. Breast cancer

   b. Withdrawal bleeding

   c. Thrombophlebitis

   d. Application site allergic reactions

8. A patient who is scheduled for a gynecologic examination and Pap smear informs the nurse that she just began her menstrual cycle. What is the best response by the nurse?

   a. "This will have no bearing on your test today."

   b. "We will proceed with the examination and reschedule your Pap smear for next week."

   c. "We will reschedule your examination when you have finished menstruating."

   d. "We will do the test and take into consideration that you are menstruating."

9. A patient informs the nurse that she believes she has premenstrual syndrome and is having physical symptoms as well as moodiness. What physical symptoms does the nurse recognize are consistent with PMS? (Select all that apply.)

   a. Fluid retention

   b. Low back pain

   c. Fever

   d. Headache

   e. Hypotension

10. A patient asks the nurse if there are any available nonsurgical options to terminate a pregnancy if she is only 2 weeks pregnant. What information should the nurse provide to the patient about a medication that blocks progesterone?

    a. Mifepristone (RU-486, Mifeprex) is used only in early pregnancy to terminate a pregnancy nonsurgically.

    b. Methotrexate is used only in early pregnancy to terminate a pregnancy nonsurgically.

    c. Clomiphene (Clomid) is used only in early pregnancy to terminate a pregnancy nonsurgically.

    d. Birth control pills can be used to terminate the pregnancy.

11. The nurse is preparing a patient for a gynecologic examination when the patient says, "I hope the exam doesn't hurt as much as intercourse with my husband does." What should the nurse document this finding as?

    a. Dysmenorrhea

    b. Dyspareunia

    c. Dysuria

    d. Dysthymia

12. The nurse is providing information at the local YMCA about screenings for breast and cervical cancer. The nurse should inform young women that they should begin their screenings at what time?

    a. Annual breast and pelvic examinations are important for all women 21 years of age or older and for those who are sexually active, regardless of age.

    b. Annual breast and pelvic examinations should begin at age 14 years old.

    c. Annual breast and pelvic examinations should begin when a woman becomes sexually active.

    d. Annual breast and pelvic examinations should be performed when a woman begins taking birth control.

13. The nurse is assisting a patient in preparing for a pelvic examination. What position will the nurse place the patient in for the examination?

    a. Left lateral

    b. Prone

    c. Jackknife

    d. Lithotomy

14. When the nurse places the patient in the stirrups for a pelvic exam she observes a bulge caused by rectal cavity protrusion. What does the nurse know this protrusion is called?

    a. Cystocele

    b. Rectocele

    c. Uterine prolapse

    d. Hemorrhoids

CHAPTER 57

Management of Patients With Female Reproductive Disorders

Learning Objectives

1. Compare the various types of vaginal infections and the signs, symptoms, and treatments of each.
2. Use the nursing process as a framework for care of the patient with a vulvovaginal infection.
3. Use the nursing process as a framework for care of the patient with genital herpes.
4. Discuss the signs and symptoms, management, and nursing care of inflammatory processes and structural disorders of the female reproductive tract.
5. Compare the signs and symptoms, management, and nursing care implications of benign and malignant conditions of the female reproductive tract.
6. Use the nursing process as a framework for care of the patient undergoing a hysterectomy.
7. Describe the nursing management of the patient undergoing radiation therapy for cancer of the female reproductive tract.

SECTION I: ASSESSING YOUR UNDERSTANDING

Activity A *Fill in the blanks.*

1. The vagina is protected against infection by its normally low pH (3.5 to 4.5), which is maintained in part by the actions of _____, the dominant bacteria in a healthy vaginal ecosystem.

2. The epithelium of the vagina is highly responsive to _____.

3. Bacterial vaginosis is characterized by a _____ odor.

4. Bacterial vaginosis is not usually considered a serious condition, although it can be associated with _____, _____ _____, _____, and _____.

5. Human papillomavirus (HPV) can be found in lesions of the _____, _____, _____, _____, _____, and _____.

6. There are more than _____ types of HPV.

7. The most common strains of HPV, 6 and 11, usually cause _____ on the vulva.

8. Women with HPV should have annual Pap smears because of the potential of HPV to cause _____.

9. At least _____ people in the United States have genital herpes infection and most have not been diagnosed.

10. There are _____ types of herpes viruses belonging to three different groups that cause infections in humans.

11. _____ is the most significant risk factor for the development of ovarian cancer.

Activity B *Briefly answer the following.*

1. What patient-teaching points may decrease/ minimize the 10 common risk factors for vulvovaginal infections?

_____

_____

2. Explain why a decrease in estrogen can lead to vaginal infections.

_____

_____

_____

3. List the treatment options available for the patient who has vulvovaginitis.

_____

_____

_____

4. Explain the extent of organ involvement with pelvic inflammatory disease (PID).

_____

_____

_____

5. Vulvovaginal candidiasis can occur at any time, although certain populations may be infected more than others. Which people are at an increased risk for this condition?

_____

_____

_____

Activity C *Match the word in Column II with its associated definition in Column I.*

Column I

____ 1. Intense burning and inflammation of the vulva

____ 2. A preferred treatment for candidiasis

____ 3. The recommended treatment for trichomoniasis

____ 4. The drug of choice for herpes genitalis

____ 5. A potential complication of toxic shock syndrome

____ 6. The downward displacement of the bladder toward the vaginal orifice

____ 7. Test used for diagnosis of cervical cancer

____ 8. Term used to describe the surgical procedure in which the uterus, cervix, and ovaries are removed

____ 9. A term used to describe vaginal bleeding

____ 10. Another name for benign tumors of the uterus

____ 11. In utero exposure to this drug increases the incidence of vaginal cancer.

____ 12. A risk factor for uterine cancer

____ 13. Exercises that strengthen the pelvic muscles

____ 14. An opening between two hollow organs

____ 15. Displacement of the uterus into the vaginal canal

____ 16. Cysts that arise from parts of the ovum

Column II

a. Fibroids

b. Fistula

c. Cystocele

d. Mycostatin

e. Acyclovir

f. Vulvodynia

g. Dermoid

h. Septic shock

i. Menorrhagia

j. Diethylstilbestrol (DES)

k. Kegel

l. Prolapse

m. Hormone replacement therapy (HRT)

n. Pap smear

o. Total hysterectomy

p. Flagyl

SECTION II: APPLYING YOUR KNOWLEDGE

Activity D *Consider the scenarios and answer the questions.*

CASE STUDY: Bacterial Vaginosis

Maryanne, a 19-year-old college student, has recently noticed increased vaginal discharge that is grey to yellowish-white in color and comes into the clinic for treatment.

1. The nurse will educate Maryanne on reduction of risk factors that cause bacterial vaginosis. What risk factors does the nurse include when educating?

_____

_____

_____

2. What does the nurse recognize is a diagnostic sign of bacterial vaginosis?

_____

3. Metronidazole (Flagyl) is prescribed to be taken twice a day for 1 week. While taking this medication, what should Maryanne be instructed to do?

_____

_____

CASE STUDY: Pelvic Inflammatory Disease

Donna is a 26-year-old graduate student who has been sexually active with multiple partners for 5 years. Last year she experienced several incidences of cervicitis. She now comes to the clinic complaining of severe lower abdominal discomfort and is walking with a shuffling gait.

1. What negative outcomes is it possible for Donna to have if she is not treated immediately?

_____

_____

2. What type of treatment does the nurse anticipate instructing Donna about?

_____

_____

3. What organisms should Donna be tested for prior to treatment?

_____

SECTION III: PRACTICING FOR NCLEX

Activity E *Answer the following questions.*

1. A patient has been diagnosed with a vaginal infection and received a prescription for metronidazole (Flagyl). The nurse knows that this is the recommended treatment for a vaginal infection caused by what organism?

a. *Candida albicans*

b. *Escherichia coli*

c. *Streptococcus*

d. *Trichomonas vaginalis*

2. A patient is diagnosed with Bartholinitis. What organism does the nurse recognize the patient is most likely infected with?

a. *Candida albicans*

b. *Chlamydia*

c. *Gardnerella vaginalis*

d. *Trichomonas vaginalis*

3. What interventions for the relief of pain and discomfort can the nurse educate the patient with a vulvovaginal infection about using? (Select all that apply.)

a. Warm perineal irrigations

b. Sitz baths

c. Cornstarch for chafed inner thighs

d. Cold compresses to the vagina

e. A vaginal douche

4. A patient has had a pessary inserted for long-term treatment of a prolapsed uterus. As part of the teaching plan, what should the nurse advise the patient to do?

a. See her gynecologist to remove and clean the pessary at regular intervals.

b. Keep the insertion site clean and dry.

c. Avoid sexual intercourse.

d. Avoid climbing stairs as much as possible.

5. A patient diagnosed with endometriosis asks for an explanation of the disease. What should the nurse explain to the patient?

   a. She has developed an infection in the lining of her uterus.

   b. Tissue from the lining of the uterus has implanted in areas outside the uterus.

   c. The lining of the uterus is thicker than usual, causing heavy bleeding and cramping.

   d. The lining of the uterus is too thin because endometrial tissue has implanted outside the uterus.

6. A patient is taking oral danazol (Danocrine), 800 mg/day, for 9 months for the treatment of endometriosis. How does the nurse describe this medication to the patient?

   a. It is a gonadotropin that decreases ovarian and pituitary stimulations.

   b. It is an antigonadotropin that increases pituitary stimulation and decreases ovarian stimulation.

   c. It is a gonadotropin that decreases pituitary stimulation and increases ovarian stimulation.

   d. It is an antigonadotropin that decreases pituitary and ovarian stimulations.

7. The nurse in the gynecology clinic is interviewing a patient who informs the nurse that her mother and aunt had carcinoma of the cervix. What does the nurse recognize are two chief symptoms of early carcinoma that the patient should be questioned about?

   a. Leukoplakia and metrorrhagia

   b. Dyspareunia and foul-smelling vaginal discharge

   c. "Strawberry" spots and menorrhagia

   d. Leukorrhea and irregular vaginal bleeding or spotting

8. The nurse is reviewing a patient's lab work and notes a stage II Pap smear result. What does this indicate for the patient?

   a. Cancer in situ

   b. Vaginal invasion

   c. Pelvic wall invasion

   d. Bladder extension

9. A perimenopausal woman informs the nurse that she is having irregular vaginal bleeding. What should the nurse encourage the patient to do?

   a. Stop taking her Premarin (hormonal therapy).

   b. See her gynecologist as soon as possible.

   c. Disregard this phenomenon because it is common during this life stage.

   d. Mention it to her physician during her next annual examination.

10. A patient has been diagnosed with a vulvar malignancy. What primary treatment for vulvar malignancy will the nurse prepare the patient for?

    a. Chemotherapy creams

    b. Laser vaporization

    c. Radiation

    d. Wide excision

11. The nurse is caring for a patient postoperatively who had a simple vulvectomy. What nursing interventions should be provided to this patient? (Select all that apply.)

    a. Cleansing the wound daily

    b. Offering a low-residue diet

    c. Positioning the patient with pillows

    d. Sitting in a warm tub of water

    e. Application of antibiotic ointment

12. A patient has a diagnosis of stage III ovarian cancer and wants to know what organs are involved. What information should be provided to the patient?

    a. The cancer involves only the ovaries.

    b. The cancer involves the ovaries with pelvic extension.

    c. The cancer involves metastases outside the pelvis.

    d. The cancer involves distant metastases.

13. A patient reports to the nurse that she has a sense of pelvic pressure and urinary problems such as incontinence, frequency, and urgency. The problem has gotten much worse since the birth of her third child. What does the nurse suspect the patient is experiencing?

a. A cystocele

b. A rectocele

c. An enterocele

d. A urinary tract infection

14. A woman who has been trying to conceive is diagnosed with fibroid tumors of the uterus and is scheduled to have a procedure using a laser through a hysteroscope passed through the cervix. What type of procedure will the nurse prepare the patient for?

a. A hysteroscopic resection of myomas

b. Laparoscopic myomectomy

c. Laparoscopic myolysis

d. Laparoscopic cryomyolysis

15. The nurse is encouraging a patient to have a cervical examination and Pap smear. It has been many years since the patient's last exam, and she was diagnosed with HPV 6 years ago. The patient states, "I am not having any trouble down there, so it is best to leave things alone." What is the best response by the nurse?

a. "Early cervical cancer rarely produces any symptoms."

b. "If you are not having any problems, then there is no reason to have one."

c. "You could have another type of sexually transmitted infection."

d. "If your insurance is paying for it, you should have an exam."

Assessment and Management of Patients With Breast Disorders

Learning Objectives

1. Describe the anatomy and physiology of the breast.
2. Identify the assessment and diagnostic studies used to diagnose breast disorders.
3. Identify and describe the pathophysiology of breast disorders, both benign and malignant.
4. Summarize evidence-based guidelines for the early detection of breast cancer.
5. Develop a plan for educating patients and consumer groups about breast self-awareness.
6. Describe the different modalities used to treat breast cancer.
7. Use the nursing process as a framework for care of the patient undergoing surgery for the treatment of breast cancer.
8. Describe the physical, psychosocial, and rehabilitative needs of the patient who has had breast surgery for the treatment of breast cancer.

SECTION I: ASSESSING YOUR UNDERSTANDING

Activity A *Fill in the blanks.*

1. The breasts are located between the _____ and _____ ribs over the pectoralis muscle from the sternum to the midaxillary line.

2. Fascial bands, called _____, support the breast on the chest wall.

3. A thorough breast examination, including instruction in breast self-examination (BSE), takes at least _____ minutes.

4. _____ is the firm enlargement of glandular tissue beneath and immediately surrounding the areola of the male.

5. Mastitis, an inflammation or infection of breast tissue, occurs most commonly in _____ women.

Activity B *Briefly answer the following.*

1. List the major risk factors for a woman to develop breast cancer.

   _____

   _____

2. Describe what role the nurse plays in BSE education.

   _____

   _____

   _____

   _____

3. When do variations in breast tissue occur?

   _____

   _____

4. List at least six causes of nipple discharge in a nonlactating woman.

_____

_____

_____

_____

5. Research suggests that there are racial disparities in cancer mortality. What are these disparities driven by?

_____

_____

Activity C *Match the term in Column II with its corresponding definition in Column I.*

Column I

____ **1.** Overdeveloped breast tissue usually seen in boys

____ **2.** Breast augmentation

____ **3.** Mammography after injection of dye

____ **4.** Breast cancer in the ductal system

____ **5.** Breast pain, usually hormonal in nature

____ **6.** Infection of breast tissue

____ **7.** Partial breast radiation

Column II

a. Galactography

b. Mastalgia

c. Paget's disease

d. Mastitis

e. Gynecomastia

f. Brachytherapy

g. Mammoplasty

SECTION II: APPLYING YOUR KNOWLEDGE

Activity D *Consider the scenario and answer the questions.*

CASE STUDY: Total Mastectomy (i.e., simple mastectomy)

Louise is 53 years old and single. The biopsy findings indicate that she has a malignancy in her breast. She is scheduled for a simple mastectomy.

1. On examination, Louise's tumor is found in the anatomic area where tumors usually develop. Where does the nurse determine that the tumor will be palpated?

_____

2. Postoperatively, what type of sensations other than discomfort might Louise feel?

_____

_____

_____

3. The nurse informs Louise that it is time to change her dressing for the first time. What preparation should the nurse provide for Louise before and during this time?

_____

_____

_____

_____

SECTION III: PRACTICING FOR NCLEX

Activity E *Answer the following questions.*

1. The nurse is educating a patient about the best time to perform BSE. When does the nurse inform her is the best time after menses to perform BSE?

   a. 3 to 4 days

   b. 5 to 7 days

   c. 8 to 9 days

   d. After the 10th day

2. The nurse is assessing the breast of a female patient and observes a prominent venous pattern on the left breast. What does the nurse understand that this can be indicative of?

   a. Increased blood supply required by a tumor

   b. Infection

   c. Ulceration of the nipple

   d. Thrombus formation

3. The nurse is assessing an older adult female who has not seen her physician in 2 years. The nurse is assisting the patient into a gown and notices that the patient has edema and pitting of the skin on the right breast. What does the nurse understand is the significance of this finding?

a. It may result from inflammation due to mastitis while the patient is breastfeeding.

b. This finding is not uncommon and is significant only when of recent origin.

c. It may result from a neoplasm blocking lymphatic drainage, giving the skin an orange-peel appearance, a classic sign of advanced breast cancer.

d. This finding is most likely related to benign cysts of the breast in the nipple area.

4. The nurse is educating a group of women at the YMCA about breast cancer. What does the nurse understand is the current trend that should be focused on rather than BSE?

a. Breast self-awareness

b. Mammography every year

c. Hormone replacement

d. Ultrasound with mammography

5. The nurse is discussing mammography with a female patient at the clinic. The patient asks at what age she should begin getting yearly mammograms. What answer should the nurse provide to the patient?

a. 35

b. 40

c. 50

d. 55

6. A patient is having a fine-needle biopsy (FNB) for a mass in the left breast. When the needle is inserted and the mass is no longer palpable, what does the nurse know has most likely occurred?

a. The mass has been absorbed into the tissues of the breast.

b. The mass may be cystic and was ruptured when the needle was inserted.

c. The mass may not have been located correctly.

d. The mass is not palpable because it is an inflammatory lesion.

7. A patient is having a biopsy that will remove the entire mass, plus a margin of surrounding tissue. What type of biopsy will be documented on the operative permit?

a. Excisional biopsy

b. Incisional biopsy

c. Core biopsy

d. Ultrasound-guided core biopsy

8. The nurse is providing preoperative instruction for a patient who will be having an excisional breast biopsy. The patient asks the nurse what type of bra should be used after the procedure. What should the nurse inform the patient?

a. The patient should avoid the use of a bra for 24 hours after the procedure.

b. The patient may wear a bra as long as it is an underwire bra.

c. The patient should wear a supportive bra after the procedure.

d. The patient will not be able to wear a bra until the sutures are removed.

9. A female patient comes to the clinic with the complaint that she is having a greenish-colored discharge from the nipple and the breast feels warm to touch. What does the nurse suspect these symptoms may indicate?

a. Infection

b. Cancer

c. A ruptured cyst

d. Blocked lymph duct

10. The nurse is assisting a patient with breastfeeding. The patient said that with her last baby, she had a problem with her nipples becoming irritated. What can the nurse suggest to the patient to prevent this problem? (Select all that apply.)

a. Daily washing with water

b. Massage with breast milk or lanolin

c. Exposure to air

d. Hot compresses

e. Aspirin

11. A patient is considering use of chemoprevention because she is at high risk for developing breast cancer. What can the nurse do to assist the patient with her decision?

a. Inform the patient that medication should not be used prophylactically due to the many side effects.

b. Inform the patient that she should take every measure available to her to prevent this disease.

c. Provide the patient with information regarding the benefits, risks, and possible side effects.

d. Provide the patient with information about bilateral mastectomy for the prevention of this disease.

12. A patient is told that she has a common form of breast cancer where the tumor arises from the duct system and invades the surrounding tissues, often forming a solid irregular mass. What type of cancer does the nurse prepare to discuss with the patient?

a. Infiltrating ductal carcinoma

b. Infiltrating lobular carcinoma

c. Medullary carcinoma

d. Mucinous carcinoma

13. A patient had a sentinel node biopsy and informs the nurse that something is very wrong with her. The patient explains that she had a bowel movement and urinated and both are a blue color. What should the nurse inform the patient?

a. The cancer may be invasive and holding on to some of the dye that is used.

b. The patient must be having a reaction to the dye that was used.

c. The dye that was used during the biopsy is safe and being excreted.

d. The physician will have to discuss this with her.

14. A patient has had a total mastectomy 12 hours ago and the nurse is assessing the surgical wound. The nurse observes ecchymosis, swelling, and tightness around the wound, and the patient states that it is painful. What does the nurse suspect has occurred?

a. The patient has developed an infection.

b. The patient has developed a hematoma.

c. The patient has developed lymphedema.

d. The patient has developed a cyst.

15. A patient is scheduled to receive radiation therapy for 6 weeks after her lumpectomy. The patient states she is worried about the side effects of the radiation. What can the nurse inform her about the side effects of the radiation?

a. "The radiation can make you very nauseated, but something will be given for nausea."

b. "The radiation can cause you to lose your hair, but you can wear a wig or scarves."

c. "The radiation can cause musculoskeletal fatigue and you may not be able to continue to work while receiving the radiation."

d. "The radiation can cause some skin breakdown towards the end of treatment in the axillary folds."

Assessment and Management of Problems Related to Male Reproductive Processes

1. Describe structures and function of the male reproductive system.
2. Discuss nursing assessment of the male reproductive system and identify diagnostic tests that complement assessment.
3. Discuss the causes and management of male sexual dysfunction.
4. Compare the types of prostatectomy with regard to advantages and disadvantages.
5. Use the nursing process as a framework for care of the patient with prostate cancer or undergoing prostatectomy.
6. Describe the nursing management of patients with testicular cancer.
7. Describe the various disorders of the penis, including pathophysiology, clinical manifestations, and management.

SECTION I: ASSESSING YOUR UNDERSTANDING

Activity A *Fill in the blanks.*

1. Two specific tests used to diagnose prostate cancer are _____ and _____.

2. The most common isolated organism that causes prostatitis is _____.

3. The most commonly used medication for estrogen therapy in the treatment of prostate cancer is _____; other hormonal therapies such as _____, _____, _____, _____, and _____ suppress testicular androgen.

4. Five major potential complications after prostatectomy are _____, _____, _____, _____, and _____.

5. Two tumor markers that may be elevated in testicular cancer are _____ and _____.

6. The testes have a dual function: _____ and secretion of the male sex hormone _____, which induces and preserves the male sex characteristics.

7. _____ and _____ often decrease in as many as two thirds of men older than 70 years of age.

8. Men older than 50 years of age are at increased risk for genitourinary tract cancers including those of the _____, _____, _____, and _____.

9. The cells within the prostate gland produce a protein called the _____ _____ which can be measured in the blood.

10. _____ occurs when semen travels toward the bladder instead of exiting through the penis, resulting in infertility.

11. _____, a complication of prostatectomy, occurs in 80% to 95% of patients.

12. _____ are the oral medications that are considered first-line therapy in the treatment of erectile dysfunction.

Activity B *Briefly answer the following.*

1. List four symptoms associated with prostatitis.

   _____

   _____

2. Name seven symptoms that a patient with benign prostatic hyperplasia might display.

   _____

   _____

   _____

   _____

3. What factors should be considered when a patient is choosing a penile implant?

   _____

   _____

   _____

   _____

Activity C *Match each disorder of the male reproductive system listed in Column II with its description listed in Column I.*

Column I

____ 1. Collection of fluid in the testes

____ 2. An obstructive complex characterized by increased urinary frequency

____ 3. Constricted foreskin of the penis

____ 4. Failure of the testes to descend into the scrotum

____ 5. Inflammation of the testes

____ 6. Abnormal dilation of the veins in the scrotum

____ 7. Inflammation of the prostate gland

____ 8. Infection of the epididymis

Column II

a. Cryptorchidism
b. Epididymitis
c. Hydrocele
d. Orchitis
e. Phimosis
f. Prostatism
g. Prostatitis
h. Variocele

SECTION II: APPLYING YOUR KNOWLEDGE

Activity D *Consider the scenario and answer the questions.*

CASE STUDY: Prostatectomy

Tom is a 65-year-old college administrator who is scheduled for a robotic-assisted laparoscopic radical prostatectomy after undergoing medical management of his prostate cancer for 1 year. Tom's wife will be accompanying him to the hospital and staying during his surgical procedure.

1. Tom asks the nurse if he will be able to have sex again. What should the nurse discuss with him?

   _____

   _____

   _____

   _____

2. The day after Tom has his surgery, he complains of a feeling of fullness in the lower abdomen and feeling as though he needs to void. He says he sees blood around his penis where the catheter is. What does the nurse determine may be occurring?

_____

_____

3. What interventions can the nurse provide to alleviate Tom's discomfort from this problem?

_____

_____

_____

SECTION III: PRACTICING FOR NCLEX

Activity E *Answer the following questions.*

1. A patient comes to the clinic with complaints of inability to sustain an erection and is prescribed a PDE-5 inhibitor, sildenafil (Viagra). What medication should the nurse caution the patient about taking with this medication?

a. Isosorbide (Isordil)

b. Lisinopril (Prinivil)

c. Diphenhydramine (Benadryl)

d. Levothyroxine (Synthroid)

2. A patient is having a DRE in the physician's office and the nurse is to assist in the examination. What can the nurse instruct the client to do to decrease the discomfort from the exam?

a. Take a deep breath and hold it when the physician inserts a gloved finger into the rectum.

b. Take a deep breath and exhale when the physician inserts a gloved finger into the rectum.

c. When bending over the examining table, point the feet outward to decrease the discomfort.

d. Inform the patient that the examination is not uncomfortable and will be over in a short period of time.

3. The nurse is demonstrating the technique for performing a testicular self-examination (TSE) to a group of men for a company health fair. One of the men asks the nurse at what age a man should begin performing TSE. What is the best answer by the nurse?

a. "It should begin in adolescence."

b. "It should begin in men over age 50."

c. "It should be performed in high-risk males over age 30."

d. "It should begin at age 40."

4. A patient comes to the emergency department and tells the nurse, "I took a pill to help me perform and then passed out." The nurse is assessing the patient and finds a nitroglycerin patch on his back. What is the first intervention the nurse must perform?

a. Take the patient's blood pressure.

b. Ask the patient to obtain a urine specimen.

c. Start an IV.

d. Administer atropine 0.5 mg.

5. A patient has demonstrated interest in obtaining a penile implant. What should the patient consider prior to making this decision? (Select all that apply.)

a. ADLs

b. Social activities

c. Expectations of the patient and his partner

d. Financial status

e. Occupation

6. A patient is planning to use a negative-pressure (vacuum) device to maintain and sustain an erection. What should the nurse caution the patient about with the use of this device?

a. Do not use the device while taking nitrates.

b. Do not leave the constricting band in place for longer than 1 hour to avoid penile injury.

c. Watch for erosion of the prosthesis through the skin.

d. Watch for the development of infection.

7. When developing an educational program for a group of adolescents about sexually transmitted infections (STIs), what should the nurse inform the group about the single greatest risk factor for contracting an STI?

   a. The type of contraception used

   b. The number of times the person has contact with a partner

   c. The number of sexual partners

   d. Where the patient lives

8. A patient is being treated for prostatitis and the nurse is providing education about the treatment. What should the nurse include in the education of this patient?

   a. Force fluids to prevent urine from backing up and distending the bladder.

   b. Take several cool baths during the day to alleviate discomfort.

   c. Be sure to take the 3-day course of antifungal medication.

   d. Avoid foods and liquids with diuretic action or that increase prostatic secretions.

9. A patient informs the nurse that his father died of prostate cancer, so he wants to know ways in which to reduce his risk factors for developing it. What education can the nurse give to the patient to decrease modifiable risk factors?

   a. Limit red meat and dairy products high in fat.

   b. Quit smoking.

   c. Avoid wearing tight pants and underwear.

   d. Monitor blood pressure.

10. A patient is suspected to have prostate cancer related to observed clinical symptoms. What definitive test can the nurse assist with to confirm a diagnosis of prostate cancer?

    a. DRE

    b. PSA

    c. Prostate biopsy

    d. Cystoscopy

11. A patient is having brachytherapy for the treatment of prostate cancer and asks the nurse if he can have sexual intercourse after radiation therapy is completed. What is the best response by the nurse?

    a. "You most likely will not be able to have sexual intercourse after radiation therapy."

    b. "You must be sure to use a condom for 2 weeks after implantation and then it will no longer be necessary."

    c. "There are no restrictions to sexual activity during radiation."

    d. "You must use a condom for at least 6 months after beginning radiation therapy."

12. A patient with an indwelling catheter after a radical prostatectomy is having bladder spasms. What medication prescribed by the physician can the nurse administer to help alleviate the discomfort?

    a. Cephalexin (Keflex)

    b. Phenazopyridine (Pyridium)

    c. Oxybutynin (Ditropan)

    d. Tadalafil (Cialis)

13. The nurse is educating a patient about performing testicular self-examination (TSE). The nurse informs the patient that the best time to perform the exam is when?

    a. In the morning when arising

    b. After exercise

    c. After a warm bath or shower

    d. At bedtime

14. A patient experiences hypotension, lethargy, and muscle spasms while receiving bladder irrigations after a transurethral resection of the prostate (TURP). What is the first action the nurse should take?

    a. Discontinue the irrigations.

    b. Increase the rate of the IV fluids.

    c. Administer a unit of packed red blood cells.

    d. Prepare the patient for an ECG.

15. What does the nurse tell the patient is the best way to decrease the risk of developing penile cancer?

    a. Avoid sexual intercourse with multiple partners.

    b. Use good genital hygiene.

    c. Use a condom when having sexual intercourse.

    d. Perform self-examinations.

Integumentary Function

Assessment of Integumentary Function

1. Identify the structures and functions of the skin.
2. Differentiate the composition and function of each skin layer: epidermis, dermis, and subcutaneous tissue.
3. Describe the normal aging process of the skin and skin changes common in older adult patients.
4. List appropriate questions that help elicit information during an assessment of the skin.
5. Describe the components of physical assessment that are most useful when examining the skin, hair, and nails.
6. Identify and describe primary and secondary skin lesions and their pattern and distribution.
7. Recognize common skin eruptions and manifestations associated with systemic disease.
8. Discuss common skin tests and procedures used in diagnosing skin and related disorders.

SECTION I: ASSESSING YOUR UNDERSTANDING

Activity A *Fill in the blanks.*

1. There are the three layers of the skin: _____, _____, and _____.

2. The epidermis is composed of three types of cells: _____, _____, and _____.

3. The epidermis is almost completely replaced every _____.

4. The subcutaneous tissue, which is primarily composed of _____ tissue, has a major role in _____ regulation.

5. The term used to describe hair loss is _____.

6. There are two types of skin glands: _____ and _____.

7. Skin needs to be exposed to sunlight to manufacture vitamin _____.

8. Jaundice can first be observed by examining the _____ and _____.

9. The nurse should know that clubbing of the nails is usually a diagnostic sign of _____.

10. _____, _____, and _____ are the major physical processes involved in loss of heat from the body to the environment.

Activity B *Briefly answer the following.*

1. Describe how the production of melanin is controlled.

_____

_____

_____

_____

2. Describe what function the hair of the skin serves.

_____

_____

_____

_____

3. What is the function of the receptor endings of nerves in the skin?

_____

_____

_____

_____

4. When assessing the skin of an older adult, what major age-related changes are seen in the skin?

_____

_____

_____

_____

Activity C *Match the description in Column II with the associated key term in Column I.*

Column I

___ **1.** Dermatosis

___ **2.** Erythema

___ **3.** Hirsutism

___ **4.** Hyperpigmentation

___ **5.** Hypopigmentation

___ **6.** Keratin

___ **7.** Melanin

___ **8.** Petechia

___ **9.** Telangiectases

___ **10.** Vitiligo

Column II

a. Pinpoint red spots that appear on the skin as a result of blood leakage into the skin

b. A localized or widespread condition characterized by destruction of the melanocytes in circumscribed areas of the skin, resulting in white patches

c. The substance responsible for coloration of the skin

d. Decrease in the melanin of the skin, resulting in a loss of pigmentation

e. Red marks on the skin caused by distention of the superficial blood vessels

f. An insoluble, fibrous protein that forms the outer layer of skin

g. Increase in the melanin of the skin, resulting in an increase in pigmentation

h. Any abnormal skin condition

i. Redness of the skin caused by congestion of the capillaries

j. The condition of having excessive hair growth

SECTION II: APPLYING YOUR KNOWLEDGE

Activity D *Consider the scenario and answer the questions.*

Paula, age 72, is being seen in the clinic for a regular checkup. She asks the nurse to check several small lesions on her back and arms. Paula has diabetes that is well controlled with diet.

1. The nurse is assessing the various lesions on Paula's back and arms. What should the nurse document about the findings?

_____

_____

2. The nurse observes dull, red bumps smaller than a pencil eraser on Paula's arms. They are bilateral and occur in linear clusters. What does the nurse determine that these lesions are?

_____

3. Why would it be important for the nurse to assess Paula's legs and feet for skin changes?

_____

_____

_____

SECTION III: PRACTICING FOR NCLEX

Activity E *Answer the following questions.*

1. The nurse is caring for an adult patient with a normal body temperature. What should the nurse know would be the approximate insensible water loss per day in this patient?
   a. 250 mL/day
   b. 600 mL/day
   c. 800 mL/day
   d. 1,000 mL/day

2. The nurse is applying a cold towel to a patient's neck to reduce body heat. How does the nurse understand that the heat is reduced?
   a. Conduction
   b. Convection
   c. Evaporation
   d. Radiation

3. The nurse is assessing the fingernails of a patient at the clinic. The nurse observes pitting on the surface of the nail. What disorder is this finding indicative of?
   a. Psoriasis
   b. Vitiligo
   c. Diabetes
   d. Melanoma

4. The nurse is caring for a patient with dark skin who is having gastrointestinal bleeding. How can the nurse determine from skin color change that shock may be present?
   a. The skin is ashen gray and dull.
   b. The skin is dusky blue.
   c. The skin is reddish pink.
   d. The skin is whitish pink.

5. The nurse assesses a dark-skinned patient who has cherry-red nail beds, lips, and oral mucosa. What does this assessment data indicate the patient may be experiencing?
   a. Anemia
   b. Carbon monoxide poisoning
   c. Polycythemia
   d. Shock

6. The nurse is assessing a patient with a primary skin lesion called a macule. What does the nurse understand is a clinical example of this lesion?
   a. Hives
   b. Impetigo
   c. Port-wine stains
   d. Psoriasis

7. The nurse examines a patient and notices a herpes simplex/zoster skin lesion. How does the nurse document this lesion?

   a. Macule

   b. Papule

   c. Vesicle

   d. Wheal

8. When assessing a patient with risk factors related to human immunodeficiency virus (HIV), what does the nurse know can be the first manifestation of the disease?

   a. Telangiectasia

   b. Ecchymosis

   c. Fluid-filled vesicles

   d. Purplish cutaneous lesions

9. A patient is visiting the physician to determine what type of allergy is causing a rash. What type of testing does the nurse anticipate the physician will schedule?

   a. Skin biopsy

   b. Skin scrapings

   c. Tzanck smear

   d. Patch test

10. The nurse is assisting with the collection of a Tzanck smear. What is the suspected diagnosis of the patient?

    a. Fungal infection

    b. Herpes zoster

    c. Psoriasis

    d. Seborrheic dermatosis

11. A patient has a serum bilirubin concentration of 3 mg/100 mL. What does the nurse observe when performing a skin assessment on this patient?

    a. Jaundice

    b. Pallor

    c. Bronzed appearance

    d. Cherry red face

12. A patient comes to the clinic and asks the nurse why the skin of the forehead, palms, and soles has a yellow-orange tint. There is no yellowing of the sclera or mucous membranes. What should the nurse question the patient regarding?

    a. "Have you been ingesting large quantities of alcohol?"

    b. "Have you been diagnosed with Addison's disease?"

    c. "Have you been in the sun a lot?"

    d. "Have you been eating a large amount of carotene-rich foods?"

13. A patient has contact dermatitis on the hand, and the nurse observes an area that is thickened and rough between the thumb and forefinger. What does the nurse know that this is significant of related to repeated scratching and rubbing?

    a. Atrophy

    b. Lichenification

    c. Keloid

    d. Scales

14. The nurse assesses a patient with silvery-white, thick scales on the scalp, elbows, and hand of a patient that bleed when picked off. What does the nurse suspect that this patient may have?

    a. Vitiligo

    b. Psoriasis

    c. Melanoma

    d. Petechia

15. The nurse observes an African-American patient with a large hypertrophied area of scar tissue on the left ear lobe. What does the nurse document this finding as?

    a. Atrophy

    b. Scar

    c. Lichenification

    d. Keloid

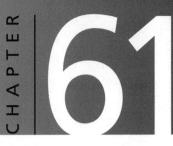

Management of Patients With Dermatologic Problems

Learning Objectives

1. Describe the general management of the patient with a wound, pruritus, or a dermatologic secretory disorder.
2. Describe the management and nursing care of the patient with infections of the skin and parasitic skin diseases.
3. Describe the management and nursing care of the patient with noninfectious inflammatory dermatoses, including contact dermatitis or psoriasis.
4. Use the nursing process as a framework for care of patients with blistering disorders, including toxic epidermal necrolysis and Stevens-Johnson syndrome.
5. Describe the management and nursing care of the patient with skin tumors (benign, malignant, and metastatic).
6. Use the nursing process as a framework for care of the patient with melanoma.
7. Compare the various types of dermatologic and plastic reconstructive procedures.
8. Describe the management and nursing care of patients undergoing plastic and cosmetic procedures.

SECTION I: ASSESSING YOUR UNDERSTANDING

Activity A *Fill in the blanks.*

1. The most common skin condition in adolescents and young adults between the ages of 12 and 35 years is _____.

2. There are three types of wound dressings: _____, _____, and _____.

3. Autolytic _____ is a process that uses the body's own digestive enzymes to break down necrotic tissue.

4. Corticosteroids are widely used in treating dermatologic conditions to provide _____, _____, and _____ effects.

5. The main secretory function of the skin is performed by the _____, which help regulate body temperature.

6. Scabies is an infestation of the skin by the itch mite _____.

7. Bullous impetigo, a deep-seated infection characterized by large, fluid-filled blisters, is caused by the bacteria _____.

8. Pemphigus vulgaris is a(n) _____ disease in which the immunoglobulin (IgG) antibody is directed against a specific cell-surface antigen in epidermal cells.

9. _____ is an important principle of psoriasis treatment.

10. There are three types of therapy indicated for the treatment of psoriasis: _____, _____, and _____.

11. _____ is the leading cause of death in people with blistering diseases.

Activity B *Briefly answer the following.*

1. List four major objectives of therapy for patients with dermatologic problems:

_____

_____

_____

2. Describe why moisture retentive dressings are efficient at removing exudate:

_____

_____

_____

3. How do cytokines work?

_____

_____

4. The nurse is applying foam dressing to an exudative sacral decubitus ulcer. After application of the foam dressing, what is important that the nurse do?

_____

_____

5. Name the potential complications of Stevens Johnson syndrome (SJS) and toxic epidermal necrolysis (TEN):

_____

_____

6. List five risk factors related to the development of melanoma:

_____

_____

_____

_____

Activity C *Match the term in Column I with the definition in Column II.*

Column I

___ 1. Comedone

___ 2. Cheilitis

___ 3. Carbuncle

___ 4. Furuncle

___ 5. Tinea

___ 6. Pyodermas

___ 7. Liniments

___ 8. Xerosis

___ 9. Santyl

___ 10. Gel

___ 11. Lidex

___ 12. Famvir

___ 13. Scabies

___ 14. Permethrin

___ 15. TEN

Column II

a. A potentially fatal skin disorder

b. An enzymatic debriding agent

c. A prescription scabicide

d. Localized skin infection involving only 1 hair follicle

e. Primary lesion of acne

f. Dry crackling skin at corners of mouth

g. Localized skin infection involving hair follicles

h. A semisolid emulsion that becomes liquid when applied to the skin or scalp

i. Most common fungal infection of skin or scalp

j. Bacterial skin infections

k. Overly dry skin

l. Lotions with added oil to soften skin

m. A topical corticosteroid with medium to high potency

n. An antiviral agent used to treat herpes zoster

o. An infestation caused by the itch mite

SECTION II: APPLYING YOUR KNOWLEDGE

Activity D *Consider the scenarios and answer the questions.*

CASE STUDY: Acne Vulgaris

Brian is a 15-year-old who has been experiencing facial eruptions of acne for about a year. The numerous lesions are inflamed and present on the face and neck. He has tried many over-the-counter medications and nothing seems to help. His father had a history of severe acne when he was a teenager.

1. What type of dietary advice can the nurse provide to Brian that may assist in preventing the "flare-ups" related to acne?

_____

_____

_____

_____

2. The physician prescribes an oral antibiotic for Brian to take for 1 month and then wants to see him at that time to determine effectiveness. What type of antibiotic is generally prescribed for treatment?

_____

3. What nursing interventions will assist Brian in coping with his acne?

_____

_____

_____

_____

CASE STUDY: Melanoma

Steve is a 26-year-old professional baseball player for a Florida farm team. He spends many hours in the sun practicing between 9:00 AM and 4:00 PM. His V-neck uniform leaves little protection for his chest. Steve had a mole on his chest for 5 years. One day last October, he noticed that the margins of the mole were elevated and palpable and the color had become darker. Since his father had melanoma when he was 32 years old, Steve decided to see a physician.

1. On examination, a circular lesion with irregular outer edges and a pinkish hue in the center is observed on Steve's chest. What type of lesion is consistent with this finding?

_____

2. What procedure does the nurse prepare the patient for to obtain confirmation of the diagnosis?

_____

3. The nurse measures the lesion and documents that it is greater than 14 mm in thickness and growing vertically. What prognosis does the nurse expect the physician will discuss with the patient after the biopsy results are returned?

_____

_____

SECTION III: PRACTICING FOR NCLEX

Activity E *Answer the following questions.*

1. The nurse is changing the dressing of a chronic wound. There is no sign of infection or heavy drainage. How long will the nurse leave the wound covered for?

   a. 6 to 12 hours

   b. 12 to 24 hours

   c. 24 to 36 hours

   d. 48 to 72 hours

2. A patient has a moisture-retentive dressing for the treatment of a sacral decubitus ulcer. How long should the nurse leave the dressing in place before replacing it?

a. 4 to 6 hours

b. 8 hours

c. 12 to 24 hours

d. 24 to 36 hours

3. The patient is advised to apply a suspension-type lotion to a dermatosis site. The nurse should advise the patient to apply the lotion how often to be effective?

a. Every hour

b. Every 3 hours

c. Every 12 hours

d. Every day at the same time

4. What should the nurse assess for to determine if a patient using corticosteroids for a dermatologic condition is having local side effects? (Select all that apply.)

a. Skin atrophy

b. Striae

c. Telangiectasia

d. Comedones

e. Ecchymosis

5. The nurse is instructing the patient in how to apply a corticosteroid cream to lesions on the arm. What intervention can the nurse instruct the patient to do to increase the absorption of the medication?

a. Apply an occlusive dressing over the site after application.

b. Make sure that the skin is slightly dehydrated so that the medication can absorb through the skin cracks.

c. Apply a thick layer of cream over the lesions so that if some rubs off, there is more to absorb.

d. Apply the medication every 2 hours.

6. The nurse should assess all possible causes of pruritus for a patient complaining of generalized pruritus. What does the nurse understand can be other causes for this condition?

a. End-stage kidney disease

b. Hypothyroidism

c. Pneumonia

d. Myasthenia gravis

7. A patient is being evaluated for nodular cystic acne. What systemic pharmacologic agent may be prescribed for the treatment of this disorder?

a. Accutane

b. Benzoyl peroxide

c. Retin-A

d. Salicylic acid

8. A patient is complaining of severe itching that intensifies at night. The nurse decides to assess the skin using a magnifying glass and penlight to look for the "itch mite." What skin condition does the nurse anticipate finding?

a. Contact dermatitis

b. Pediculosis

c. Scabies

d. Tinea corporis

9. A patient is diagnosed with psoriasis after developing scales on the scalp, elbows, and behind the knees. The patient asks the nurse where this was "caught." What is the best response by the nurse?

a. Psoriasis is an inflammatory dermatosis that results from a superficial infection with *Staphylococcus aureus*.

b. Psoriasis comes from dermal abrasion.

c. Psoriasis is an inflammatory dermatosis that results from an overproduction of keratin.

d. Psoriasis results from excess deposition of subcutaneous fat.

10. The nurse is assessing a patient for psoriatic lesions after treatment with a nonsteroidal cream. What type of lesion does the nurse know is characteristic of psoriasis?

a. Red, raised patch covered with silver scales

b. Cluster of pustules

c. Group of raised vesicles

d. Pattern of bullae that rupture and form a scaly crust

11. A patient is being treated for chronic venous stasis ulcers of the lower extremities. What medication does the nurse understand will increase peripheral blood flow by decreasing the viscosity of blood and assist with the healing of the ulcers?

a. Heparin

b. Warfarin (Coumadin)

c. Aspirin

d. Pentoxifylline (Trental)

12. A patient is diagnosed with seborrheic dermatitis on the face and is prescribed a corticosteroid preparation for use. What should the nurse educate the patient about regarding use of the steroid on the face?

a. Use very warm water to clean the face prior to applying the medication.

b. Avoid using the medication around the eyelids because it may cause cataracts and glaucoma.

c. Wash the face several times a day and reapply the medication.

d. Scrape the scaly patches off prior to applying the medication.

13. A patient has developed a boil on the face and the nurse observes the patient squeezing the boil. What does the nurse understand is a potential severe complication of this manipulation?

a. Scarring

b. Brain abscess

c. Erythema

d. Cellulitis

14. The nurse is caring for a patient with extensive bullous lesions on the trunk and back. Prior to initiating skin care, what is a priority for the nurse to do?

a. Wash the lesions vigorously.

b. Rupture the bullous lesions.

c. Administer analgesic pain medication.

d. Apply cold compresses.

15. The nurse is assessing a patient with TEN. What assessment data would indicate that the patient may be progressing to keratoconjunctivitis? (Select all that apply.)

a. Skin peeling on eyelids

b. Pruritus of the eyes

c. Burning of the eyes

d. Dryness of the eyes

e. Blurred optic discs

Management of Patients With Burn Injury

Learning Objectives

1. Discuss the incidence of burn injury in the United States.
2. Describe the factors that affect the severity of burn injury.
3. Describe the local and systemic effects of a major burn injury.
4. Identify priorities of care and potential complications for each phase of burns.
5. Identify fluid replacement requirements during the emergent/resuscitative and acute phases of a burn injury.
6. Discuss the nurse's role in burn wound management during the acute/intermediate phase of burn care.
7. Use the nursing process as a framework of care for the patient with burns during the emergent/resuscitative and rehabilitation phases of burn care.
8. Describe the psychosocial challenges associated with burn injuries and identify strategies for intervention.

SECTION I: ASSESSING YOUR UNDERSTANDING

Activity A *Fill in the blanks.*

1. The two age groups that have increased morbidity and mortality from burn injuries are _____ and _____.

2. Burns that exceed _____ of the total body surface area (TBSA) are considered major burn injuries and produce both a local and a systemic inflammatory response.

3. _____ is the immediate consequence of ensuing fluid loss and results in decreased perfusion and oxygen delivery.

4. Burn injuries are classified according to _____ and _____.

5. Two pulmonary complications that occur secondary to inhalation injuries are _____ and _____.

6. The leading cause of death in thermally injured patients is _____.

7. The resuscitation goal of fluid replacement therapy, postburn injury, is a urinary output of _____ to _____ for adults.

8. The three major bacteria responsible for infection in burn centers are _____, _____, and _____.

9. Three commonly used topical antibacterials for skin care are _____, _____, and _____.

10. Four signs of postburn sepsis include _____, _____, _____, and _____.

Activity B *Briefly answer the following.*

1. Explain why the survival rate for burn victims has increased significantly over the last 80 years.

_____

_____

_____

2. What are the three zones of burn injury and what areas are involved with each?

_____

_____

_____

3. What two detrimental effects does radiation injury have?

_____

_____

4. What is the pathophysiology of carbon monoxide poisoning?

_____

_____

5. What types of general emergency procedures should be employed at the burn scene?

_____

_____

_____

6. What does the depth of burn injury depend on?

_____

_____

7. When a patient sustains inhalation injury below the vocal cords, what is the usual cause?

_____

_____

8. The nurse is performing a secondary survey for a patient who sustained severe burns. What does this entail?

_____

_____

9. Describe the measures that can be taken to avoid the development of hypertrophic and keloid scars after a burn injury.

_____

_____

_____

_____

10. Discuss why congestive heart failure is a potential complication of an acute burn.

_____

_____

_____

Activity C *Match the term in Column I with the associated definition in Column II.*

Column I

____ 1. Xenograft

____ 2. Debridement

____ 3. Eschar

____ 4. Fasciotomy

____ 5. Contracture

____ 6. Homograft

____ 7. Escharotomy

Column II

a. Graft transferred from one human (living or cadaveric) to another human; also called allograft

b. Graft obtained from an animal of a species other than that of the recipient (e.g., pigskin); also called a heterograft

c. Devitalized tissue resulting from a burn or wound

d. Shrinkage of burn scar through collagen maturation

e. Incision made through the fascia to release constriction of underlying muscle

f. Removal of foreign material and devitalized tissue until surrounding healthy tissue is exposed

g. Linear excision made through eschar to release constriction of underlying tissue

SECTION II: APPLYING YOUR KNOWLEDGE

Activity D *Consider the scenario and answer the questions.*

Brad, a 22-year-old, sustained full-thickness burns on his anterior chest, face, and neck when he was trying to start a charcoal fire to prepare dinner for his father. His father sprayed him with water from a hose and took him to a hospital emergency department 3 miles away. On arrival, Brad was semiconscious and in respiratory distress. Brad is determined to weigh 72 kg.

1. Upon arrival at the emergency department, what indicators does the nurse have that Brad may have an inhalation injury as well as the severe burns?

   _____

   _____

   _____

2. What does the nurse prepare to assist with due to the Brad's immediate condition?

   _____

   _____

3. According to the rule of 9's, Brad has been burned over 13.5% of his body. According to the American Burn Association (ABA) fluid resuscitation guide, how much fluid should he receive in the first 24 hours after the burn injury?

   _____

   _____

SECTION III: PRACTICING FOR NCLEX

Activity E *Answer the following questions.*

1. The nurse is caring for a patient who sustained a full-thickness burn to his arm when he was scalded with boiling water. How did the nurse determine that the patient's burns are full-thickness burns?

   a. Classification by the appearance of blisters

   b. Identification by the destruction of the dermis and epidermis

   c. Not associated with edema formation

   d. Usually very painful because of exposed nerve endings

2. The nurse is caring for a patient who has sustained severe burns to 50% of the body. The nurse is aware that fluid shifts during the first week of the acute phase of a burn injury cause massive cell destruction. What should the nurse report immediately when reviewing laboratory studies?

   a. Hypernatremia

   b. Hypokalemia

   c. Hyperkalemia

   d. Hypercalcemia

3. What laboratory value observed by the nurse is unexpected during the fluid remobilization phase of a major burn?

   a. Hematocrit level of 45%

   b. A pH of 7.20, PaO_2 of 38 mm Hg, and bicarbonate level of 15 mEq/L

   c. Serum potassium level of 3.2 mEq/L

   d. Serum sodium level of 140 mEq/L

4. The nurse is caring for a patient who sustained a major burn. What serious gastrointestinal disturbance should the nurse monitor for that frequently occurs with a major burn?

   a. Diverticulitis

   b. Hematemesis

   c. Paralytic ileus

   d. Ulcerative colitis

5. A person suffers leg burns from spilled charcoal lighter fluid. A family member extinguishes the flames. While waiting for an ambulance, what should the burned person do?

   a. Have someone assist him into a bath of cool water, where he can wait for emergency personnel.

   b. Lie down, have someone cover him with a blanket, and cover his legs with petroleum jelly.

   c. Remove his burned pants so that the air can help cool the wound.

   d. Sit in a chair, elevate his legs, and have someone cut his pants off around the burned area.

6. The nurse in the emergency department receives a patient who sustained a severe burn injury. What is the priority action by the nurse in this situation?

   a. Establish a patent airway.

   b. Insert an indwelling catheter.

   c. Replace fluids.

   d. Administer pain medication.

7. A sample consensus formula for fluid replacement recommends that a balanced salt solution be administered in the first 24 hours of a burn in the range of 2 to 4 mL/kg/% of burn, with 50% of the total given in the first 8 hours postburn. A 176-lb (80-kg) man with a 30% burn should receive a minimum of how much fluid replacement in the first 8 hours?

   a. 1,200 mL

   b. 2,400 mL

   c. 3,600 mL

   d. 4,800 mL

8. The nurse is monitoring for fluid and electrolyte changes in the emergent phase of burn injury for a patient. Which of the following will be an expected outcome? (Select all that apply.)

   a. Base-bicarbonate deficit

   b. Elevated hematocrit level

   c. Potassium deficit

   d. Sodium deficit

   e. Magnesium deficit

9. During the acute phase of burn injury, the nurse knows to assess for signs of potassium shifting during what time frame?

   a. Within 24 hours

   b. Between 24 and 48 hours

   c. At the beginning of the third day

   d. Beginning on day 4 or day 5

10. The nurse is planning the care of a patient with a major burn. What outcome will the nurse understand will be optimal during fluid replacement?

    a. A urinary output of 10 mL/hr

    b. A urinary output of 30 mL/hr

    c. A urinary output of 80 mL/hr

    d. A urinary output of 100 mL/hr

11. What are the expected findings in the fluid remobilization phase that the nurse should monitor for? (Select all that apply.)

    a. Hemodilution

    b. Increased urinary output

    c. Metabolic alkalosis

    d. Sodium deficit

    e. Hypoglycemia

12 The nurse is providing wound care for a client with burns to the lower extremities. Which topical antibacterial agent carries a side effect of leukopenia that the nurse should monitor for within 48 hours after application?

    a. Cerium nitrate solution

    b. Gentamicin sulfate

    c. Sulfadiazine, silver (Silvadene)

    d. Mafenide (Sulfamylon)

13. The nurse knows that which topical antibacterial agent does not penetrate eschar?

    a. Acticoat

    b. Mafenide acetate

    c. Silver nitrate 0.5%

    d. Silver sulfadiazine 1%

14. The nurse is applying an occlusive dressing to a burned foot. What position should the foot be placed in after application of the dressing?

    a. Adduction

    b. Dorsiflexion

    c. External rotation

    d. Plantar flexion

15. A patient will be receiving biologic dressings. The nurse understands that biologic dressings, which use skin from living or recently deceased humans, are known by what name?

    a. Autografts

    b. Heterografts

    c. Homografts

    d. Xenografts

16. The nurse is administering an analgesic to a patient with major burns. What is the recommended route for administration for this patient?

a. Intramuscular

b. Intravenous

c. Oral

d. Subcutaneous

17. To meet early nutritional demands for protein, a 198-lb (90-kg) burned patient will need to ingest a minimum of how much protein every 24 hours?

a. 90 g/day

b. 110 g/day

c. 180 g/day

d. 270 g/day

Sensory Function

Assessment and Management of Patients With Eye and Vision Disorders

Learning Objectives

1. Identify significant eye structures and describe their functions.
2. Specify assessment and diagnostic findings used in the evaluation of ocular disorders.
3. Describe assessment and management strategies for patients with low vision and blindness.
4. Identify the pharmacologic actions and nursing management of common ophthalmic medications.
5. Discuss clinical features, assessment and diagnostic findings, and medical or surgical management of glaucoma, cataracts, and other ocular disorders.
6. Describe the nursing management of patients with glaucoma, cataracts, and ocular trauma.
7. Discuss general discharge education for patients after ocular surgery.

SECTION I: ASSESSING YOUR UNDERSTANDING

Activity A *Fill in the blanks.*

1. Normal intraocular pressure is _____.

2. The second leading cause of irreversible blindness in the world is _____.

3. Two significant changes in the optic nerve that occur in patients with glaucoma are _____ and _____.

4. The most common laser surgeries for glaucoma are _____ and _____.

5. According to the World Health Organization, the leading cause of blindness in the world is _____.

6. An initial treatment for a splash injury to the eye would be _____.

7. Three microorganisms that most commonly cause bacterial conjunctivitis are: _____, _____, and _____.

8. A characteristic sign of viral conjunctivitis is _____.

9. One of the most serious ocular consequences of diabetes is _____.

10. The most common cause of retinal inflammation in patients with AIDS is _____.

11. A healthy tear is composed of three layers: _____, _____, and _____.

12. The nurse is assessing a patient for ptosis, which is defined as _____.

Activity B *Briefly answer the following.*

1. Describe how the nurse would assess a patient's visual acuity.

_____

_____

2. What nursing measures are important to educate the patient about when performing tonometry?

_____

_____

3. When is the Amsler grid test used?

_____

_____

Activity C

PART I

Match the characteristic or function of the eye listed in Column II with its associated structure listed in Column I.

Column I

____ **1.** Choroid

____ **2.** Lens

____ **3.** Pupil

____ **4.** Retina

____ **5.** Vitreous humor

____ **6.** Cornea

____ **7.** Sclera

____ **8.** Iris

____ **9.** Uvea

____ **10.** Limbus

Column II

a. Maintains the form of the eyeball

b. Area where most of the blood vessels for the eye are located

c. Degree of convexity modified by contraction and relaxation of the ciliary muscles

d. Contractile membrane between the cornea and lens

e. Transparent part of the fibrous coat of the eyeball

f. Accommodates to the intensity of light by dilating or contracting

g. White part of the eye

h. The pigmented, vascular coating of the eye

i. The edge of the cornea where it joins the sclera

j. Contains nerve endings that transmit visual impulses to the brain

PART II

Match the term listed in Column II with its associated definition listed in Column I.

Column I

____ **1.** Excessive production of tears

____ **2.** Another term for an external hordeolum

____ **3.** Term for the right eye

____ **4.** A term used to describe an inflammatory condition of the uveal tract

____ **5.** Another term for nearsightedness

____ **6.** An inflammatory condition affecting the iris

____ **7.** Inflammation of the cornea

____ **8.** A loss of cornea substance or tissue as a result of inflammation

____ **9.** Abnormal sensitivity to light

____ **10.** Term for the left eye

____ **11.** Absence of the lens

____ **12.** Uneven curvature of the cornea

____ **13.** Drooping of the upper eyelid

____ **14.** A tear in the eye tissue

____ **15.** A condition in which one eye deviates from the object at which the person is looking

Column II

a. Iritis

b. Keratitis

c. Photophobia

d. Aphakia

e. Oculus dexter

f. Ptosis

g. Epiphora

h. Strabismus

i. Laceration

j. Ulcer

k. Oculus sinister

l. Uveitis

m. Astigmatism

n. Sty

o. Myopia

SECTION II: APPLYING YOUR KNOWLEDGE

Activity D *Consider the scenario and answer the questions.*

CASE STUDY: Cataract Surgery

Marcella is a 75-year-old single woman who has had progressive diminished vision and increased difficulty with night driving. Her physician suspects that Marcella has a cataract and does a complete eye examination and history.

1. During the health history, the nurse collects data that would indicate whether Marcella has any common factors that contribute to cataract development. What would these factors be?

   _____

   _____

2. Marcella informed the nurse of visual symptoms she has been having. Which symptoms would the nurse recognize as significant for cataracts?

   _____

   _____

3. It is determined that Marcella has cataracts, and she has agreed to have surgery to remove them. When the nurse is providing postoperative education, what is important for the nurse to tell Marcella about side lying?

   _____

   _____

SECTION III: PRACTICING FOR NCLEX

Activity E *Answer the following questions.*

1. An older adult patient informs the nurse, "I don't see as well as I used to." What should the nurse explain to the patient about why vision becomes less efficient with age? (Select all the apply.)
   a. There is a decrease in pupil size.
   b. There is slowing of accommodation.
   c. There is an increase in lens opaqueness.
   d. Most older patients develop glaucoma.
   e. The optic nerve begins to degenerate.

2. During a routine eye examination, a patient complains that she is unable to read road signs at a distance when driving her car. What should the patient be assessed for?
   a. Astigmatism
   b. Anisometropia
   c. Myopia
   d. Presbyopia

3. It is determined that a patient is legally blind and will be unable to drive any longer. Legal blindness refers to a best-corrected visual acuity (BCVA) that does not exceed what reading in the better eye?
   a. 20/50
   b. 20/100
   c. 20/150
   d. 20/200

4. A patient is suspected of having glaucoma. What reading of IOP would demonstrate an increase resulting from optic nerve damage?
   a. 0 to 5 mm Hg
   b. 6 to 10 mm Hg
   c. 11 to 20 mm Hg
   d. 21 mm Hg or higher

5. The nurse at the eye clinic is caring for a patient with suspected glaucoma. What complaint would be significant for a diagnosis of glaucoma?
   a. A significant loss of central vision
   b. Diminished acuity
   c. Pain associated with a purulent discharge
   d. The presence of halos around lights

6. The nurse is performing an assessment of the visual fields for a patient with glaucoma. When assessing the visual fields in acute glaucoma, what would the nurse expect to find?
   a. Clear cornea
   b. Constricted pupil
   c. Marked blurring of vision
   d. Watery ocular discharge

7. The nurse is educating a patient with glaucoma about medications. What medications will the nurse educate the patient about that decrease aqueous production? (Select all that apply.)
   a. Alpha-adrenergic agonists
   b. Carbonic anhydrase inhibitors
   c. Beta-blockers
   d. Miotics
   e. Calcium channel blockers

8. A patient has had cataract extractions and the nurse is providing discharge instructions. What should the nurse encourage the patient to do at home?
   a. Maintain bed rest for 1 week.
   b. Lie on the stomach while sleeping.
   c. Avoid bending the head below the waist.
   d. Lift weights to increase muscle strength.

9. A patient is being seen in the ophthalmology clinic for a suspected detached retina. What clinical manifestations does the nurse recognize as significant for a retinal detachment? (Select all that apply.)
   a. A visual field of floating particles
   b. A definite area of blank vision
   c. Momentary flashes of light
   d. Pain
   e. Halos around the eyes

10. An older adult patient has noticed a significant amount of vision loss in the last few years. What does the nurse recognize as the most common cause of visual loss in older adults?
    a. Macular degeneration
    b. Ocular trauma
    c. Retinal vascular disease
    d. Uveitis

11. A patient is brought into the emergency department with chemical burns to both eyes. What is the priority action of the nurse for this patient's care?
    a. Administering local anesthetics and antibacterial drops for 24 to 36 hours
    b. Applying hot compresses at 15-minute intervals
    c. Flushing the lids, conjunctiva, and cornea with tap water or normal saline
    d. Cleansing the conjunctiva with a small cotton-tipped applicator

12. A patient comes to the clinic with a suspected eye infection. The nurse recognizes that the patient most likely has conjunctivitis, as evidenced by what symptom?
    a. Blurred vision
    b. Elevated IOP
    c. A mucopurulent ocular discharge
    d. Severe pain

13. What type of medication would the nurse use in combination with mydriatics to dilate the patient's pupil?
    a. Anti-infectives
    b. Corticosteroids
    c. Cycloplegics
    d. NSAIDs

14. A patient is to have an angiography done using fluorescein as a contrast agent to determine if the patient has macular edema. What laboratory work should the nurse monitor prior to the angiography?
    a. BUN and creatinine
    b. AST and ALT
    c. Hemoglobin and hematocrit
    d. Platelet count

15. The nurse is administering an ophthalmic ointment to a patient with conjunctivitis. What disadvantage of the application of an ointment does the nurse explain to the patient?
    a. It does not work as rapidly as eye drops do.
    b. Blurred vision results after application.
    c. It has a lower concentration than eye drops.
    d. It has more side effects than eye drops.

CHAPTER 64

Assessment and Management of Patients With Hearing and Balance Disorders

1. Describe the anatomy and physiology of the ear.
2. Describe methods used to assess hearing and to diagnose hearing and balance disorders.
3. List the manifestations that may be exhibited by a person with a hearing disorder.
4. Identify ways to communicate effectively with a person with a hearing disorder.
5. Differentiate problems of the external ear from those of the middle ear and inner ear.
6. Compare the various types of surgical procedures used for managing middle ear disorders and appropriate nursing care.
7. Use the nursing process as a framework of care for patients undergoing mastoid surgery.
8. Use the nursing process as a framework of care for patients with vertigo.
9. Describe the different types of inner ear disorders, including the clinical manifestations, diagnosis, and management.

SECTION I: ASSESSING YOUR UNDERSTANDING

Activity A *Fill in the blanks.*

1. The organ of hearing is known as the
   _____.

2. Mechanical vibrations are transformed into neural activity so that sounds can be differentiated by the _____.

3. A sensorineural (perceptive) hearing loss results from impairment of the _____ cranial nerve.

4. The critical level of loudness that most people (without a hearing loss) are comfortable with is a decibel (dB) reading of _____ dB.

5. Severe hearing loss is associated with a decibel loss in the range of _____ to _____ dB.

6. A hearing loss that is a manifestation of an emotional disturbance is known a _____ hearing loss.

7. The minimum noise level known to cause noise-induced hearing loss, regardless of duration, is _____ to _____ dB.

8. It is projected that by 2050, _____% of people over age 55 will have some form of hearing loss.

9. A facial nerve neuroma is a tumor on the _____ nerve.

10. An acoustic neuroma is a benign tumor of the _____ nerve.

Activity B *Briefly answer the following.*

1. Describe how sound is conducted and transmitted.

_____

_____

_____

_____

2. What three tests are used to evaluate gross auditory acuity?

_____

_____

_____

3. When assessing hearing and balance, what should be included?

_____

_____

_____

4. Name the three characteristics that are important when evaluating hearing.

_____

_____

_____

5. A patient is having a tympanogram. What significance does this test have?

_____

_____

_____

Activity C *Match the term in Column I with the definition in Column II.*

Column I

____ **1.** Dizziness

____ **2.** Vertigo

____ **3.** Exostoses

____ **4.** Nystagmus

____ **5.** Otalgia

____ **6.** Otorrhea

____ **7.** Otosclerosis

____ **8.** Presbycusis

____ **9.** Rhinorrhea

____ **10.** Tinnitus

Column II

a. Illusion of movement in which the individual or the surroundings are sensed as moving

b. Progressive hearing loss associated with aging

c. Sensation of fullness or pain in the ear

d. Drainage from the nose

e. Subjective perception of sound with internal origin; unwanted noises in the head or ear

f. A condition characterized by abnormal spongy bone formation around the stapes

g. Involuntary rhythmic eye movement

h. Altered sensation of orientation in space

i. Small, hard, bony protrusions in the lower posterior bony portion of the ear canal

j. Drainage from the ear.

SECTION II: APPLYING YOUR KNOWLEDGE

Activity D *Consider the scenarios and answer the questions.*

CASE STUDY: Mastoid Surgery: Postoperative Care

Amber is a 73-year-old grandmother who is scheduled for mastoid surgery to remove a cholesteatoma, a cystlike sac filled with keratin debris, which was large enough to occlude the ear canal.

1. The patient is informed that she will have a mastoid pressure dressing in place after surgery. The nurse tells Amber that the dressing will be removed at what time?

_____

_____

_____

2. Although infrequent, what type of nerve damage should the nurse assess for and immediately report to the physician?

_____

_____

_____

3. What should the nurse inform the patient are indicators of infection and should be reported immediately to the physician?

_____

_____

CASE STUDY: Ménière's Disease

David is a 42-year-old lawyer who travels internationally. He has recently been diagnosed with Ménière's disease.

1. What does the nurse recognize are classic symptoms that are diagnostic for Ménière's disease?

_____

_____

_____

2. The nurse is educating the patient with Ménière's disease about a dietary regimen. What foods should the nurse include for the patient to avoid or limit?

_____

_____

3. The nurse cautions David about taking certain medications that will increase the dizziness or tinnitus. Which medications should be avoided?

_____

_____

SECTION III: PRACTICING FOR NCLEX

Activity E *Answer the following questions.*

1. The nurse is performing an assessment of a patient's ears. When looking at the tympanic membrane, the nurse observes a healthy membrane. What should the appearance be?

    a. Pearly gray and translucent

    b. White and cloudy

    c. Pink with white exudate

    d. Dark yellow with cerumen

2. The nurse is assessing the auricles of a patient. When the left auricle is manipulated, the patient complains of pain. What does this finding indicate?

    a. The patient may have seborrheic dermatitis.

    b. The patient may have an inner ear infection.

    c. The patient may have acute external otitis.

    d. The patient may have acute otitis media.

3. The nurse is examining the area behind the patient's auricle and sees a flaky scaliness. What disorder does the nurse suspect the patient has?

    a. Sebaceous cysts

    b. Seborrheic dermatitis

    c. Tophi

    d. Acute external otitis

4. A nursing student is learning how to adequately use an otoscope to examine the ear. What method should the instructor educate the student to use when examining with an otoscope?

   a. Otoscope should be held in the examiner's right hand, in a pencil-hold position, with the examiner's hand braced against the patient's face.

   b. Otoscope should be held in the examiner's left hand, with a full hand grasp to be able to guide the scope into the internal ear.

   c. Otoscope should be held in the examiner's dominant hand, with a full hand grasp to be able to guide the scope into the internal ear.

   d. Otoscope should be held in the examiner's left hand, in a pencil-hold position, with the examiner's hand braced against the patient's face.

5. A patient comes to the clinic with some hearing loss. The physician is unable to observe the tympanic membrane due to the accumulation of cerumen. What intervention can the nurse provide so that observation can be made?

   a. The nurse can remove the wax with a cerumen curette.

   b. The ear can be irrigated with cool water until all of the wax is removed.

   c. The nurse can instill a small amount of mineral oil into the canal and have the patient return for removal of the wax.

   d. The nurse can instill mineral oil into the canal and immediately irrigate to remove the adherent wax.

6. A patient is scheduled to have an auditory brain stem response in 2 days. What does the nurse instruct the patient to do in preparation for the test?

   a. Shave several areas on the scalp where the electrodes will be placed.

   b. Do not eat or drink 8 hours prior to testing.

   c. Wash and rinse hair before test but do not apply any other hair products.

   d. Omit daily medications prior to testing.

7. A patient with vertigo is scheduled to have an electronystagmography in 2 weeks. What will the nurse instruct the patient to do prior to the test?

   a. Withhold caffeine and alcohol 48 hours before the test.

   b. Withhold blood pressure medication 24 hours before the test.

   c. Withhold vestibular suppressants 48 hours before the test.

   d. Do not eat or drink anything 12 hours before testing.

8. A patient has been diagnosed with a fungal infection causing external otitis. What is the most common fungal infection in the ear?

   a. *Staphylococcus aureus*

   b. *Aspergillus*

   c. *Pseudomonas*

   d. *Streptococcus*

9. A patient has been treated for external otitis for the second time during the summer months. What education can be provided for the patient to reduce the risk of developing this problem? (Select all that apply.)

   a. Do not clean the external canal with cotton-tipped applicators.

   b. Irrigate the ears daily with a warm saline solution.

   c. Avoid getting the ear wet when swimming or showering.

   d. Use an antiseptic otic preparation after swimming, unless there is a history of tympanic membrane perforation.

   e. Ensure that cerumen is absent from the external canal by irrigating once a week after instilling mineral oil.

10. A patient has serous otitis media with significant hearing loss in the right ear. The patient states, "I have not been able to hear for 2 months." What procedure does the nurse anticipate preparing the patient for?

    a. Irrigation of the ear

    b. Myringotomy

    c. Removal of cerumen with a cerumen curette

    d. Instillation of otic solution

11. The nurse is talking with a patient diagnosed with Ménière's disease about the patient's symptoms. What symptom does the patient inform the nurse is the most troublesome?

a. Nausea

b. Diarrhea

c. Tinnitus

d. Vertigo

12. The nurse is caring for a patient with Ménière's disease who is hospitalized with severe vertigo. What medication does the nurse anticipate administering to shorten the attack?

a. Meclizine (Antivert)

b. Furosemide (Lasix)

c. Cortisporin otic solution

d. Gentamicin (Garamycin) intravenously

13. A patient is complaining of ringing in the left ear and hearing loss in the same ear, but does not have any associated dizziness or vertigo. What should this patient be assessed for?

a. Otitis media

b. Acoustic neuroma

c. Labyrinthitis

d. Tinnitus

14. The nurse is talking to a family member of a hearing-impaired patient and the patient states, "I know you are talking about me. You are just whispering so that I will not hear what you are saying." What does the nurse recognize this statement indicates?

a. False pride

b. Indecision

c. Insecurity

d. Suspiciousness

15. The nurse is developing a plan of care for a patient with severe vertigo. What expected outcome statement would be a priority for this patient?

a. Patient will experience no falls due to balance disorder.

b. Patient will take medications as prescribed.

c. Patient will perform exercises as prescribed.

d. Patient will have decreased fear and anxiety.

Neurologic Function

Assessment of Neurologic Function

Learning Objectives

1. Describe the structures and functions of the central and peripheral nervous systems.
2. Differentiate between pathologic changes that affect motor control and those that affect sensory pathways.
3. Compare the functioning of the sympathetic and parasympathetic nervous systems.
4. Describe the significance of physical assessment to the diagnosis of neurologic dysfunction.
5. Describe changes in neurologic function associated with aging and their impact on neurologic assessment findings.
6. Describe diagnostic tests used for assessment of suspected neurologic disorders and the related nursing implications.

SECTION I: ASSESSING YOUR UNDERSTANDING

Activity A *Fill in the blanks.*

1. _Serotonin_ is a neurotransmitter that helps control mood and sleep.

2. Parkinson's disease is caused by an imbalance in the neurotransmitter known as _Dopamine_.

3. A person's personality and judgment are controlled by the area of the brain known as the _Frontal_ lobe.

4. The lobe of the cerebral cortex that is responsible for the understanding of language and music is the _temporal_ lobe.

5. Voluntary muscle control is governed by a vertical band of "motor cortex" located in the _Frontal_ lobe.

6. The sleep–wake cycle regulator and the site of the hunger center is known as the _hypothalamus_

7. The "master gland" is also known as the _Pituitary_ gland.

8. The major receiving and communication center for afferent sensory nerves is the _thalamus_

9. The normal adult produces about _150_ mL of cerebrospinal fluid daily from the ventricles.

10. The preganglionic fibers of the sympathetic neurons are located in the segments of the spinal cord identified as _C8_ to _L3_

11. The parasympathetic division of the autonomic nervous system yields impulses that are mediated by the secretion of _acetylcholine_, the dominant neurotransmitter in parasympathetic nervous system functions.

12. The brain center responsible for balancing and coordination is the _Cerebellum_.
    striae

Activity B *Briefly answer the following.*

1. What is the function of the blood–brain barrier?

   Endothelial cells of the brain capillaries forms tight junction to macromolecules & many compounds

2. Describe the role and functions of the autonomic nervous system.

   Regulates the activities of internal organs, and also responsible for homeostasis

3. Name the principle signs of lower motor neuron disease.

   Flaccid Paralysis & atrophy of the muscles

4. What clinical manifestations occur when there is destruction or dysfunction in the basal ganglia?

   Leads to muscle rigidity, changing Posture & movement

Activity C **Neurotransmitters and Nervous System Response**

Match the nervous system response listed in Column II with the neurotransmitter listed in Column I.

Column I

E   1. Gamma-aminobutyric acid

F   2. Enkephalin

D   3. Norepinephrine

C   4. Dopamine

A   5. Acetylcholine

B   6. Serotonin

Column II

a. Primarily excitatory; can produce vagal stimulation of heart

b. Inhibits pain pathways and can control sleep

c. Affects behavior, attention, and fine movement

d. Excitatory response, mostly affecting moods

e. Muscle and nerve inhibitory transmissions

f. Excitatory; inhibits pain transmission

Cranial Nerves

Next to each cranial nerve listed by number, write the appropriate corresponding terminology in Column I and a major associated function in Column II. The answers for the first cranial nerve are provided as an example.

Nerve No.	Column I	Column II
I	Olfactory	Smell
II		
III		
IV		
V		
VI		
VII		
VIII		
IX		
X		
XI		
XII		

SECTION II: APPLYING YOUR KNOWLEDGE

Activity D *Consider the scenario and answer the questions.*

CASE STUDY: Mental Status

Grace, an 82-year-old woman, is brought to the clinic by her son, who informs the nurse that his mother is not "as sharp" as she has been and has been forgetting to take some of her medication. The son asks that his mother be "checked out."

1. What intervention does the nurse provide when assisting Grace to change into a gown and to sit on the examining table?

   _____

   _____

2. After the physician examines Grace, laboratory studies and a CT scan of the brain are ordered. When providing instruction to Grace and her son, what will the nurse do in order to ensure that the instructions are understood?

_____

_____

_____

_____

3. How would the nurse differentiate delirium from dementia in assessing Grace?

_____

_____

_____

_____

SECTION III: PRACTICING FOR NCLEX

Activity E *Answer the following questions.*

1. A patient arrives to have an MRI done in the outpatient department. What information provided by the patient warrants further assessment to prevent complications related to the MRI?

  a. "I am trying to quit smoking and have a patch on."

  b. "I have been trying to get an appointment for so long."

  c. "I have not had anything to eat or drink since 3 hours ago."

  d. "My legs go numb sometimes when I sit too long."

2. A patient is scheduled for an electroencephalogram (EEG) in the morning. What food on the patient's tray should the nurse remove prior to the test?

  a. Orange juice

  b. Toast

  c. Coffee

  d. Eggs

3. The nurse is assisting with a lumbar puncture and observes that when the physician obtains CSF, it is clear and colorless. What does this finding indicate?

  a. A subarachnoid hemorrhage

  b. An overwhelming infection

  c. A normal finding; the fluid will be sent for testing to determine other factors

  d. Local trauma from the insertion of the needle

4. A patient had a lumbar puncture 3 days ago in the outpatient clinic and calls the nurse with complaints of a throbbing headache. What can the nurse educate the patient to do for relief of the discomfort? (Select all that apply.)

  a. Limit the amount of fluid to decrease cerebral edema.

  b. Force fluids (unless contraindicated).

  c. Get plenty of bed rest.

  d. Take some over-the-counter analgesics.

  e. Walk around.

5. A patient is having a lumbar puncture and the physician has removed 20 mL of cerebrospinal fluid. What nursing intervention is a priority after the procedure?

  a. Early ambulation

  b. Have the patient lie flat for 6 hours.

  c. Have the patient lie flat for 1 hour and then sit for 1 hour before ambulating.

  d. Have the patient lie in a semi-Fowler's position with the head of the bed at 30°.

6. The nurse is performing an assessment of cranial nerve function and asks the patient to cover one nostril at a time to see if the patient can smell coffee, alcohol, and mint. The patient is unable to smell any of the odors. The nurse is aware that the patient has a dysfunction of which cranial nerve?

  a. CN I

  b. CN II

  c. CN III

  d. CN IV

7. The nurse obtains a Snellen eye chart when assessing cranial nerve function. Which cranial nerve is the nurse testing when using the chart?

   a. CN I

   b. CN II

   c. CN III

   d. CN IV

8. A patient is being tested for a gag reflex. When the nurse places the tongue blade to the back of the throat, there is no response elicited. What dysfunction does the nurse determine the patient has?

   a. Dysfunction of the spinal accessory nerve

   b. Dysfunction of the acoustic nerve

   c. Dysfunction of the facial nerve

   d. Dysfunction of the vagus nerve

9. A patient sustained a head injury during a fall and has changes in personality and affect. What part of the brain does the nurse recognize has been affected in this injury?

   a. Frontal lobe

   b. Parietal lobe

   c. Occipital lobe

   d. Temporal lobe

10. A patient who has suffered a stroke is unable to maintain respiration and so is intubated and placed on mechanical ventilator support. What portion of the brain is most likely responsible for the inability to breathe?

    a. Frontal lobe

    b. Occipital lobe

    c. Parietal lobe

    d. Brain stem

11. A patient has expressive speaking aphasia after having a stroke. Which portion of the brain does the nurse know has been affected?

    a. Temporal lobe

    b. Inferior posterior frontal areas

    c. Posterior frontal area

    d. Parietal-occipital area

12. The nurse is assessing the pupils of a patient who has had a head injury. What does the nurse recognize as a parasympathetic effect?

    a. Dilated pupils

    b. Constricted pupils

    c. One pupil is dilated and the opposite pupil is normal

    d. Roth's spots

13. The nurse is caring for a patient who was involved in a motor vehicle accident and sustained a head injury. When assessing deep tendon reflexes (DTR), the nurse observes diminished or hypoactive reflexes. How will the nurse document this finding?

    a. 0

    b. 1+

    c. 2+

    d. 3+

14. The nurse is performing a neurologic assessment and requests that the patient stand with eyes open and then closed for 20 seconds to assess balance. What type of test is the nurse performing?

    a. Weber test

    b. Rinne test

    c. Romberg test

    d. Watch-tick test

15. A patient comes to the emergency department with severe pain in the face that was stimulated by brushing the teeth. What cranial nerve does the nurse understand can cause this type of pain?

    a. III

    b. IV

    c. V

    d. VI

66

Management of Patients With Neurologic Dysfunction

Learning Objectives

1. Describe the causes, clinical manifestations, and medical management of various neurologic dysfunctions.
2. Use the nursing process as a framework for care of the multiple needs of the patient with altered level of consciousness.
3. Identify the early and late clinical manifestations of increased intracranial pressure.
4. Use the nursing process as a framework for care of the patient with increased intracranial pressure.
5. Describe the indications for intracranial or transsphenoidal surgery.
6. Use the nursing process as a framework for care of the patient undergoing intracranial or transsphenoidal surgery.
7. Identify the various types and causes of seizures.
8. Use the nursing process to develop a plan of care for the patient experiencing seizures.
9. Identify the causes, clinical manifestations, and medical and nursing management of the patient experiencing headaches.

SECTION I: ASSESSING YOUR UNDERSTANDING

Activity A *Fill in the blanks.*

1. A patient has a lesion affecting the pons, resulting in paralysis and the inability to speak, but has vertical eye movements and lid elevation. This patient is suffering from _____.

2. Three major potential complications in a patient with a depressed level of consciousness (LOC) are _____, _____, and _____.

3. The earliest sign of increased ICP is _____ _____.

4. Three primary complications of increased ICP are _____, _____, and _____.

5. The primary, lethal complication of ICP is _____.

6. Nursing postoperative management includes detecting and reducing _____, relieving _____, preventing _____, and monitoring _____ and _____.

7. The leading cause of seizures in the elderly is
_____.

8. A major potential complication of epilepsy is
_____.

Activity B *Briefly answer the following.*

1. What is meant by an "altered level of consciousness"?

_____

_____

_____

_____

2. List five potential collaborative problems for a patient with an altered LOC.

_____

_____

_____

3. When the nurse performs a neurologic examination, what should be included?

_____

_____

_____

_____

4. If a patient with an altered LOC requires suctioning, what intervention is a priority for the nurse to provide?

_____

_____

5. What is the optimal way to determine the level of a patient's alertness?

_____

_____

_____

_____

Activity C *Match the neurologic dysfunction in Column II with its associated nursing intervention found in Column I. Some answers may be used more than once.*

Column I

___ 1. Assist with daily active or passive range of motion.

___ 2. Elevate the head of the bed 30 degrees.

___ 3. Institute a bowel-training program.

___ 4. Maintain dorsiflexion to affected area.

___ 5. Place the patient in a lateral position.

Column II

a. Footdrop

b. Incontinence

c. Impaired cough reflex

d. Keratitis

e. Paralyzed diaphragm

f. Paralyzed extremity

SECTION II: APPLYING YOUR KNOWLEDGE

Activity D *Consider the scenario and answer the questions.*

CASE STUDY: Optimizing Cerebral Perfusion Pressure

Alex, a 32-year-old male, was riding his motorcycle without a helmet through the woods and hit a large log, ejecting him over the handlebars and into a tree. He was unconscious when his friends found him and called the rescue squad. He has had a craniotomy to relieve an epidural hematoma and is in the neurologic intensive care unit (ICU).

1. In order to optimize cerebral perfusion pressure (CPP) and decrease intracranial pressure (ICP), in what position should the nurse maintain Alex?

_____

_____

_____

_____

2. What intervention can the nurse provide to avoid having Alex perform the Valsalva maneuver?

_____

_____

_____

_____

3. When the nurse plans Alex's care, how can his needs be met in order to prevent a rise in ICP and a decrease in CPP?

_____

_____

SECTION III: PRACTICING FOR NCLEX

Activity E *Answer the following questions.*

1. The nurse is caring for a patient with an altered LOC. What is the first priority of treatment for this patient?
   a. Assessment of pupillary light reflexes
   b. Determination of the cause
   c. Positioning to prevent complications
   d. Maintenance of a patent airway

2. A nurse assesses the patient's LOC using the Glasgow Coma Scale. What score indicates severe impairment of neurologic function?
   a. 3
   b. 6
   c. 9
   d. 12

3. A patient has a severe neurologic impairment from a head trauma. What does the nurse recognize is the type of posturing that occurs with the most severe neurologic impairment?
   a. Decerebrate
   b. Decorticate
   c. Flaccid
   d. Rigid

4. The nurse is caring for a patient in the neurologic ICU who sustained head trauma in a physical altercation. What would the nurse know is an optimal range of ICP for this patient?
   a. 8 to 15 mm Hg
   b. 0 to 10 mm Hg
   c. 20 to 30 mm Hg
   d. 25 to 40 mm Hg

5. A patient is admitted to the hospital with an ICP reading of 20 mm Hg and a mean arterial pressure of 90 mm Hg. What would the nurse calculate the CPP to be?
   a. 50 mm Hg
   b. 60 mm Hg
   c. 70 mm Hg
   d. 80 mm Hg

6. A nurse caring for a patient with head trauma will be monitoring the patient for Cushing's triad. What will the nurse recognize as the symptoms associated with Cushing's triad? (Select all that apply.)
   a. Bradycardia
   b. Bradypnea
   c. Hypertension
   d. Tachycardia
   e. Pupillary constriction

7. What does the nurse recognize as the earliest sign of serious impairment of brain circulation related to increasing ICP?
   a. A bounding pulse
   b. Bradycardia
   c. Hypertension
   d. Lethargy and stupor

8. The nurse is caring for a patient with increased ICP. As the pressure rises, what osmotic diuretic does the nurse prepare to administer?
   a. Glycerin
   b. Isosorbide
   c. Mannitol
   d. Urea

9. A nurse is assessing a patient's urinary output as an indicator of diabetes insipidus. The nurse knows that an hourly output of what volume over 2 hours may be a positive indicator?

   a. 50 to 100 mL/h

   b. 100 to 150 mL/h

   c. 150 to 200 mL/h

   d. More than 200 mL/h

10. When educating a patient about the use of antiseizure medication, what should the nurse inform the patient is a result of long-term use of the medication in women?

    a. Anemia

    b. Osteoarthritis

    c. Osteoporosis

    d. Obesity

11. The nurse is called to attend to a patient having a seizure in the waiting area. What nursing care is provided for a patient who is experiencing a convulsive seizure? (Select all that apply.)

    a. Loosening constrictive clothing

    b. Opening the patient's jaw and inserting a mouth gag

    c. Positioning the patient on his or her side with head flexed forward

    d. Providing for privacy

    e. Restraining the patient to avoid self-injury

12. The nurse is educating a patient with a seizure disorder. What nutritional approach for seizure management would be beneficial for this patient?

    a. Low in fat

    b. Restricts protein to 10% of daily caloric intake

    c. High in protein and low in carbohydrate

    d. At least 50% carbohydrate

13. The nurse is caring for a patient postoperatively after intracranial surgery for the treatment of a subdural hematoma. The nurse observes an increase in the patient's blood pressure from the baseline and a decrease in the heart rate from 86 to 54. The patient has crackles in the bases of the lungs. What does the nurse suspect is occurring?

    a. Increased ICP

    b. Exacerbation of uncontrolled hypertension

    c. Infection

    d. Increase in cerebral perfusion pressure

14. A patient 3 days postoperative from a craniotomy informs the nurse, "I feel something trickling down the back of my throat and I taste something salty." What priority intervention does the nurse initiate?

    a. Give the patient some mouthwash to gargle with.

    b. Request an antihistamine for the postnasal drip.

    c. Ask the patient to cough to observe the sputum color and consistency.

    d. Notify the physician of a possible cerebrospinal fluid leak.

15. A patient had a small pituitary adenoma removed by the transsphenoidal approach and has developed diabetes insipidus. What pharmacologic therapy will the nurse be administering to this patient to control symptoms?

    a. Mannitol

    b. Furosemide (Lasix)

    c. Vasopressin

    d. Phenobarbital

CHAPTER 67

Management of Patients With Cerebrovascular Disorders

Learning Objectives

1. Describe the incidence and social impact of cerebrovascular disorders.
2. Identify the risk factors for cerebrovascular disorders and related measures for prevention.
3. Compare the various types of cerebrovascular disorders: their causes, clinical manifestations, and medical management.
4. Apply the principles of nursing management to the care of a patient in the acute stage of an ischemic stroke.
5. Use the nursing process as a framework for care of a patient recovering from an ischemic stroke.
6. Use the nursing process as a framework for care of a patient with a hemorrhagic stroke.
7. Identify essential elements for family education and preparation for home care of the patient who has had a stroke.

SECTION I: ASSESSING YOUR UNDERSTANDING

Activity A *Fill in the blanks.*

1. The primary cerebrovascular disorder in the United States is _____, which is also called a(n) _____ to emphasize the urgency of its occurrence.

2. Since 1996, thrombolytic therapy with recombinant plasminogen activator (t-PA) for ischemic stroke has significantly decreased poststroke symptoms. However, the treatment challenge is that the therapy has to be given within _____ hours.

3. As a cause of death in the United States, stroke currently ranks _____.

4. The main surgical procedure for managing transient ischemic attacks (TIAs) is

   _____.

5. _____ is the most common cause of cerebrovascular disease.

6. The most common motor dysfunction of a stroke is _____.

7. Hemorrhagic strokes are caused by bleeding into _____, _____, or

   _____.

8. Potential complications of a hemorrhagic stroke include _____,

   _____, _____, or

   _____.

9. The most common cause of intracerebral hemorrhage is _____.

10. Stroke is divided into two categories: _____ and _____.

Activity B *Briefly answer the following.*

1. A patient has a cardioembolic stroke. What is the most common cardiac dysrhythmia that is observed on the monitor?

   _____

   _____

2. Name the most common type of ischemic strokes:

   _____

   _____

   _____

3. The risk of coronary heart disease and stroke has decreased in women on the Dietary Approaches to Stop Hypertension (DASH) diet. What does this dietary regimen consist of?

   _____

   _____

   _____

4. Describe how thrombolytic agents treat ischemic stroke:

   _____

   _____

Activity C *Match the clinical manifestations of specific neurologic deficits listed in Column II with the associated cause listed in Column I.*

Column I	Column II
____ **1.** Ataxia	**a.** Difficulty judging distances
____ **2.** Receptive aphasia	**b.** Unaware of the borders of objects
____ **3.** Dysphagia	**c.** Double vision
____ **4.** Homonymous hemianopsia	**d.** Staggering, unsteady gait
____ **5.** Loss of peripheral vision	**e.** Difficulty in swallowing
____ **6.** Expressive aphasia	**f.** Difficulty with proprioception
____ **7.** Diplopia	**g.** Unable to form words that are understandable
____ **8.** Paresthesia	**h.** Unable to comprehend the spoken word

SECTION II: APPLYING YOUR KNOWLEDGE

Activity D *Consider the scenario and answer the questions.*

Mrs. Coe, a 51-year-old woman, is brought into the emergency department by her husband. Her husband states, "She began slurring her words about 30 minutes ago," and he noticed that her mouth is turned down on the left side. He recognized that she was exhibiting signs of a stroke and brought her in immediately for treatment.

1. Mrs. Coe was immediately taken for a CT scan of the brain and it was determined that she suffered an ischemic stroke. The physician writes orders to initiate t-PA. What should be done prior to initiating therapy?

   _____

   _____

2. Mrs. Coe weighs 72 kg. How much t-PA will the nurse administer in the first minute as a bolus dose?

   _____

   _____

   _____

3. After the nurse administers the t-PA, what common side effect is it important that Mrs. Coe be monitored for?

   _____

   _____

   _____

SECTION III: PRACTICING FOR NCLEX

Activity E *Answer the following questions.*

1. The nurse knows that symptoms associated with a TIA, usually a precursor of a future stroke, usually subside in what period of time?

   a. 1 hour

   b. 3 to 6 hours

   c. 12 hours

   d. 24 to 36 hours

2. A stroke victim is experiencing memory loss and impaired learning capacity. The nurse knows that brain damage has most likely occurred in which lobe?

   a. Frontal

   b. Occipital

   c. Parietal

   d. Temporal

3. A patient is brought to the emergency department with a possible stroke. What initial diagnostic test for a stroke, usually performed in the emergency department, would the nurse prepare the patient for?

   a. 12-lead electrocardiogram

   b. Carotid ultrasound study

   c. Noncontrast computed tomogram

   d. Transcranial Doppler flow study

4. An emergency department nurse understands that a 110-lb recent stroke victim will receive at least the minimum dose of recombinant tissue plasminogen activator (t-PA). What minimum dose will the patient receive?

   a. 50 mg

   b. 60 mg

   c. 85 mg

   d. 100 mg

5. A patient is exhibiting classic signs of a hemorrhagic stroke. What complaint from the patient would be an indicator of this type of stroke?

   a. Numbness of an arm or leg

   b. Double vision

   c. Severe headache

   d. Dizziness and tinnitus

6. The nurse is caring for a patient having a hemorrhagic stroke. What position in the bed will the nurse maintain this patient?

   a. High-Fowler's

   b. Prone

   c. Supine

   d. Semi-Fowler's

7. A patient has had a large ischemic stroke and is hospitalized in the neurologic intensive care unit. What interventions will be provided for this patient to decrease intracranial pressure? (Select all that apply.)

   a. Administering mannitol

   b. Maintaining the partial pressure of carbon dioxide (PaCO$_2$) within a range of 30 to 35 mm Hg

   c. Administering heparin to induce anticoagulation

   d. Administering supplemental oxygen if the oxygen saturation is below 88%

   e. Elevating the head of the bed 30 degrees

8. A patient having an acute stroke with no other significant medical disorders has a blood glucose level of 420 mg/dL. What significance does the hyperglycemia have for this patient?

   a. The patient has new onset diabetes.

   b. This is significant for poor neurologic outcomes.

   c. The patient has developed diabetes insipidus due to the location of the stroke.

   d. The patient has liver failure.

9. A patient had a carotid endarterectomy yesterday and when the nurse arrived in the room to perform an assessment, the patient states, "All of a sudden, I am having trouble moving my right side." What concern should the nurse have about this complaint?

   a. A thrombus formation at the site of the endarterectomy

   b. This is a normal occurrence after an endarterectomy and would not be a concern.

   c. Bleeding from the endarterectomy site

   d. Surgical wound infection

10. A patient is in the acute phase of an ischemic stroke. How long does the nurse know that this phase may last?

    a. Up to 2 weeks

    b. Up to 1 week

    c. 1 to 3 days

    d. Up to 24 hours

11. When should the nurse plan the rehabilitation of a patient who is having an ischemic stroke?

   a. The day before the patient is discharged

   b. After the patient has passed the acute phase of the stroke

   c. After the nurse has received the discharge orders

   d. The day the patient has the stroke

12. A patient who has suffered a stroke begins having complications regarding spasticity in the lower extremity. What ordered medication does the nurse administer to help alleviate this problem?

   a. Diphenhydramine (Benadryl)

   b. Lioresal (Baclofen)

   c. Heparin

   d. Pregabalin (Lyrica)

13. A patient suffering a stroke is having a difficult time forming words. What would the nurse document this finding as?

   a. Ataxia

   b. Arthralgia

   c. Dysphagia

   d. Dysarthria

14. After having a stroke, a patient has cognitive deficits. What are the cognitive deficits the nurse recognizes the patient has as a result of the stroke? (Select all that apply.)

   a. Poor abstract reasoning

   b. Decreased attention span

   c. Short- and long-term memory loss

   d. Expressive aphasia

   e. Paresthesias

15. What clinical manifestations does the nurse recognize when a patient has had a right hemispheric stroke?

   a. Left visual field deficit

   b. Aphasia

   c. Slow, cautious behavior

   d. Altered intellectual ability

Management of Patients With Neurologic Trauma

Learning Objectives

1. Describe the mechanisms of injury, clinical signs and symptoms, diagnostic testing, and treatment options for patients with traumatic brain and spinal cord injuries.
2. Describe the nursing management of patients with brain injury.
3. Use the nursing process as a framework for care of patients with traumatic brain injury.
4. Identify the population at risk for spinal cord injury.
5. Describe the clinical features and management of the patient with neurogenic shock.
6. Discuss the pathophysiology of autonomic dysreflexia and describe the appropriate nursing interventions.
7. Use the nursing process as a framework for care of patients with spinal cord injury.

SECTION I: ASSESSING YOUR UNDERSTANDING

Activity A *Fill in the blanks.*

1. The cranial vault contains three main components: _____, _____, and _____.

2. According to the _____, the cranial vault is a closed system, and if one of the three components increases in volume, at least one of the other two must decrease in volume, or the pressure will increase.

3. Skull fractures are classified by type and location. Types include _____, _____, and _____ skull fractures, while location fractures include _____, _____, and _____ skull fractures.

4. A _____ is used to diagnose a skull fracture.

5. The most serious brain injury that can develop within the cranial vault is a
_____.

6. The four signs of a rapidly expanding, acute subdural hematoma that would require immediate surgical intervention are
_____, _____, _____, and _____.

7. The three cardinal signs of brain death are _____, _____, and _____.

8. A _____ after head injury is a temporary loss of neurologic function with no apparent structural damage.

9. The three criteria used to assess level of consciousness (LOC) using the Glasgow Coma Scale (GCS) are _____, _____, and _____.

10. Complications after traumatic head injuries can be classified according to _____, _____, and _____.

11. The five vertebrae most commonly involved in spinal cord injuries are the _____, _____, _____, _____, and _____.

Activity B *Briefly answer the following.*

1. Describe the characteristic clinical manifestations of Brown-Séquard syndrome.

_____

_____

2. Name the four most common causes of traumatic brain injury (TBI).

_____

_____

3. What is the difference between primary and secondary brain injury?

_____

_____

_____

4. A patient sustains a grade 1 head injury. Describe the clinical manifestations that would be seen with this type of injury:

_____

_____

5. When a patient sustains a head injury and is admitted to the hospital for observation, what will be monitored?

_____

_____

Activity C *Match the segmental sensorimotor function in Column II with the injury level in Column I.*

Column I

____ **1.** C1

____ **2.** C2–C3

____ **3.** C4

____ **4.** C5

____ **5.** C6

____ **6.** C7–C8

____ **7.** T1–T5

____ **8.** T6–T10

____ **9.** T11–L5

____ **10.** S1–S5

Column II

a. Full foot, leg, ankle control

b. Full elbow extension, wrist plantar flexion

c. Requires continuous ventilation

d. Knee flexion and ankle dorsiflexion

e. Full head and neck control

f. Independent of mechanical ventilation for short periods

g. Full hand and finger control

h. Good head and neck sensation and motor control

i. Fully innervated shoulder

j. Abdominal muscle control, partial good balance

SECTION II: APPLYING YOUR KNOWLEDGE

Activity D *Consider the scenario and answer the questions.*

CASE STUDY: Spinal Cord Injury

Bill, a 38-year-old man who was drinking heavily at a party, got into his car and drove home against the advice of friends. While driving, he crossed the opposite lane, swerved to get back into his lane, and hit a street sign. He was ejected from the vehicle and a passing motorist who witnessed the event called 911. After stabilization at the scene and transport to the emergency department, it was determined that Bill sustained a complete C-6 fracture as well as a fractured left femur. He has been in the hospital for 3 weeks.

1. Bill states to the nurse, "I will never be able to do anything for myself anymore. I will have to live in a nursing home where someone will take care of me." What level of independence can the nurse expect that Bill will have after rehabilitation?

_____

2. When the nurse educates Bill about prevention of complications after going home, what does the nurse include?

_____

_____

_____

_____

3. What dietary information should Bill be educated about in order to maintain a healthy lifestyle and prevent complications?

_____

_____

_____

_____

SECTION III: PRACTICING FOR NCLEX

Activity E *Answer the following questions.*

1. A patient sustained a head trauma in a diving accident and has a cerebral hemorrhage located within the brain. What type of hematoma is this classified as?

   a. An epidural hematoma

   b. An extradural hematoma

   c. An intracerebral hematoma

   d. A subdural hematoma

2. A patient comes to the emergency department with a large scalp laceration after being struck in the head with a glass bottle. After assessment of the patient, what does the nurse do before the physician sutures the wound?

   a. Irrigates the wound to remove debris

   b. Administers an oral analgesic for pain

   c. Administers acetaminophen (Tylenol) for headache

   d. Shaves the hair around the wound

3. The nurse in the emergency department is caring for a patient brought in by the rescue squad after falling from a second-story window. The nurse assesses ecchymosis over the mastoid and clear fluid from the ears. What type of skull fracture is this indicative of?

   a. Occipital skull fracture

   b. Temporal skull fracture

   c. Frontal skull fracture

   d. Basilar skull fracture

4. While riding a bicycle in a race, a patient fell into a ditch and sustained a head injury. Another cyclist found the patient lying unconscious in the ditch and called 911. What type of concussion does the patient most likely have?

   a. Grade 1 concussion

   b. Grade 2 concussion

   c. Grade 3 concussion

   d. Grade 4 concussion

5. While stopped at a stop sign, a patient's car was struck from behind by another vehicle. The patient sustained a cerebral contusion and was admitted to the hospital. During what time period after the injury will the effects of injury peak?

   a. 6 to 8 hours

   b. 18 to 36 hours

   c. 12 to 24 hours

   d. 48 to 72 hours

6. A patient brought to the hospital after a skiing accident was unconscious for a brief period of time at the scene, then woke up disoriented and refused to go to the hospital for treatment. The patient became very agitated and restless, then quickly lost consciousness again. What type of TBI is suspected in this situation?

   a. Epidural hematoma

   b. Acute subdural hematoma

   c. Chronic subdural hematoma

   d. Grade 1 concussion

7. The nurse is caring for a patient in the emergency department with a diagnosed epidural hematoma. What procedure will the nurse prepare the patient for?

   a. Hypophysectomy

   b. Application of Halo traction

   c. Burr holes

   d. Insertion of Crutchfield tongs

8. A patient sustained a head injury and has been admitted to the neurosurgical intensive care unit (ICU). The patient began having seizures and was administered a sedative-hypnotic medication that is ultra-short acting and can be titrated to patient response. What medication will the nurse be monitoring during this time?

   a. Lorazepam (Ativan)

   b. Midazolam (Versed)

   c. Phenobarbital

   d. Propofol (Diprivan)

9. The nurse is planning the care of a patient with a TBI in the neurosurgical ICU. In developing the plan of care, what interventions should be a priority? (Select all that apply.)

   a. Making nursing assessments

   b. Setting priorities for nursing interventions

   c. Anticipating needs and complications

   d. Initiating rehabilitation

   e. Ensuring that the patient regains full brain function

10. The nurse is planning to provide education about prevention in the community YMCA due to the increase in numbers of spinal cord injuries (SCIs). What predominant risk factors does the nurse understand will have to be addressed? (Select all that apply.)

    a. Young age

    b. Male gender

    c. Older adult

    d. Substance abuse

    e. Low-income community

11. For a patient with an SCI, why is it beneficial to administer oxygen to maintain a high partial pressure of oxygen (PaO_2)?

    a. So that the patient will not have a respiratory arrest

    b. Because hypoxemia can create or worsen a neurologic deficit of the spinal cord

    c. To increase cerebral perfusion pressure

    d. To prevent secondary brain injury

12. A patient was body surfing in the ocean and sustained a cervical spinal cord fracture. A halo traction device was applied. How does the patient benefit from the application of the halo device?

    a. It is the only device that can be applied for stabilization of a spinal fracture.

    b. It allows for stabilization of the cervical spine along with early ambulation.

    c. It is less bulky and traumatizing for the patient to use.

    d. The patient can remove it as needed.

13. A patient with a C7 spinal cord fracture informs the nurse, "My head is killing me!" The nurse assesses a blood pressure of 210/140 mm Hg, heart rate of 48 and observes diaphoresis on the face. What is the first action by the nurse?

    a. Place the patient in a sitting position.

    b. Call the physician.

    c. Assess the patient for a full bladder.

    d. Assess the patient for a fecal impaction.

14. A patient has developed autonomic dysreflexia and all measures to identify a trigger have been unsuccessful. What medication can the nurse provide as ordered by the physician to decrease the blood pressure?

    a. Nifedipine (Procardia) sublingual

    b. Furosemide (Lasix) IV administered rapidly

    c. Hydralazine hydrochloride (Apresoline) IV administered slowly

    d. Bumex rapid bolus IV

15. A patient has an S5 spinal fracture from a fall. What type of assistive device will this patient require?

    a. Voice or sip-n-puff controlled electric wheelchair

    b. Electric or modified manual wheelchair, needs transfer assistance

    c. Cane

    d. The patient will be able to ambulate independently.

Management of Patients With Neurologic Infections, Autoimmune Disorders, and Neuropathies

Learning Objectives

1. Differentiate among the infectious disorders of the nervous system according to causes, manifestations, medical care, and nursing management.
2. Describe the pathophysiology, clinical manifestations, and medical and nursing management of multiple sclerosis, myasthenia gravis, and Guillain-Barré syndrome.
3. Use the nursing process as a framework for care of patients with multiple sclerosis and Guillain-Barré syndrome.
4. Describe disorders of the cranial nerves, their manifestations, and indicated nursing interventions.
5. Use the nursing process as a framework for care of the patient with a cranial nerve disorder.

SECTION I: ASSESSING YOUR UNDERSTANDING

Activity A *Fill in the blanks.*

1. The infectious disorders of the nervous system are _____, _____, _____, _____, and _____.

2. Classic clinical features of Guillain-Barré syndrome (GBS) are _____ and _____.

3. The most common cause of acute encephalitis in the United States is _____. The two medications of choice for this disorder are _____ and _____.

4. The three diagnostic tests used to support diagnosis of Creutzfeldt–Jakob are _____, _____, and _____.

5. The primary pathology of multiple sclerosis (MS) is damage to the _____.

6. Disease-modifying therapies that are available to treat MS include _____ therapies and _____ agents.

7. Myasthenia gravis is considered an autoimmune disease in which antibodies are directed against _____.

8. The majority of patients with myasthenia gravis exhibit these two clinical signs: _____ and _____.

9. _____ and _____ are the bacteria responsible for the majority of cases of bacterial meningitis in adults.

10. _____ with _____ is the clinical feature unique to the patient with St. Louis encephalitis.

Activity B *Briefly answer the following.*

1. The nurse is using a bedside risk scoring system for an adult patient with bacterial meningitis. Name five risks for an unfavorable outcome:

_____

_____

_____

2. Explain what *demyelination* refers to in reference to MS.

_____

_____

_____

3. What strategies can the nurse educate the patient with MS about to avoid the disabling effects of fatigue?

_____

_____

_____

_____

Activity C *Match the cranial nerve listed in Column II with its associated clinical disorder listed in Column I. Answers may be used more than once.*

Column I

___ 1. Optic neuritis

___ 2. Pituitary tumor

___ 3. Brain stem ischemia

___ 4. Trigeminal neuralgia

___ 5. Bell's palsy

___ 6. Herpes zoster

___ 7. Ménière's syndrome

___ 8. GBS

___ 9. Vagal body tumors

___ 10. Sinus tract tumor

Column II

a. I

b. II

c. IV

d. V

e. VI

f. VII

g. VIII

h. X

SECTION II: APPLYING YOUR KNOWLEDGE

Activity D *Consider the scenario and answer the questions.*

CASE STUDY: Multiple Sclerosis

Toni, a 32-year-old mother of two, has had MS for 5 years. She is currently enrolled in a school of nursing. Her husband is supportive and helps with the care of their preschool sons. Toni has been admitted to the acute care facility for diagnostic studies related to symptoms of visual disturbances.

1. Toni is enrolled full time in the nursing program and has classroom and clinical activities 4 days per week. What should the nurse educate Toni about regarding the cause of relapsing episodes of MS?

_____

_____

_____

_____

2. Toni is prescribed IV prednisolone 1 g IV daily for 3 to 5 days, followed by an oral taper of prednisone. What will the nurse educate Toni about regarding the side effects of the medication?

_____

_____

3. The nurse is aware that MS may be affecting Toni in other areas. What should the nurse assess for during Toni's hospitalization?

_____

_____

_____

SECTION III: PRACTICING FOR NCLEX

Activity E *Answer the following questions.*

1. A college student goes to the infirmary with a fever, headache, and a stiff neck. The nurse suspects the student may have meningitis and has the student transferred to the hospital. If the diagnosis is confirmed, what should the nurse institute for those who have been in contact with this student? (Select all that apply.)

  a. Administration of rifampin (Rifadin)

  b. Administration of ciprofloxacin hydrochloride (Cipro)

  c. Administration of ceftriaxone sodium (Rocephin)

  d. Amoxicillin (Amoxil)

  e. Rofecoxib (Vioxx)

2. A patient has been diagnosed with meningococcal meningitis at a community living home. When should prophylactic therapy begin for those who have had close contact with the patient?

  a. Within 24 hours after exposure

  b. Within 48 hours after exposure

  c. Within 72 hours after exposure

  d. Therapy is not necessary prophylactically and should only be used if the person develops symptoms.

3. The nurse caring for a patient with bacterial meningitis is administering dexamethasone (Decadron) that has been ordered as an adjunct to antibiotic therapy. When does the nurse know is the appropriate time to administer this medication?

  a. 1 hour after the antibiotic has infused and daily for 7 days

  b. 15 to 20 minutes before the first dose of antibiotic and every 6 hours for the next 4 days

  c. 2 hours prior to the administration of antibiotics for 7 days

  d. It can be administered every 6 hours for 10 days.

4. The nurse is caring for a patient admitted to the hospital with a brain abscess that developed from an untreated case of otitis media. What assessment data is a priority to alert the nurse to changes in intracranial pressure?

  a. Level of consciousness

  b. Peripheral pulses

  c. Sensory perception

  d. Crackles bilaterally

5. The nurse is administering the IV antiviral medication ganciclovir (Cytovene) to the patient with HSV-1 encephalitis. What is the best way for the nurse to administer the medication to avoid crystallization of the medication in the urine?

  a. Administer the medication rapidly over 15 minutes with 100 mL of normal saline.

  b. Dilute the medicine in 500 mL of lactated Ringer's solution.

  c. Administer via slow IV over 1 hour.

  d. Administer in a drip over 4 hours.

6. The nurse is volunteering for a Red Cross blood drive and is taking the history of potential donors. Which volunteer would the nurse know will not be allowed to donate blood?

  a. A donor with a history of hypertension with a blood pressure of 140/90 mm Hg

  b. A donor who is taking medication for benign prostatic hyperplasia

  c. A donor who moved to the United States from Canada

  d. A donor who was in college in England for 1 year

7. A patient diagnosed with MS 2 years ago has been admitted to the hospital with another relapse. The previous relapse followed a complete recovery with the exception of occasional vertigo. What type of MS does the nurse recognize this patient most likely has?

   a. Benign

   b. Primary progressive

   c. Relapsing-remitting (RR)

   d. Disabling

8. The nurse is caring for a patient with MS who is having spasticity in the lower extremities that decreases physical mobility. What interventions can the nurse provide to assist with relieving the spasms? (Select all that apply.)

   a. Have the patient take a hot tub bath to allow muscle relaxation.

   b. Demonstrate daily muscle stretching exercises.

   c. Apply warm compresses to the affected areas.

   d. Allow the patient adequate time to perform exercises.

   e. Assist with a rigorous exercise program to prevent contractures.

9. The nurse is assisting with administering a Tensilon test to a patient with ptosis. If the test is positive for myasthenia gravis, what outcome does the nurse know will occur?

   a. Thirty seconds after administration, the facial weakness and ptosis will be relieved for approximately 5 minutes.

   b. After administration of the medication, there will be no change in the status of the ptosis or facial weakness.

   c. The patient will have recovery of symptoms for at least 24 hours after the administration of the Tensilon.

   d. Eight hours after administration, the acetylcholinesterase begins to regenerate the available acetylcholine and will relieve symptoms.

10. During a Tensilon test to determine if a patient has myasthenia gravis, the patient complains of cramping and becomes diaphoretic. Vital signs are BP 130/78, HR 42 and respiration 18. What intervention should the nurse prepare to do?

    a. Place the patient in the supine position.

    b. Administer diphenhydramine (Benadryl) for the allergic reaction.

    c. Administer atropine to control the side effects of edrophonium.

    d. Call the rapid response team because the patient is preparing to arrest.

11. A patient with myasthenia gravis is in the hospital for treatment of pneumonia. The patient informs the nurse that it is very important to take pyridostigmine bromide (Mestinon) on time. The nurse gets busy and does not administer the medication until after breakfast. What outcome will the patient have related to this late dose?

    a. The muscles will become fatigued and the patient will not be able to chew food or swallow pills.

    b. There should not be a problem, since the medication was only delayed by about 2 hours.

    c. The patient will go into cardiac arrest.

    d. The patient will require a double dose prior to lunch.

12. A patient suspected of having GBS has had a lumbar puncture for cerebrospinal fluid (CSF) evaluation. When reviewing the laboratory results, what does the nurse find that is diagnostic for this disease?

    a. Glucose in the CSF

    b. Elevated protein levels in the CSF

    c. Red blood cells present in the CSF

    d. White blood cells in the CSF

13. The nurse is caring for a patient with GBS in the intensive care unit and is assessing the patient for autonomic dysfunction. What interventions should be provided in order to determine the presence of autonomic dysfunction?

    a. Assess the respiratory rate and oxygen saturation.

    b. Assess the blood pressure and heart rate.

    c. Assess the peripheral pulses.

    d. Listen to the bowel sounds.

14. The nurse is caring for a patient in the emergency department with an onset of pain related to trigeminal neuralgia. What subjective data stated by the patient does the nurse determine triggered the paroxysms of pain?

 a. "I was sitting at home watching television."

 b. "I was putting my shoes on."

 c. "I was brushing my teeth."

 d. "I was taking a bath."

15. A patient with Bell's palsy says to the nurse, "It doesn't hurt anymore to touch my face. How am I going to get muscle tone back so I don't look like this anymore?" What interventions can the nurse suggest to the patient?

 a. Suggest massaging the face several times daily, using a gentle upward motion, to maintain muscle tone.

 b. Suggest applying cool compresses on the face several times a day to tighten the muscles.

 c. Inform the patient that the muscle function will return as soon as the virus dissipates.

 d. Tell the patient to smile every 4 hours.

CHAPTER 70

Management of Patients With Oncologic or Degenerative Neurologic Disorders

Learning Objectives

1. Describe brain and spinal cord tumors: their classification, pathophysiology, clinical manifestations, diagnosis, and medical and nursing management.
2. Use the nursing process as a framework for care of patients with nervous system metastases or primary brain tumor.
3. Identify the pathophysiologic processes responsible for various degenerative neurologic disorders.
4. Use the nursing process as a framework for care of patients with Parkinson's disease.
5. Identify resources for patients and families with oncologic and degenerative neurologic disorders.
6. Use the nursing process as a framework for care of patients following a cervical diskectomy.

SECTION I: ASSESSING YOUR UNDERSTANDING

Activity A *Fill in the blanks.*

1. The majority of metastatic lesions to the brain occur from six areas: _____, _____, _____, _____, _____, and _____.

2. The three most common systemic signs of increased intracranial pressure (ICP) are _____, _____, and _____.

3. The three common focal or localized symptoms of increased ICP are _____, _____, and _____.

4. A spinal cord tumor located within the spinal cord is classified as _____.

5. Five degenerative disorders of the central and peripheral nervous system are _____, _____, _____, _____, and _____.

6. The four cardinal signs of Parkinson's disease are _____, _____, _____, and _____.

7. The five chief symptoms of amyotrophic lateral sclerosis are _____, _____, _____, _____, and _____.

8. Two common characteristics of muscular dystrophies are _____ and _____.

9. Cervical disk herniation usually occurs at the _____ or _____ interspaces.

10. Two major collaborative problems for patients with a cervical diskectomy would be _____ and _____.

Activity B *Briefly answer the following.*

1. Describe the physiologic changes that result from the infiltration of tissue subsequent to the growth of a brain tumor:

_____

_____

_____

2. Describe the various classifications of brain tumors based on their pathophysiology:

_____

_____

_____

3. What is the difference between primary and secondary brain tumors?

_____

_____

_____

4. Describe the process of stereotactic biopsy and its benefits in the diagnosis of brain tumors:

_____

_____

_____

_____

5. When a patient is diagnosed with Parkinson's disease, what clinical manifestation is present at diagnosis?

_____

_____

Activity C *Match the neurologic disorder listed in Column II with its associated description listed in Column I.*

Column I

____ **1.** Impaired ability to execute voluntary movements

____ **2.** Rapid, jerky, purposeless movements of extremities or facial muscles

____ **3.** A sensation of "pins and needles"

____ **4.** Restlessness and agitation

____ **5.** Disease of the spinal nerve root

____ **6.** Minute and illegible handwriting

____ **7.** Very slow voluntary movements and speech

____ **8.** Abnormal voice quality caused by incoordination of speech muscles

Column II

a. Akathisia

b. Bradykinesia

c. Chorea

d. Dyskinesia

e. Dysphonia

f. Micrographia

g. Paresthesia

h. Radiculopathy

SECTION II: APPLYING YOUR KNOWLEDGE

Activity D *Consider the scenarios and answer the questions.*

CASE STUDY: Parkinson's Disease

Charles is a 76-year-old retired professional golfer. He has recently been diagnosed as having Parkinson's disease.

1. Why is it important for the nurse to ensure that Charles be started on an exercise regimen as part of his treatment plan? What types of exercises might the nurse recommend and why?

_____

_____

_____

_____

2. Charles will be started on a chemotherapy program using carbidopa/levodopa. Why will carbidopa be added to the levodopa?

_____

_____

3. The nurse is developing a plan of care for Charles. What goals does the nurse set for him?

_____

_____

_____

CASE STUDY: Huntington's Disease

Mike is a 49-year-old television producer who has been diagnosed as having Huntington's disease. He lives alone in a penthouse apartment and is extremely busy and successful in his business. He has no living relatives. He is experiencing uncontrollable movements and has difficulty feeding himself. He recently started chemotherapy with haloperidol (Haldol).

1. What does the nurse recognize as the most prominent features that Mike has related to the diagnosis of Huntington's disease?

_____

_____

_____

_____

2. Mike has informed the nurse that he has no relatives or close friends who would be able to assist with his care. What information should Mike receive about resources to help with his options?

_____

_____

3. Mike has been prescribed a selective serotonin reuptake inhibitor (SSRI) included with other medications. What benefit will the SSRI have for him during his disease?

_____

_____

_____

_____

SECTION III: PRACTICING FOR NCLEX

Activity E *Answer the following questions.*

1. A patient is diagnosed with an intracerebral tumor. The nurse knows that the diagnosis may include which of the following? (Select all that apply.)

 a. Astrocytoma

 b. Ependymoma

 c. Medulloblastoma

 d. Meningioma

 e. Acoustic neuroma

2. A nurse knows that a patient exhibiting seizurelike movements localized to one side of the body most likely has what type of tumor?

 a. A cerebellar tumor

 b. A frontal lobe tumor

 c. A motor cortex tumor

 d. An occipital lobe tumor

3. An older adult patient exhibiting clinical manifestations of a brain tumor is admitted to the hospital for testing. What tumor types does the nurse know are commonly seen in the older adult?

 a. Anaplastic astrocytoma

 b. Cerebral metastasis from other sites

 c. Glioblastoma multiforme

 d. Medulloblastoma

4. A patient is exhibiting bradykinesia, rigidity, and tremors related to Parkinson's disease. The nurse understands that these symptoms are directly related to what decreased neurotransmitter level?

 a. Acetylcholine

 b. Dopamine

 c. Serotonin

 d. Phenylalanine

5. The nurse is caring for a patient with Parkinson's disease and is preparing to administer medication. What does the nurse administer to the patient that is considered the most effective drug currently given for the tremor of Parkinson's?

a. Requip

b. Levodopa

c. Symmetrel

d. Permax

6. A patient with a brain tumor is complaining of headaches that are worse in the morning. What does the nurse know could be the reason for the morning headaches?

a. Increased intracranial pressure

b. Dehydration

c. Migraines

d. The tumor is shrinking.

7. A patient is diagnosed with a spinal cord tumor and has had a course of radiation and chemotherapy. Two months after the completion of the radiation, the patient complains of severe pain in the back. What is pain an indicator of in a patient with a spinal cord tumor?

a. Lumbar sacral strain

b. The development of a skin ulcer from the radiation

c. Hematoma formation

d. Spinal metastasis

8. The nurse is performing an assessment for a patient in the clinic with Parkinson's disease. The nurse determines that the patient's voice has changed since the last visit and is now more difficult to understand. How should the nurse document this finding?

a. Dysphagia

b. Dysphonia

c. Hypokinesia

d. Micrographia

9. A patient with Parkinson's disease is experiencing an on-off syndrome. What does the nurse recognize that the patient's clinical symptoms will be?

a. The patient will have unilateral resting tremors and then will have a period of no tremors present.

b. The patient will have a slow, shuffling gait and then will be able to move at a faster pace.

c. The patient will have a period when medication with levodopa will be unnecessary.

d. The patient will have periods of near immobility, followed by a sudden return of effectiveness of the medication.

10. A patient with Parkinson's disease asks the nurse what can be done to prevent problems with bowel elimination. What would be an intervention that would assist this patient with a regular stool pattern?

a. Take psyllium (Metamucil) daily.

b. Take a laxative whenever bloating is experienced.

c. Adopt a diet with moderate fiber intake.

d. Adopt a high-fiber diet.

11. The daughter of a patient with Huntington's disease asks the nurse what the risk is of her inheriting the disease. What is the best response by the nurse?

a. "The disease is not hereditary and therefore there is no risk to you."

b. "If one parent has the disorder, there is an 75% chance that you will inherit the disease."

c. "If one parent has the disorder, there is a 50% chance that you will inherit the disease."

d. "The disease is inherited and all offspring of a parent will develop the disease."

12. The nurse is caring for a patient with Huntington's disease in the long-term care facility. What does the nurse recognize as the most prominent symptom of the disease that the patient exhibits?

a. Rapid, jerky, involuntary movements

b. Slow, shuffling gait

c. Dysphagia and dysphonia

d. Dementia

13. A patient with Huntington's disease is prescribed medication to reduce the chorea. What medication will the nurse administer that is the only drug approved for the treatment of this symptom?

a. Tetrabenazine (Xenazine)

b. Carbamazepine (Tegretol)

c. phenobarbital

d. Diazepam (Valium)

14. A patient is diagnosed with amyotrophic lateral sclerosis, also known as ALS or Lou Gehrig's disease. The nurse understands that the symptoms of the disease will begin in what way?

a. Ascending paralysis

b. Numbness and tingling in the lower extremities

c. Weakness starting in the muscles supplied by the cranial nerves

d. Jerky, uncontrolled movements in the extremities

15. A patient with amyotrophic lateral sclerosis asks if the nurse has heard of a drug that will prolong the patient's life. The nurse knows that there is a medication that may prolong the life by 3 to 6 months. What medication is the patient referring to?

a. Baclofen (Lioresal)

b. Riluzole (Rilutek)

c. dantrolene sodium (Dantrium)

d. diazepam (Valium)

Acute Community-Based Challenges

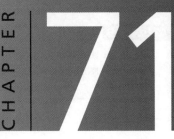

Management of Patients With Infectious Diseases

Learning Objectives

1. Differentiate between colonization, infection, and disease.
2. Identify federal and local resources available to the nurse seeking information about infectious diseases.
3. Identify the benefits of vaccines recommended for health care workers.
4. Identify standard and transmission-based precautions and discuss the elements of these standards.
5. Describe the concept and the nursing management of emerging infectious diseases.
6. Use the nursing process as a framework for care of patients with sexually transmitted infections (STIs).
7. Describe home health care measures that reduce the risk of infection.
8. Use the nursing process as a framework for care of patients with infectious diseases.

SECTION I: ASSESSING YOUR UNDERSTANDING

Activity A *Fill in the blanks.*

1. More than ____ vaccines are currently licensed in the United States (Centers for Disease Control and Prevention [CDC], 2012c).

2. Health care workers should be immune to _____, _____, _____, _____, _____, _____, and _____.

3. The rehydration goal for moderate dehydration is to deliver about _____ over 4 hours.

4. The two primary agencies involved in setting guidelines about infection prevention are the _____ and the _____.

5. Two bacteria that are part of normal skin flora are _____ and _____; _____ and _____, which are considered transient flora, have increased pathogenic potential.

6. The three primary organisms responsible for health care–associated infections (HAI) potential are _____, _____, and _____.

7. Immunosuppressed adults should be vaccinated for _____ and _____.

8. Portals of entry of STI-causing microorganisms and sites of infection include the _____, as well as the mucosal linings of the _____, _____, _____, _____, and _____.

Activity B *Briefly answer the following.*

1. Describe the chain of essential events necessary for an infection to occur.

_____

_____

_____

2. What is the difference between an infectious disease and an infection?

_____

_____

3. What is the most frequent cause of bacterial infections in health care institutions?

_____

_____

4. What is the most important aspect of reducing the risk of bloodborne infection?

_____

_____

5. A patient has been admitted to the hospital with active tuberculosis infection. What precautions will be provided for this patient?

_____

_____

_____

_____

Activity C *Match the disease or condition listed in Column II with its associated causative organism listed in Column I.*

Column I

_____ 1. Varicella zoster

_____ 2. *Neisseria gonorrhoeae*

_____ 3. Hepatitis B virus

_____ 4. *Staphylococcus aureus*

_____ 5. Epstein-Barr virus

_____ 6. Salmonella species

_____ 7. *Streptococcus pneumoniae*

_____ 8. *Microsporum* species

Column II

a. Chickenpox

b. Bloodborne hepatitis

c. Diarrheal disease

d. Gonorrhea

e. Impetigo

f. Mononucleosis

g. Pneumococcal pneumonia

h. Ringworm

SECTION II: APPLYING YOUR KNOWLEDGE

Activity D *Consider the scenario and answer the questions.*

Kallie, a 23-year-old woman, was informed by her boyfriend that he had been treated for the STI gonorrhea (*Neisseria gonorrhoeae*) at the local clinic about 2 weeks ago but was reluctant to tell her. Kallie thought that she had a mild urinary tract infection because of burning when urinating.

1. Kallie goes to the clinic for diagnosis and treatment. Besides gonorrhea, what else should she be tested for?

_____

2. Kallie asks the nurse what would have happened if her boyfriend had not told her about the infection. What can the nurse inform her that the complications would be?

_____

_____

3. What test will be performed to confirm a definitive diagnosis of gonorrhea?

_____

_____

4. What education should the nurse provide to Kallie in order to decrease the possibility of contracting another STI?

_____

_____

_____

SECTION III: PRACTICING FOR NCLEX

Activity E *Answer the following questions.*

1. The nurse is trying to determine if a patient admitted to the hospital the previous day has a bacterial wound infection. What laboratory study should the nurse review to obtain this information?

   a. The complete blood count (CBC)

   b. Microbiology report

   c. MRI report

   d. Chemistry studies

2. The nurse is discussing childhood immunization recommendations with a pediatric patient's parent. Where would the nurse find the most current information on this topic?

   a. The World Health Organization

   b. The Joint Commission

   c. CDC

   d. The Occupational Safety Health Administration

3. After providing care for a patient with *Clostridium difficile,* the nurse is preparing to wash the hands before leaving the room. What is the best method of cleaning the hands in order to prevent spreading the bacteria?

   a. Remove gloves and wash the hands with soap and water.

   b. Remove gloves and use Hibiclens solution to wash hands.

   c. Remove gloves and use Betadine solution prior to washing hands with soap and water.

   d. Use an alcohol-based solution to clean hands.

4. The nurse is caring for a patient with a meningococcus infection. What type of precautions should be used for this patient?

   a. Airborne

   b. Contact

   c. Droplet

   d. Standard

5. The nurse is providing an education program to reduce the incidence of infection currently on the rise in the community. What areas should the nurse focus on when presenting this program? (Select all that apply.)

   a. Regulated health practices

   b. Sanitation techniques

   c. The use of antibiotics to prevent infections

   d. Immunization programs

   e. Swimming in the community pool

6. A pregnant patient asks the nurse if it is all right for her take the varicella immunization for entrance into nursing school. What is the best response by the nurse?

   a. "If you will be working in the health care field, you must take the immunization."

   b. "It is not recommended that pregnant women take the live virus. You should wait until after your child is born."

   c. "It is not a live virus, so it should be fine."

   d. "You will have to delay entrance into the nursing program if they force you to take it."

7. A patient has developed chicken pox and asks the nurse what the incubation period would be. What should the nurse inform the patient?

   a. It is 24 to 48 hours.

   b. It is 2 to 3 days.

   c. It is 7 to 10 days.

   d. It is 10 to 21 days.

8. A patient is admitted with severe dehydration related to diarrhea. The patient was hiking in the mountains during a camping trip and drank water from a mountain stream without purifying. What does the nurse know is the most likely cause of this diarrhea?

   a. *Giardia lamblia*

   b. *Calicivirus*

   c. *Escherichia coli*

   d. *Shigella*

9. The nurse is admitting a patient with severe diarrhea. What is the most important element of assessment for this patient?

   a. Stool color

   b. Hydration status

   c. Bowel sounds

   d. Appetite

10. A patient comes to the clinic with complaints of a painless sore on her lip 2 weeks after she had oral sex with her boyfriend. The nurse observes a chancre on the lips and the physician orders testing for syphilis. If results are positive, what is the likely stage the patient is in?

    a. Primary

    b. Secondary

    c. Latency

    d. Tertiary

11. The nurse has received several laboratory studies back at the clinic. Which of these results should be reported to the local health department?

    a. Wound infection with MRSA

    b. Positive influenza

    c. Positive gonorrhea

    d. Positive mononucleosis

12. An adolescent informs the school nurse that she is afraid of contracting an STI but her boyfriend does not want to use condoms. What is the best response by the nurse?

    a. "You are too young to be having sex at all."

    b. "If he won't use a condom, then he doesn't care about you."

    c. "The use of condoms is one of the best ways to reduce the risk of acquiring an STI."

    d. "I can understand your concern and you should bring him here so that I can talk with him about STIs."

13. After attending a conference at a hotel for several days, a patient is having symptoms suspected of being related to Legionnaires' disease. When making a bed assignment for this patient, how should the assignment be made?

    a. The patient should be placed in a private room on droplet precautions.

    b. The patient should be placed in a negative pressure room.

    c. The patient should be placed in a private room on airborne precautions.

    d. The patient can be placed in a semiprivate room because the disease is not transmitted from person to person.

14. A nurse has heard that there have been three cases of pertussis in the community and wants to make sure his or her inoculations are up to date. What action should the nurse take?

    a. Have a single-dose Tdap administered.

    b. It is not necessary to be inoculated since there is a slim chance of acquiring the disease.

    c. Take a series of 3 Tdap 3 months apart.

    d. Have a Tdap administered and 6 months later have another.

15. A family will be staying in a cabin by a lake and, upon arriving, observes rodent droppings on the floor in the kitchen. What is the best way for the family to clean up in order to avoid contracting hantavirus from the feces?

    a. Sweep up all of the droppings and then apply a bleach solution.

    b. Vacuum the droppings and then apply a bleach solution.

    c. Apply a bleach solution prior to sweeping or vacuuming the floor.

    d. Sweep the droppings in a pile and then vacuum them up.

CHAPTER 72

Emergency Nursing

1. Describe emergency care as a collaborative, holistic approach that includes the patient, the family, and significant others.
2. Discuss priority emergency measures instituted for the patient with an emergency condition.
3. Identify the priorities of care for the patient with intra-abdominal injuries and multiple injuries.
4. Compare and contrast the emergency management of patients with heat stroke, frostbite, and hypothermia.
5. Specify the similarities and differences of the emergency management of patients with swallowed or inhaled poisons, skin contamination, and food poisoning.
6. Discuss the emergency management of patients with drug overdose, those with acute alcohol intoxication, and those who have been sexually assaulted.
7. Differentiate between the emergency care of patients who are overactive, those who are violent, those who are depressed, and those who are suicidal.

SECTION I: ASSESSING YOUR UNDERSTANDING

Activity A *Fill in the blanks.*

1. The _____ survey focuses on stabilizing life-threatening conditions.

2. According to the _____, every emergency department (ED) with a Medicare provider agreement must perform a medical screening examination on all patients arriving with an emergency medical complaint if their acute signs and symptoms could result in serious injury or death if left untreated.

3. A patient with a foreign body airway obstruction typically demonstrates the inability to

   _____, _____, or _____. With complete obstruction, permanent brain injury will occur in _____ minutes.

4. In the case of gunfire in the ED, _____ is a priority.

5. The cardinal manifestations of heat cramps include _____, particularly in the shoulders, abdomen, and lower extremities; _____, and _____ (ENA, 2013).

6. The second most common cause of unintentional death in children younger than 14 years of age is _____.

7. The most common victims of snakebites are those between the ages of _____ and _____ years of age.

8. Antivenin to treat snakebites must be administered within a time frame of _____ to _____ hours.

9. Depending on the severity of a snakebite, antivenin is diluted in _____ mL to _____ mL of _____.

Activity B *Briefly answer the following.*

1. Describe the indications for endotracheal intubation.

   _____

   _____

   _____

   _____

2. Why is lactated Ringer's solution initially useful as fluid replacement for a patient experiencing hypovolemic shock?

   _____

   _____

   _____

   _____

3. Name three of the risk factors of upper airway obstruction in the older adult.

   _____

   _____

   _____

   _____

4. When the nurse is performing a rapid neurologic assessment in the ED, what mnemonic is helpful?

   _____

   _____

   _____

   _____

5. Name and define the three categories commonly used in triage in the ED.

   _____

   _____

   _____

   _____

Activity C *Match the wound in Column I with the definition given in Column II.*

Column I

___ 1. Laceration

___ 2. Avulsion

___ 3. Abrasion

___ 4. Ecchymosis

___ 5. Hematoma

___ 6. Stab

___ 7. Cut

___ 8. Patterned

Column II

a. Incision of the skin with well-defined edges, usually caused by a sharp instrument; this type of wound is typically deeper than long

b. Denuded skin

c. Incision of the skin with well-defined edges, usually longer than deep

d. Tumorlike mass of blood trapped under the skin

e. Wound representing the outline of the object (e.g., steering wheel) causing the wound

f. Blood trapped under the surface of the skin

g. Skin tear with irregular edges and vein bridging

h. Tearing away of tissue from supporting structures

SECTION II: APPLYING YOUR KNOWLEDGE

Activity D *Consider the scenario and answer the questions.*

CASE STUDY: Heat Stroke

Carson, a 42-year-old man, was on top of a roof fixing several loose shingles in 95-degree weather. His wife came outside to bring him something to drink and found him lying on the roof. When she called his name, he appeared not to understand her and lay there looking around. She immediately called the rescue squad and they were able to transport him to the hospital. Carson had a temperature of 106.2°F upon arrival to the ED.

1. What other clinical manifestations does the nurse anticipate finding with Carson's diagnosis of heat stroke?

   _____

   _____

   _____

   _____

2. What should the nurse prepare to do to prevent complications related to Carson's heat stroke?

_____

_____

_____

_____

3. Why is it important for the nurse to monitor Carson's urine output at least every hour?

_____

_____

SECTION III: PRACTICING FOR NCLEX

Activity E *Answer the following questions.*

1. An adolescent is brought to the ED after a vehicular accident and is pronounced dead on arrival (DOA). When the parents arrive at the hospital, what is the priority action by the nurse?

a. Ask them to sit in the waiting room until she can spend time alone with them.

b. Speak to both parents together and encourage them to support each other and express their emotions freely.

c. Speak to one parent at a time in a private setting so that each can ventilate feelings of loss without upsetting the other.

d. Ask the emergency physician to medicate the parents so that they can handle their child's unexpected death quietly and without hysteria.

2. A triage nurse in the ED determines that a patient with dyspnea and dehydration is not in a life-threatening situation. What triage category will the nurse choose?

a. Delayed

b. Emergent

c. Immediate

d. Urgent

3. The nurse in the ED is triaging patients during the shift. What does the nurse know is the first priority in treating any patient in the ED?

a. Controlling hemorrhage.

b. Establishing an airway.

c. Obtaining consent for treatment.

d. Restoring cardiac output.

4. The nurse is caring for a patient in the ED who is breathing but unconscious. In order to avoid an upper airway obstruction, the nurse is inserting an oropharyngeal airway. How would the nurse insert the airway?

a. At an angle of 90 degrees

b. Upside down and then rotated 180 degrees

c. With the concave portion touching the posterior pharynx

d. With the convex portion facing upward

5. The nurse received a patient from a motor vehicle accident who is hemorrhaging from a femoral wound. What is the initial nursing action for the control of the hemorrhage?

a. Apply a tourniquet.

b. Apply firm pressure over the involved area or artery.

c. Elevate the injured part.

d. Immobilize the area to control blood loss.

6. The nurse is admitting a patient with a penetrating abdominal injury from a knife wound. What should the nursing measures for a penetrating abdominal injury include? (Select all that apply.)

a. Assessing for manifestations of hemorrhage

b. Covering any protruding viscera with sterile dressings soaked in normal saline solution

c. Looking for any associated chest injuries

d. Exploring the abdominal wound with a gloved finger

e. Irrigating the wound with normal saline and a syringe

7. A patient has experienced blunt abdominal trauma from a motor vehicle crash. The nurse assesses the patient, knowing that which organ is the most frequently injured solid abdominal organ?

   a. Duodenum

   b. Large bowel

   c. Liver

   d. Pancreas

8. A patient is brought to the ED by a friend, who states that a tree fell on the patient's leg and crushed it while they were cutting firewood. What priority actions should the nurse perform? (Select all that apply.)

   a. Applying a clean dressing to protect the wound

   b. Elevating the site to limit the accumulation of fluid in the interstitial spaces

   c. Inserting an indwelling catheter

   d. Splinting the wound in a position of rest to prevent motion

   e. Performing a fasciotomy

9. For a patient who is experiencing multiple injuries, which sequence of medical or nursing management would the nurse identify as a priority?

   a. Assess for head injuries, control hemorrhage, establish an airway, prevent hypovolemic shock.

   b. Control hemorrhage, prevent hypovolemic shock, establish an airway, assess for head injuries.

   c. Establish an airway, control hemorrhage, prevent hypovolemic shock, assess for head injuries.

   d. Prevent hypovolemic shock, assess for head injuries, establish an airway, control hemorrhage.

10. A female patient was sexually assaulted when leaving work. When assisting with the physical examination, what nursing interventions should be provided? (Select all that apply.)

    a. Have the patient shower or wash the perineal area before the examination.

    b. Assess and document any bruises and lacerations.

    c. Record a history of the event, using the patient's own words.

    d. Label all torn or bloody clothes and place each item in a separate brown bag so that any evidence can be given to the police.

    e. Ensure that the police are present when the examination is performed.

11. A patient with frostbite to both lower extremities from exposure to the elements is preparing to have rewarming of the extremities. What intervention should the nurse provide prior to the procedure?

    a. Administer an analgesic as ordered.

    b. Massage the extremities.

    c. Elevate the legs.

    d. Apply a heat lamp.

12. A patient brought to the ED by the rescue squad after getting off a plane at the airport is complaining of severe joint pain, numbness, and an inability to move the arms. The patient was on a diving vacation and went for a last dive this morning before flying home. What is a priority action by the nurse?

    a. Ensure a patent airway and that the patient is receiving 100% oxygen.

    b. Send the patient for a chest x-ray.

    c. Send the patient to the hyperbaric chamber.

    d. Draw labs for a chemistry panel.

13. A nurse is working as a camp nurse during the summer. A camp counselor comes to the clinic after receiving a snakebite on the arm. What is the first action by the nurse?

    a. Apply ice to the area.

    b. Apply a tourniquet to the arm above the bite.

    c. Have the patient lie down and place the arm below the level of the heart.

    d. Make an incision and suck the venom out.

14. The nurse is administering antivenin to a patient who was bitten on the arm by a poisonous snake. What intervention provided by the nurse is required prior to the procedure and every 15 minutes after?

   a. Administer diphenhydramine (Benadryl).

   b. Administer cimetidine (Tagamet).

   c. Measure the circumference of the arm.

   d. Assess peripheral pulses.

15. A patient was bitten by a tick 3 months ago and is now having muscle aches as well as joint pain and swelling. The patient is having difficulty with self-care and requires assistance with activities of daily living (ADLs). What stage of Lyme disease does the nurse recognize the patient is in?

   a. Stage I

   b. Stage II

   c. Stage III

   d. Stage IV

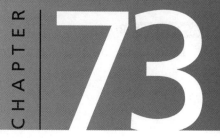

Terrorism, Mass Casualty, and Disaster Nursing

1. Identify the necessary components of an emergency operations plan.
2. Discuss how triage in a disaster differs from triage in an emergency department.
3. Evaluate the different levels of personal protection and decontamination procedures that may be necessary during an event involving mass casualties or weapons of mass destruction.
4. Describe the physical injuries that may occur after blast events and isolation precautions necessary for bioterrorism agents.
5. Identify the differences among the various chemical agents used in terrorist events, their effects, and the decontamination and treatment procedures that are necessary.
6. Determine the injuries associated with varying levels of radiation or chemical exposure and the associated decontamination processes.

SECTION I: ASSESSING YOUR UNDERSTANDING

Activity A *Fill in the blanks.*

1. An example of a biological weapon of mass destruction is _____; an example of a chemical weapon of mass destruction is _____.

2. Four federal agencies that provide disaster assistance are _____ _____, _____, _____, and _____.

3. Only three states and the District of Columbia have locations for Disaster Medical Assistance Teams. These states are _____, _____, and _____.

4. _____ is a key component of disaster management.

5. Two biological agents most likely to be used during a terrorist attack are _____ and _____.

6. Exposure to anthrax, without clinical signs and symptoms of the disease, requires a 60-day treatment with one of two antibiotics: _____ or _____. The mortality rate associated with respiratory distress is _____.

7. Cremation is preferred for all deaths due to smallpox because the virus can survive in scabs for up to _____ years.

Activity B *Briefly answer the following.*

1. Describe the Incident Command System.

_____

_____

_____

2. Describe five factors that influence an individual's response to disaster.

_____

_____

_____

_____

3. Explain why patients who are most critically ill, with a high mortality rate, would be assigned a low triage priority in a disaster situation.

_____

_____

_____

_____

4. Name at least four cultural variables that health care providers need to consider in any disaster situation in which a large number of diverse religious and ethnic groups of patients need to be treated.

_____

_____

_____

5. Name and describe each of the four effects that a blast wave has on a victim.

_____

_____

_____

_____

Activity C **Triage Categories During a Mass Casualty Incident (MCI)**

Match the color category in Column II with the condition in Column I. Colors may be used more than once.

Column I		Column II
_____	1. Fractured humerus	Red
_____	2. C-1 spinal transection	Yellow
_____	3. Third-degree burns over 25% total body surface area (TBSA)	Green
		Black
_____	4. Hemothorax	
_____	5. Radiation exposure with seizures 24 hours after exposure	
_____	6. Burn to hand	
_____	7. Depression	
_____	8. Maxillofacial wound without airway compromise	
_____	9. Sucking chest wound	
_____	10. Open femur fracture	
_____	11. Third-degree burns over 75% TBSA	
_____	12. Penetrating head wound with ice pick	
_____	13. Stable abdominal wound without hemorrhage	
_____	14. Soft-tissue injury of lower extremity with adequate collateral circulation	

SECTION II: APPLYING YOUR KNOWLEDGE

Activity D *Consider the scenario and answer the questions.*

A train derailment caused the injuries of 34 people, with injuries ranging from minor to critical. All patients have been brought to the local emergency department (ED) for treatment. Physicians have been called from their offices to assist with caring for the wounded and nurses have been called in to assist with the disaster.

1. What should the triage team be sure to do in order to make sure that all patients have been identified?

   _____

   _____

   _____

2. What does the nurse understand is the primary principle in a disaster when there are several critical patients?

   _____

   _____

   _____

3. What should the nurse ensure is in place in order to control the overload of patients, visitors, and EMS personnel in the ED?

   _____

   _____

SECTION III: PRACTICING FOR NCLEX

Activity E *Answer the following questions.*

1. The nurse is assisting in a disaster caused by a massive tornado that has destroyed much of the community. This disaster will require statewide and federal assistance. What classification would the disaster be?
   a. Level I
   b. Level II
   c. Level III
   d. Level IV

2. The Department of Homeland Security issues a code "blue" relative to a situation. What does the nurse know that this indicates?
   a. Perceived low risk
   b. Guarded risk
   c. Possible risk but ill-defined
   d. High risk with no specific site

3. The NATO triage system uses color-coded tagging to identify severity of injuries. A patient with survivable but life-threatening injuries (i.e., incomplete amputation) would be tagged with which color?
   a. Black
   b. Green
   c. Red
   d. Yellow

4. The nurse is triaging people that have been involved in a bus accident. A triaged patient with psychological disturbances would be tagged with which color?
   a. Black
   b. Green
   c. Red
   d. Yellow

5. A triaged patient with a significant injury that can wait several hours for treatment would be assigned what priority?
   a. Priority 1
   b. Priority 2
   c. Priority 3
   d. Priority 4

6. Several patients that have been involved in a bombing are unlikely to survive. What priority are these patients given during triage?
   a. Priority 1
   b. Priority 2
   c. Priority 3
   d. Priority 4

7. A patient was involved in an avalanche that killed many people on a ski trip, including the patient's brother. The nurse is educating the patient about recognition of stress reactions and ways to manage stress. What type of process is the nurse introducing to the patient?

a. Defusing

b. Debriefing

c. Preparedness

d. Demobilization

8. The nurse receives a call from EMS personnel that they are bringing in eight patients who have been exposed to a chemical after a spill. The patients have been "washed off." After the initial assessment, what should be done?

a. Remove clothing and jewelry and rinse the patients off with water.

b. Have the patients wash with soap and water and then rinse.

c. Treat the patients for any burned areas from the chemical since they have already been decontaminated.

d. Start an IV with lactated Ringer's solution at 125 mL/h.

9. A patient was brought into the ED after sustaining injuries due to an explosion while welding. The patient is breathing but has an oxygen saturation of 90%, a respiratory rate of 32, and is coughing. What is the priority action by the nurse?

a. Administer oxygen at 2 L/min via nasal cannula.

b. Administer oxygen with a nonrebreather mask.

c. Start an IV of normal saline solution at 125 mL/h.

d. Obtain a chest x-ray.

10. A patient is suspected to have an air embolus after being in close proximity to an explosion at a sports arena. What position should the nurse place the patient in to prevent migration of the embolus?

a. Supine with head of the bed at 30 degrees

b. High-Fowler's position

c. Prone left lateral position

d. Lithotomy

11. A patient was suspected of being in direct contact with anthrax but is exhibiting no signs or symptoms. What type of prophylaxis does the nurse know this patient will have to take?

a. Penicillin G IM for 1 dose

b. Rocephin (Ceftriaxone) IV for 7 days

c. Ciprofloxacin (Cipro) for 60 days

d. Erythromycin for 2 weeks

12. A patient is being brought into the ED who is probably infected with anthrax. The nurse should ensure what level of personal protective equipment to wear for everyone who will come in contact with the patient?

a. Level A

b. Level B

c. Level C

d. Level D

13. A soldier is preparing to enter an area in which there is a high risk for chemical exposure to a nerve agent. What should the soldier be given prior to entering this area?

a. Mark I automatic injectors that contain 2 mg atropine and 600 mg pralidoxime chloride

b. Mark I automatic injectors that contain an antiseizure medication such as carbamazepine

c. Mark I automatic injector filled with morphine 10 mg

d. Mark I automatic injector filled with cyanide

14. A nuclear reactor overheated, releasing radiation throughout the plant. A worker close to reactor received at least 800 rads and has had an onset of vomiting, bloody diarrhea, and, when brought to the hospital, was in shock. What is this patient's predicted survival?

a. Possible

b. Probable

c. Likely

d. Improbable

15. The nurse is triaging patients from a 10-car pile-up on the interstate and assesses a patient with a sucking chest wound. What category should this patient be placed in?

a. Priority 1

b. Priority 2

c. Priority 3

d. Priority 4

Answers

CHAPTER 1

SECTION I: ASSESSING YOUR UNDERSTANDING

Activity A

1. infectious diseases, trauma, obesity, and bioterrorism
2. hypertension, heart disease, diabetes, and cancer
3. care mapping, multidisciplinary action plans (MAPs), clinical guidelines, and algorithms
4. nurse practitioner, clinical nurse specialist, certified nurse-midwife, and certified registered anesthetist

Activity B

1. Refer to chapter heading "Nursing Defined" under "The Health Care Industry and the Nursing Profession" in the text for phenomena.
2. Six significant changes are: an increase in the aging population, increased cultural diversity, the changing patterns of diseases, increased technology, increased consumer expectations, and higher costs for health care.
3. Human responses requiring nursing intervention should include self-image changes, impaired ventilation, and anxiety and fear. Answer may also include pain and discomfort, grief, and impaired functioning in areas such as rest and sleep.
4. Four major concepts supporting wellness are: the capacity to perform to the best of one's ability; the flexibility of adjusting and adapting to various situations; a reported feeling of well-being; and a feeling of "harmony," that everything is together.
5. In Maslow's hierarchy of needs, needs are ranked as follows. Refer to Figure 1-1 in the text.

Need	Example
Physiologic	Food and water
Safety and security	Financial security
Belongingness and affection	Companionship
Esteem and self-respect	Recognition by society
Self-actualization	Achieved potential in an area
Self-fulfillment	Creativity (painting)
Knowledge and understanding	Information and explanation
Aesthetics	Attractive environment

6. Answer should include six of these seven: stress, improper diet, lack of exercise, smoking, illicit drugs, high-risk behaviors (including risky sexual practices), and poor hygiene.
7. Nursing care must be culturally competent, appropriate, and sensitive to cultural differences.
8. Evidence-based practice includes using current literature and research, outcomes assessment, and standardized plans of care (clinical guidelines and pathways, algorithms) to improve patient care.
9. Clinical pathways are tools for tracking a patient's progress toward positive outcomes within a specific period of time. Pathways include tests, treatments, activities, medications, consultations, and education within a set time period to achieve desired outcomes.
10. Care mapping is more beneficial than a clinical pathway when a patient's complex condition defies prediction and a specific timeframe for achieving outcomes is excluded.
11. Managed care is characterized by prenegotiated payment rates, mandatory precertification, utilization review, limited choice of provider, and fixed-price reimbursement.
12. Case management is a system in which one person or team coordinates the care for the patient and family. The goals include quality care, appropriate and timely care delivery, and cost reduction.
13. The central idea of community-oriented nursing practice is that nursing intervention can promote wellness, reduce the spread of illness, and improve the health status of groups of citizens or the community at large. Its emphasis is on primary, secondary, and tertiary prevention. Community-based nursing occurs in a variety of settings within the community, including home settings, and is directed toward people and families.

Activity C

1. **Flow Chart: Radial Pulse Assessment**

   Refer to your knowledge of fundamental skills.

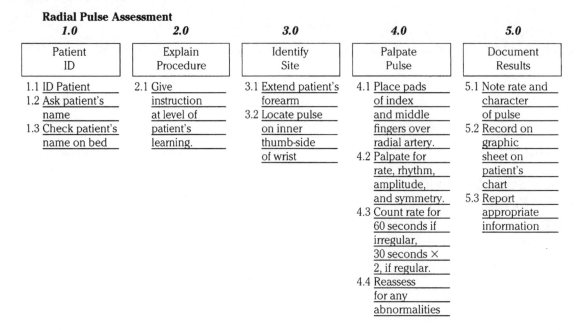

Radial Pulse Assessment

1.0	2.0	3.0	4.0	5.0
Patient ID	Explain Procedure	Identify Site	Palpate Pulse	Document Results
1.1 ID Patient 1.2 Ask patient's name 1.3 Check patient's name on bed	2.1 Give instruction at level of patient's learning.	3.1 Extend patient's forearm 3.2 Locate pulse on inner thumb-side of wrist	4.1 Place pads of index and middle fingers over radial artery. 4.2 Palpate for rate, rhythm, amplitude, and symmetry. 4.3 Count rate for 60 seconds if irregular, 30 seconds × 2, if regular. 4.4 Reassess for any abnormalities	5.1 Note rate and character of pulse 5.2 Record on graphic sheet on patient's chart 5.3 Report appropriate information

2. **Flow Chart: CQI Cause and Effect Diagram: Delayed Medication**

CQI Cause and Effect Diagram: Delayed Medication

Possible Causes

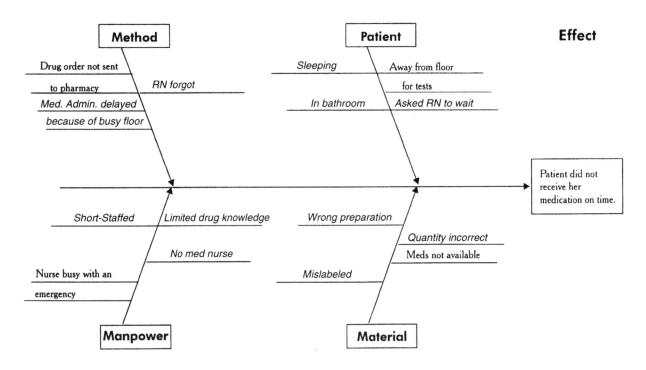

SECTION II: APPLYING YOUR KNOWLEDGE

Activity D

1. a   **2.** b   **3.** a, c, e

SECTION III: PRACTICING FOR NCLEX

Activity E

1. d   **2.** a   **3.** d   **4.** b   **5.** c
6. c   **7.** c   **8.** d   **9.** a, b, c   **10.** c

CHAPTER 2

SECTION 1: ASSESSING YOUR UNDERSTANDING

Activity A

1. Community-based care
2. individuals, families
3. Hypertension, diabetes, obesity
4. self-care, preventive care, continuity of care, collaboration
5. palliative
6. schedule, location
7. Occupational Safety and Health Act (OSHA)

Activity B

1. federal legislation, tighter insurance regulations, decreasing hospital revenues, alternate health care delivery systems
2. Nurses will need to be expert, independent decision makers who are self-directed; flexible; adaptable; and competent in critical thinking, physical assessment, health education, and basic nursing care.
3. promoting and maintaining the health of individuals and families, preventing and minimizing the progression of disease, improving the quality of life.
4. Skilled nursing services may include intravenous therapy, injections, parenteral nutrition, venipuncture, catheter insertion, pressure ulcer and wound care, and ostomy care.
5. call the patient to obtain permission for a visit, schedule the visit, and verify the address
6. During the initial home visit, the patient is evaluated and a plan of care is established.
7. Nursing responsibilities include direct patient care, assessment and screening, treatment (acute, chronic, or emergency conditions), referral to other agencies, and health education.
8. Answer should include six of the following: trauma, tuberculosis, upper respiratory tract infections, poor nutrition and anemia, lice, scabies, peripheral vascular disease, hypothermia, arthritis, skin disorders, dental and foot problems, sexually transmitted infections, and mental illness.
9. *Primary* prevention focuses on health promotion and disease prevention (e.g., diabetic counseling). *Secondary* prevention focuses on health maintenance, early detection, and prompt intervention

(e.g., health care screening). *Tertiary* prevention focuses on minimizing deterioration and improving the quality of life (e.g., health care screening, rehabilitation).
10. Because hospitals are reimbursed at a fixed rate per diagnosis-related group (DRG), patients are being discharged prior to full recovery. This issue is compounded by the growth in the aging population.
11. **Tele-health** is an emerging trend in home health care; this facilitates exchange of information via telephone or computers between patients and nurses regarding health information such as blood glucose readings, vital signs, and cardiac parameters (Stanhope & Lancaster, 2012). Use of a broad spectrum of computer and Internet resources, such as Web cams, also facilitates exchange of information.

SECTION II: APPLYING YOUR KNOWLEDGE

Activity C

CASE STUDY: Assessing the Need for a Home Visit

Refer to chapter heading "Home Health Visits" and Chart 2-3, Assessing the Home Environment, in the text to complete the case study.

SECTION III: PRACTICING FOR NCLEX

Activity D

1. a   **2.** b   **3.** c   **4.** d   **5.** c
6. c

CHAPTER 3

SECTION I: ASSESSING YOUR UNDERSTANDING

Activity A

1. confidentiality, use of restraints, trust, refusing care, end-of-life concerns
2. Living will, durable power of attorney
3. self-reasoning

Activity B

1. A strong formal and informal foundation of knowledge; a willingness to pursue or ask questions; and an ability to develop solutions that are new, even if different from the current set of standards.
2. Answer may include active thinker, fair, independent and open-minded, persistent, empathic, honest, organized and systematic, proactive, flexible, realistic, humble, logical, curious, and insightful. Critical thinkers are good communicators and are committed to excellence.
3. Analysis, evaluation, explanation, inference, interpretation, and self-regulation.
4. Critical thinking is influenced by the culture, attitude, and experiences of the individual, who sees the situation through the lens of her or his experiences.

5. A *moral dilemma* is a conflict between two or more moral principles (choose between the lesser of two evils). A *moral problem* occurs when moral claims/principles are competing but one claim/principle is dominant. *Moral uncertainty* occurs when there is confusion about a principle and there is a strong feeling that something is not right. *Moral distress* results when constraints stand in the way of pursuing the correct action.

6. Nursing practice encompasses the protection, promotion, and optimization of health and abilities, prevention of illness and injury, alleviation of suffering through the diagnosis and treatment of human response, and advocacy in the care of individuals, families, communities, and populations.

7. A "durable power of attorney" exists when a person identifies another person to make health care decisions on his or her behalf.

8. Suggested statements include: "Please tell me what brought you to the hospital," "Please tell me what you think your needs are," and "Please tell me about your past history."

9. A *nursing diagnosis* identifies actual or potential health problems that guide nurses in the development of a plan of care and is amenable to resolution by nursing actions. *Collaborative problems* are potential problems or complications that are medical in origin and require collaborative interventions with the physician and the health care team. The nursing diagnosis and collaborative problems are the patient's nursing problems. A medical diagnosis identifies diseases, conditions, or pathology that can be medically managed. Refer to Figure 3-2 in the text.

10. Expected outcomes of nursing intervention should be stated in behavioral terms and should be realistic as well as measurable. Expected behavioral outcomes serve as the basis for evaluating the effectiveness of nursing intervention.

Activity C

Refer to Figures 3-1 and 3-2, and Charts 3-7, Steps of the Nursing Process, and 3-8, Nursing Outcomes Classification, in the text.

1. N	**2.** N	**3.** C	**4.** C	**5.** N
6. N	**7.** C	**8.** C	**9.** N	**10.** C

Activity D

PART I: Critical Thinking

Refer to Chart 3-2, The Inquiring Mind: Critical Thinking in Action, in the text.

1. e	**2.** g	**3.** f	**4.** d	**5.** a
6. c	**7.** b			

PART II: Ethical Principles

Refer to Chart 3-3, Common Ethical Principles, in the text.

1. d	**2.** e	**3.** b	**4.** f	**5.** a
6. c				

SECTION II: APPLYING YOUR KNOWLEDGE

Activity E

CASE STUDY: Ethical Analysis

Assessment

Your answer should include the conflict between the nurse's professional obligation to provide treatment to all and the unpleasant outcome of choosing "the lesser of two evils."

Planning

You should be able to analyze the medical and political data that influence the treatment options. Because of the vast numbers of infected citizens relative to available treatment, not everyone can be cared for.

Implementation

You need to carefully analyze the outcomes of both theories for your decision making. There is no right or wrong answer. You just need to support your decision with an ethical theory.

Evaluation

Your evaluation needs to show logical sequencing of problem solving based on an ethical theory. There is no right or wrong response.

SECTION III: PRACTICING FOR NCLEX

Activity F

1. d	**2.** c	**3.** b	**4.** d	**5.** a
6. a	**7.** d	**8.** a, b, c	**9.** c	**10.** b
11. a, b, c	**12.** d	**13.** c	**14.** a	**15.** a
16. d	**17.** b			

CHAPTER 4

SECTION I: ASSESSING YOUR UNDERSTANDING

Activity A

1. Significant factors include the availability of health care outside the hospital setting, the employment of diverse health care providers to accomplish care management goals, and the increased use of alternative strategies other than the traditional approaches to care.

2. People with a chronic illness need as much health care information as possible to actively participate in and assume responsibility for the management of their own care. Health education can help the patient adapt to illness and cooperate with a treatment regimen. The goal of health education is to teach people to maximize their health potential.

3. Answer may include five of the following: medication compliance; maintaining a healthy diet; increasing daily exercise; self-monitoring for signs of illness; practicing good overall hygiene; seeking

health screenings and evaluations; and performing therapeutic, preventive measures.

4. *Adherence* implies that a patient makes one or more lifestyle changes to carry out specific activities to promote and maintain health.

5. Factors influencing adherence include demographic variables such as age, sex, and education; illness variables such as the severity of illness and the effects of therapy; psychosocial variables such as intelligence and attitudes toward illness; financial variables; and therapeutic regimen variables.

6. Choice, establishment of agreed upon goals, and the quality of the patient–provider relationship

7. Refer to the "Transtheoretical Model of Change" adapted from Miller (2009) and DiClemente (2007). Refer to Table 4-2, Stages in the Transtheoretical Model of Change, in the text.

8. The teaching–learning process requires the active involvement of teacher and learner, in an effort to reach the desired outcome: a change in behavior. The teacher serves as a facilitator of learning.

9. Answer may include six of the following: The elderly have difficulty adhering to a therapeutic regimen because of increased sensitivity to medications, difficulty in adjusting to change and stress, financial constraints, forgetfulness, inadequate support systems, lifetime habits of self-medication, visual impairments, hearing deficits, and mobility limitations.

10. the elderly's ability to draw inferences, apply information, understand major teaching points

11. The effects of a learning situation are influenced by a person's physical, emotional, and experiential readiness to learn. *Physical readiness* implies the physical ability of a person to attend to a learning situation. Basic physiologic needs are met so that higher-level needs can be addressed. *Emotional readiness* involves the patient's motivation to learn and can be encouraged by providing realistic goals that can be easily achieved so that self-esteem needs can be met. A person needs to be ready to accept the emotional changes (anxiety, stress) that accompany behavior modification resulting from the learning process. *Experiential readiness* refers to a person's past experiences that influence his or her approach to the learning process. Previous positive feedback and improved self-image reinforce experiential readiness.

12. lecture method, group teaching, demonstrations, use of teaching aids, reinforcement, and follow-up

13. increase the quality and years of healthy life for people and eliminate health disparities among various segments of the population

14. demographics and disease factors, barriers, resources, and perceptual factors.

15. improves the function of the circulatory system and the lungs; decreases cholesterol and low-density lipoprotein levels; decreases body weight by increasing calorie expenditure; delays degenerative changes such as osteoporosis; improves flexibility and overall muscle strength and endurance

Activity B

1. Health education is an independent function of nursing practice that is a primary responsibility of the nursing profession.

2. Although diseases in children and those of an infectious nature are of utmost concern, the largest groups of people today who need health education are those with chronic illnesses and disabilities.

3. Patients are encouraged to adhere to their therapeutic regimen. Adherence connotes active, voluntary, collaborative patient *efforts*, whereas compliance is a more passive role.

4. Evaluation should be continuous throughout the teaching process so that the information gathered can be used to improve teaching activities.

5. The elderly usually experience significant gains from health promotion activities.

6. About 80% of those older than 65 years of age have one or more chronic illnesses.

SECTION II: APPLYING YOUR KNOWLEDGE

Activity C

1. The variables of choice, establishment of mutual goals, and quality of the patient–provider relationship directly influence the behavioral changes that can result from patient education. These factors are directly linked to motivation for learning.

2. Using a learning contract or agreement can be a motivator for learning; positive reinforcement is provided as the person moves from one goal to the next.

SECTION III: PRACTICING FOR NCLEX

Activity D

1. b	2. a, b, e	3. a, b, e	4. b	5. a
6. a	7. a	8. a	9. b	10. a
11. a	12. c			

CHAPTER 5

SECTION I: ASSESSING YOUR UNDERSTANDING

Activity A

1. obtaining a patient health history, performing a physical examination

2. Answer may include the following: patterns of sleep, exercise, nutrition, recreation, and personal habits such as smoking, the use of illicit drugs, alcohol, and caffeine.

3. heart disease, cancer, stroke

4. iron, folate, calcium

Activity B

1. The nurse needs to establish rapport, put the patient at ease, encourage honest communication, make eye contact, and listen carefully.

2. When an atmosphere of mutual trust and confidence exists between an interviewer and a patient, the patient becomes more open and honest, and is more likely to share personal concerns and problems.

3. The term *chief complaint* refers to that issue that brings the patient to the attention of the health care provider. When documenting a patient's chief complaint, exact words should be recorded in quotation marks.

4. Answer may include six of the following: cancer, hypertension, heart disease, diabetes, epilepsy, mental illness, tuberculosis, kidney disease, arthritis, allergies, asthma, alcoholism, and obesity.

5. Fruits, vegetables, grains, proteins, dairy, oils

6. *Negative nitrogen balance* occurs when nitrogen output (urine, feces, perspiration) exceeds nitrogen intake (food). When this happens, tissue is breaking down faster than it is being replaced.

7. Refer to Chart 5-2, Factors Associated With Potential Nutritional Deficits.

Activity C
PART I

a. Inspection
b. Inspection
c. Palpation
d. Palpation
e. Percussion
f. Auscultation
g. Auscultation
h. Palpation

PART II

Refer to Table 5-1, Physical Indicators of Nutritional Status, in the text.

1. h   **2.** c   **3.** d   **4.** e   **5.** g
6. b

SECTION II: APPLYING YOUR KNOWLEDGE

Activity D
CASE STUDY: Calculating a Healthy Diet
PART I: Estimate Ideal Body Weight

1. b, medium frame (her height-to-wrist circumference ratio is 10.4)
2. 125 lb, lose 50 lb (refer to Chart 5-8, Calculating Ideal Body Weight, in the text).
3. 29, overweight

PART II: Calculate a Balanced Diet

1. 50 kg
2. 1418
3. 1985 (1418 + 567)
4. 993 calories from carbohydrates, 595 calories from fat, 397 calories from protein
5. 248 g of carbohydrates, 66 g of fat, 99 g of protein

PART III: Design a Healthy Diet

1. 1 ½ cups
2. 2 ½ cups
3. 3-ounce equivalents

4. 5-ounce equivalents
5. 3 cups

SECTION III: PRACTICING FOR NCLEX

Activity E

1. b, d, e   **2.** a, c, d   **3.** d   **4.** b   **5.** b
6. c   **7.** b, c, d   **8.** a, b, c **9.** b   **10.** a
11. d   **12.** a   **13.** a   **14.** a   **15.** a

CHAPTER 6

SECTION I: ASSESSING YOUR UNDERSTANDING

Activity A

1. challenging, damaging, threatening
2. dead, diseased, injured
3. hypothalamus
4. synthesize enzymes, transform energy, grow and reproduce
5. level of education
6. constancy, homeostasis, stress, and adaptation
7. blood pressure, acid–base balance, blood glucose levels, body temperature, fluids and electrolyte balance
8. redness, heat, swelling, pain, loss of function

Activity B

1. When the body suffers an injury, the response is *maladaptive* if the defense mechanisms have a negative effect on health.

2. *Hyperpnea* is the body's development of rapid breathing after intense exercise in response to an accumulation of lactic acid in muscle tissue and a deficit of oxygen.

3. Examples of acute, *time-limited* stressors may include taking an examination, giving a speech, or driving in a snowstorm. Examples of chronic, *enduring* stressors may include poverty, a handicap or disability, or living with an alcoholic.

4. Examples of day-to-day stressors may include traffic jam, sick child, missed appointment, car would not start, train is late. Examples of major events affecting large groups of people could include earthquakes, wars, terrorism, events of history. Examples of infrequent, significant events in an individual's life would include marriage, birth, death, retirement.

5. Adolph Meyer, in the 1930s, first showed a correlation between illness and critical life events. A Recent Life Changes Questionnaire (RLCQ) was developed by Holmes and Rahe (1967) that assigned numerical values to life events requiring a change in an individual's life pattern. A correlation was seen between illness and the number of stressful events; the higher the numerical value, the greater the chance for becoming ill.

6. Cognitive appraisal refers to the evaluation of an event relative to what is at stake and what coping resources are available. External resources consist

of money to purchase services and materials and social support systems that provide emotional and esteem support.

7. Hans Selye stated that "stress is essentially the rate of wear and tear on the body." He also defined stress as being a "nonspecific response" of the body regardless of the stimulus producing the response.

8. Answer should include six of the following: hypertension, diseases of the heart and blood vessels, kidney diseases, rheumatic and rheumatoid arthritis, inflammation of the skin and eyes, infections, allergic and hypersensitivity diseases, nervous and mental diseases, sexual dysfunction, digestive diseases, metabolic diseases, and cancer.

9. Answer can include anxiety, ineffective coping patterns, impaired thought processes, disrupted relationships, impaired adjustment, ineffective coping, social isolation, risk for spiritual distress, decisional conflict.

10. People with positive energy and a healthy outlook on life typically perceive stressors as interesting, challenging, meaningful, and opportunities for change and growth.

11. Refer to chapter heading "Stress: Threats to the Steady State" in the text.

Activity C

1. b	**2.** a	**3.** a	**4.** a	**5.** b
6. a	**7.** b	**8.** a		

SECTION II: APPLYING YOUR KNOWLEDGE

Activity D

1. The goal of relaxation training is to produce a response that counters the stress response. When this goal is achieved, the action of the hypothalamus adjusts, decreasing sympathetic and parasympathetic nervous system activity.

2. Commonly used techniques include progressive muscle relaxation, the Benson Relaxation Response, and relaxation with guided imagery. Other relaxation techniques include meditation, breathing techniques, massage, Reiki, music therapy, biofeedback, and the use of humor.

3. The different relaxation techniques share four similar elements: (1) a quiet environment, (2) a comfortable position, (3) a passive attitude, and (4) a mental device (something on which to focus one's attention, such as a word, phrase, or sound).

SECTION III: PRACTICING FOR NCLEX

Activity E

1. b	**2.** c	**3.** a	**4.** a, c, d	**5.** a
6. a, b, c	**7.** b	**8.** d	**9.** c	**10.** a, c, d
11. d	**12.** a, c, d	**13.** b, c, d	**14.** a, b, d	**15.** a
16. d				

CHAPTER 7

SECTION I: ASSESSING YOUR UNDERSTANDING

Activity A

1. Madeleine Leininger
2. skin color, religion, geographic area
3. culture-specific, culture-universal
4. biomedical or scientific view, naturalistic or holistic perspective, magico-religious view
5. Spanish
6. allows for restructuring, can be accommodated, is congruent.

Activity B

1. The four basic characteristics of culture are: it is learned from birth through language and socialization, it is shared by all members of the same cultural group, it is influenced by specific environmental and technical factors, and it is dynamic and ever changing.

2. *Culturally competent nursing care* is effective, individualized care that shows respect for the dignity, personal rights, preferences, beliefs, and practices of people receiving care while acknowledging the biases of the caregiver and preventing that bias from interfering with care.

3. Four examples of American subcultures are Black/African American, Hispanic/Latino Americans, Asian/Pacific Islanders, and Native Americans (American Indians and Alaska Natives).

4. Answer should include five of the following subcultural groupings: religion, occupation, age, sexual orientation, geographic location, gender, and disability.

5. *Culturally competent or congruent nursing care* refers to the delivery of interventions within the cultural context of the patient. It involves the integration of attitudes, knowledge, and skills to enable nurses to deliver care in a culturally sensitive manner.

6. Four strategies include changing the subject, non-questioning, inappropriate laughter, and nonverbal cues.

7. Catholics, Mormons, Buddhists, Jews, and Muslims routinely abstain from eating as part of their religious practice.

8. The yin and yang theory of illness proposes that the seat of energy in the body is within the autonomic nervous system, where balance is maintained between the key opposing forces. Yin represents the female and negative forces, whereas yang represents the male positive energy.

Activity C

1. e	**2.** c	**3.** a	**4.** d	**5.** b
6. a	**7.** c	**8.** a	**9.** e	**10.** c

SECTION II: APPLYING YOUR KNOWLEDGE

Activity D

1. Greet the patient using the last or complete name. Avoid being too casual or familiar. Point to yourself and say your name. Smile. Proceed in an unhurried manner. Pay attention to any effort by the patient or family to communicate. Speak in a low, moderate voice. Avoid talking loudly. Repeat and summarize frequently. Use audiovisual aids when feasible.
2. A patient who is Muslim does not eat pork or pork products.

SECTION III: PRACTICING FOR NCLEX

Activity E

1. a	**2.** b	**3.** c	**4.** b	**5.** a
6. a	**7.** d	**8.** d	**9.** d	**10.** b

CHAPTER 8

SECTION I: ASSESSING YOUR UNDERSTANDING

Activity A

1. genotype; phenotype
2. chromosomes; autosomes; sex chromosomes; X chromosomes; one X and one Y chromosome; one sex chromosome of each pair
3. 80%, 50%
4. Down syndrome
5. 1 in every 160, 50%
6. Hemochromatosis (iron overload)
7. Genomics
8. 46
9. Sickle cell anemia
10. Neural tube defects
11. heart disease, diabetes, arthritis

Activity B

1. *Genomic medicine* encompasses the recognition that multiple genes work in concert with environmental influences, resulting in the appearance and expression of disease.
2. See Chart 8-1, Essential Nursing Competencies for Genetics and Genomics.
3. Answer may include five of the following: heart disease, high blood pressure, cancer, osteoarthritis, neural tube defects, spina bifida, and anencephaly.
4. *Pharmacogenetics* involves the use of genetic testing to identify genetic variations that relate to the safety and efficacy of medications and gene-based treatments.
5. Nursing activities may include collecting and helping interpret relevant family and medical histories, identifying patients and families who need genetic evaluation and counseling, offering genetics information and resources, collaborating with the genetic specialist, and participating in management of patient care.

Activity C

PART I: Terminology

1. e	**2.** h	**3.** f	**4.** a	**5.** g
6. d	**7.** b	**8.** a		

PART II: Adult-Onset Disorders

1. b	**2.** c	**3.** e	**4.** d	**5.** a
6. a	**7.** d	**8.** f		

SECTION II: APPLYING YOUR KNOWLEDGE

Activity D

1. Maggie has an increased risk of pregnancy loss and of having children with an unbalanced chromosomal arrangement, which may result in physical or mental disabilities.
2. The nurse may suggest that Maggie and Josh explore prenatal counseling and testing.
3. FISH is used to detect small abnormalities and to characterize chromosomal rearrangements.

SECTION III: PRACTICING FOR NCLEX

Activity E

1. a	**2.** c	**3.** a	**4.** c	**5.** a
6. a	**7.** c	**8.** b	**9.** a	**10.** a

CHAPTER 9

SECTION I: ASSESSING YOUR UNDERSTANDING

Activity A

1. use of tobacco, use of alcohol, improper diet, physical inactivity
2. 43% (about 125 million of 288 million)
3. obesity, hypertension, diabetes
4. developmental, acquired, age-associated

Activity B

1. the presence of a prolonged course, the inability of a condition to resolve spontaneously, and the unlikely or rare possibility of a cure
2. Refer to chapter heading "Implications of Managing Chronic Conditions" in the text.
3. Answers may include: preventing the occurrence of other chronic conditions; alleviating and managing symptoms; preventing, adapting, and managing disabilities; preventing and managing crises and complications; adapting to repeated threats and progressive functional loss; living with isolation and loneliness.
4. The Trajectory Model refers to the path or course of action taken by the ill person, the ill person's family, health professionals, and others to manage the course of the illness.
5. A *disability* is an umbrella term for impairments, activity limitations, participation restrictions, and environmental factors. An *impairment* is a loss or abnormality in body structure or physiologic function.

6. Refer to chapter heading "Overview of Chronicity" in the text.
7. Refer to chapter heading "Federal Legislation" in the text.

Activity C

1. Explain that medical conditions are associated with psychological and social problems that can affect body image and alter lifestyles.
2. Explain that chronic conditions have acute, stable, and unstable periods; flare-ups; and remissions. Each phase requires different types of management.
3. Explain that complying with a therapeutic treatment plan requires time, knowledge, and a long-term commitment to prevent the incidence of complications.
4. Explain that the whole family experiences stress and caretaker fatigue. Social changes that can occur include loss of income, role reversals, and altered socialization activities.

SECTION II: APPLYING YOUR KNOWLEDGE

Activity D

Refer to Table 9-2, Phases in the Trajectory Model of Chronic Illness, in the text.

Step 1: The nurse uses assessment to determine specific problems and the trajectory phase of the chronic illness. For example, the nurse determines whether any musculoskeletal deficiencies are evident, whether fatigue is interfering with activities of daily living (ADLs), and whether the patient is emotionally capable of coping with the diagnosis.

Step 2: The nurse interacts with the family and the medical team to establish and prioritize specific collaborative goals of management and support. For example, the nurse, working with the physician and physical therapist, designs an exercise program that will maximize current musculoskeletal strength while preventing excessive stress on major joints.

Step 3: The nurse can help the patient and family define a plan of action; i.e., draft a list of activities, exercises, and rest periods that can support established goals. The nurse can also identify specific criteria to be used to measure progress toward goal attainment. For example, the patient can keep a daily record of pain and joint stiffness, participation in work activities, and time allocated for recreation. The nurse can review the plan periodically with the patient.

Step 4: The nurse plans specific interventions to provide care. The nurse can help with direct care (i.e., range of motion [ROM] exercises, applications of warm compresses, adjustments to the environment). The nurse can recommend referrals to counseling or agencies that can help provide services. The nurse can help the family work together to determine a lifelong approach to treatment and support.

Step 5: The nurse follows up to determine if the problem, along with treatment and management interventions, is being resolved and whether there is adherence to the plan. The nurse identifies environmental, social, and psychological factors that may facilitate or hinder goal achievement. For example, the nurse could explore the time commitment and types of activities required for child care and how they affect the patient. Does the patient have support from extended family members? Can the patient adjust her work schedule if necessary? Are there any associated systemic conditions that may compromise a plan of care, such as renal problems or swollen joints?

SECTION III: PRACTICING FOR NCLEX

Activity E

1. b   2. a   3. b   4. a   5. b
6. c   7. a   8. b   9. c   10. d

CHAPTER 10

SECTION I: ASSESSING YOUR UNDERSTANDING

Activity A

1. erythema, reactive hyperemia, tissue ischemia, anoxia
2. sacrum, heels
3. streptococci, staphylococci, *Pseudomonas aeruginosa, Escherichia coli*
4. 3 g/mL, 1.25–1.5 g/kg/day
5. Braden, Norton
6. external rotation of the hip, plantar flexion of the foot (foot drop)
7. prolonged bed rest, lack of exercise, incorrect positioning in bed, the weight of the bedding
8. three
9. osteomyelitis
10. carbonated soft drinks, milkshakes, alcoholic beverages, tomato juice, citrus fruit juices

Activity B

1. The three goals of rehabilitation are to restore the patient's ability to function independently or at a pre-illness or pre-injury level, maximize independence, and prevent secondary disability.
2. Stroke recovery and traumatic brain injury, spinal cord injury, orthopedic, cardiac, pulmonary, pediatric, comprehensive pain management, and rehabilitation are specialty rehabilitation programs accredited by CARF.
3. Refer to chapter heading "The Patient With Self-Care Deficits in Activities of Daily Living" in the text.
4. Answer should include *five of the following eight diagnoses:* impaired physical mobility, activity intolerance, risk for injury, risk for disuse syndrome, impaired walking, impaired wheelchair

mobility, and impaired bed mobility. Answer should also include *four of the following five goals:* absence of contracture and deformity, maintenance of muscle strength and joint mobility, independent mobility, increased activity tolerance, and prevention of further disability.

5. Answer should include four of the following: impaired physical mobility, activity intolerance, risk for injury, risk for disuse syndrome, impaired walking, impaired wheelchair mobility, and impaired bed mobility.

6. Weakened muscles, joint contractures, and deformity are common complications associated with prolonged immobility.

7. Exercises are passive, active-assistive, active, resistive, and isometric or muscle setting. Nursing activities are described in Table 10-1 in the text.

8. Refer to Chart 10-6, Risk Factors—Pressure Ulcers, in the text.

9. Refer to Figure 10-5 in the text.

10. Eschar does not permit free drainage of the tissue.

Activity C

1. e   **2.** a   **3.** b   **4.** d   **5.** f
6. c

SECTION II: APPLYING YOUR KNOWLEDGE

Activity D

CASE STUDY: Assisted Ambulation: Crutches

1. push-ups performed in a sitting position
2. 49 inches
3. 8 to 10 inches
4. 3-point gate

SECTION III: PRACTICING FOR NCLEX

Activity E

1. d   **2.** b   **3.** a, b, c   **4.** a   **5.** a
6. b   **7.** c   **8.** d   **9.** d   **10.** c
11. a   **12.** a   **13.** a, b, c   **14.** a, b, c

CHAPTER 11

SECTION I: ASSESSING YOUR UNDERSTANDING

Activity A

1. calcium
2. macular degeneration
3. thinking, problem solving; verbal skills
4. Depression
5. Falls
6. Medicare

Activity B

1. *Geriatric syndromes* refer to common conditions found in the elderly that tend to be multifactorial and do not fall under discrete disease categories, such as falls, delirium, frailty, dizziness, and urinary incontinence.

2. myocardial hypertrophy, fibrosis, valvular stenosis, decreased pacemaker cells, reduced stroke volume

3. decreased cardiac output, decreased perfusion of the liver

4. pneumonia, urinary tract infections, tuberculosis, gastrointestinal infections, skin infections

5. *Continuing care retirement communities* (CCRCs) provide three levels of living arrangements and care and provide for "aging in place." CCRCs consist of independent single-dwelling houses or apartments for people who can manage all of their day-to-day needs; assisted living apartments for those who need limited assistance with their daily living needs; and skilled nursing services when continuous nursing assistance is required. CCRCs usually contract for a large down payment before the resident moves into the community. This payment gives a person or couple the option of residing in the same community from the time of total independence through the need for assisted or skilled nursing care. Decisions about living arrangements and health care can be made before any decline in health status occurs. CCRCs also provide continuity at a time in an older adult's life when many other factors, such as health status, income, and availability of friends and family members, may be changing.

6. Refer to chapter heading "Cognitive Aspects of Aging" in the text.

7. A comprehensive assessment that begins with a thorough medication history, including use of alcohol, recreational drugs, and over-the-counter and herbal medications, is essential. It is best to ask the patient or reliable informants to provide all medications for review. Assessing the patient's understanding of when and how to take each medication as well as the purpose of each medication allows the nurse to assess the patient's knowledge about and compliance with the medication regimen. The patient's beliefs and concerns about the medications should be identified, including beliefs on whether a given medication is helpful.

8. Refer to Table 11-3, Summary of Differences Between Dementia and Delirium, in the text.

9. Refer to chapter heading "Alzheimer's Disease" in the text.

10. Refer to chapter heading "Health Care Costs of Aging" in the text.

11. Refer to chapter heading "Ethical and Legal Issues Affecting the Older Adult" in the text.

12. Refer to chapter heading "Ethical and Legal Issues Affecting the Older Adult" in the text.

SECTION II: APPLYING YOUR KNOWLEDGE

Activity C

CASE STUDY: Loneliness

1. a deterioration of self-concept, a loss of self-esteem, extensive grief over frequently occurring losses

2. applying ointment to the skin several times a day, avoiding overexposure to the sun, patting the skin dry instead of rubbing it with a towel

3. The sense of smell diminishes as a result of neurologic changes and environmental factors such as smoking, medications, and vitamin B_{12} deficiencies. The ability to recognize sweet, sour, bitter, or salty foods diminishes over time, altering satisfaction with food. Salivary flow does not decrease in healthy adults, but about 30% of older people may experience a dry mouth as a result of medications and diseases. Difficulties with chewing and swallowing are generally associated with lack of teeth and disease.

4. 60 g

5. Keep personal items stored at a level between her hips and her eyes, make certain that all her shoes fit securely, avoid climbing and bending.

CASE STUDY: Alzheimer's Disease

1. providing a calm and predictable environment

2. Maintaining personal dignity and autonomy is still an important part of Thomas's life.

3. Alzheimer's support groups are available. Socializing with old friends may be comforting. Alzheimer's disease does not eliminate the need for intimacy.

4. pneumonia, malnutrition, and dehydration

CASE STUDY: Dehydration

1. Make sure that the environmental temperature is adequate, palpate Vera's skin periodically to assess for warmth, and place extra blankets at Vera's bedside in case she becomes cold, especially in the evening.

2. Offer the patient the use of the bedpan or bedside commode frequently. Immediately change wet pads and use skin barrier cream to avoid redness and breakdown.

3. Sitting in a rocking chair discourages hypostatic pulmonary congestion, increases pulmonary ventilation, and improves venous return through contraction of the calf muscles.

SECTION III: PRACTICING FOR NCLEX

Activity D

| 1. a | 2. a, c, d | 3. a | 4. c | 5. a |
| 6. b | 7. c | 8. a | 9. c | 10. b, d, e |

CHAPTER 12

SECTION I: ASSESSING YOUR UNDERSTANDING

Activity A

1. duration, location, etiology
2. Acute, chronic (nonmalignant), cancer-related
3. pain threshold; pain tolerance
4. longer than 6 months
5. respiratory depression; 24; 6 and 12
6. enkephalin

Activity B

1. Refer to Chart 12-2, Patient Education—Educating Patients and Their Families How to Use a Pain Rating Scale, in the text.

2. the suppression of immune function that promotes tumor growth

3. histamine, bradykinin, acetylcholine, serotonin, substance P

4. past experiences with pain, anxiety, culture, age, gender, genetics, expectations about pain relief

5. Factors include intensity, timing, location, quality, personal meaning of pain, aggravating and alleviating factors, and pain behaviors.

6. tachycardia, hypertension, tachypnea, pallor, diaphoresis, mydriasis, hypervigilance, increased muscle tone

7. *Balanced analgesia* refers to the use of more than one form of analgesia concurrently to obtain more pain relief with fewer side effects.

8. A *placebo effect* occurs when a person responds to a medication or treatment because of an expectation that the treatment will work rather than the treatment's actually effectiveness.

9. Answer may include massage, thermal therapies, transcutaneous electrical, distraction, relaxation techniques, guided imagery, and music therapy.

10. Acute pain lasts from seconds to 3 to 6 weeks (e.g., appendectomy, ankle sprain). Chronic, persistent, nonmalignant pain lasts 6 months or longer (e.g., rheumatoid arthritis, fibromyalgia). Cancer-related pain can be directly associated with the cancer and/or the result of cancer treatment (e.g., ovarian and lung cancer).

11. Refer to Chart 12-4, Use of Opioids, in the text.

12. See the section "Opioid Analgesic Agents" in the text.

13. Refer to chapter heading "Patient-Controlled Analgesia" in the text.

14. Distraction, which involves focusing the patient's attention on something other than the pain, reduces the perception of pain by stimulating the descending control system. This results in the transmission of fewer painful stimuli to the brain.

Activity C

| 1. f | 2. j | 3. a | 4. h | 5. b |
| 6. g | 7. c | 8. i | 9. e | 10. d |

SECTION II: APPLYING YOUR KNOWLEDGE

Activity D

CASE STUDY: Pain Experience

1. It will be brief in duration.

2. Muscle tension

3. Promoting relaxation, playing music or watching a video, using cutaneous stimulation.

4. Clarify that Courtney knows what type of pain signals a problem, remind her that acute pain may persist for several days, review methods of pain management.

SECTION III: PRACTICING FOR NCLEX

Activity E

1. b	**2.** b	**3.** c	**4.** a	**5.** a
6. a	**7.** c	**8.** c	**9.** b	**10.** b
11. d	**12.** c, d, e	**13.** d	**14.** c	**15.** c
16. d	**17.** d	**18.** c	**19.** a	

CHAPTER 13

SECTION I: ASSESSING YOUR UNDERSTANDING

Activity A

1. 66%, potassium; intravascular, interstitial, transcultural; sodium; 50%, 6 L; plasma. (Refer to Table 13-1, Approximate Major Electrolyte Content in Body Fluids, in the text.)
2. bones; soft tissue
3. 7.35 to 7.45
4. 6.8 on the lower range, 7.8 on the upper range
5. 1.5 L
6. 8 mEq/L
7. 95%
8. osmolality, affects the movement of water between fluid compartments
9. thirst, antidiuretic hormone, renin–angiotensin aldosterone system
10. muscle contraction and the transmission of nerve impulses
11. bicarbonate-carbonic acid buffer system
12. tetany

Activity B

PART I

1. *Osmotic pressure* is the amount of hydrostatic pressure needed to stop the flow of water by osmosis. It is primarily determined by the concentration of solutes.
2. *Urine specific gravity* measures the kidney's ability to excrete or conserve water. *Blood urea nitrogen,* made up of urea, is an end product of protein (muscle and dietary) metabolism by the liver. Creatinine, as the end product of muscle metabolism, is a better indicator of renal function than blood urea nitrogen.
3. *Baroreceptors,* which are responsible for monitoring the circulating volume, are small nerve receptors that detect changes in pressure within blood vessels. *Osmoreceptors* sense changes in sodium concentration.
4. Calcium levels are primarily regulated by the combined actions of parathyroid hormone and vitamin D.
5. metastatic calcification of soft tissue, joints, and arteries
6. Na × 2 = glucose divided by 18 + BUN divided by 3
7. Intense supervision is required because only small volumes are needed to elevate the serum sodium from dangerously low levels.
8. Answer may include dyspnea, cyanosis, a weak pulse, hypotension, unresponsiveness, and pain (chest, shoulder, low back).

PART II

1.

a. Low	**b.** Low	**c.** High	**d.** High	**e.** High
f. Low	**g.** High	**h.** Low	**i.** Low	**j.** High
k. High	**l.** Low			

2.

a. Low	**b.** High	**c.** Low	**d.** Low	**e.** High
f. Low	**g.** Low	**h.** Low	**i.** Low	**j.** High
k. Low	**l.** High			

3.

a. High	**b.** Low	**c.** High	**d.** High	**e.** Low
f. High	**g.** Low	**h.** Low		

4.

a. Low	**b.** High	**c.** Low	**d.** Low	**e.** Low

5.

a. Low	**b.** High	**c.** Low	**d.** Low	**e.** High

6.

a. R-ACID	**b.** M-ACID	**c.** M-ACID	**d.** R-ACID
e. R-ALKA	**f.** R-ACID	**g.** M-ACID	**h.** M-ALKA
i. M-ALKA	**j.** R-ALKA		

Activity C

1. f	**2.** d	**3.** c	**4.** b	**5.** a
6. e				

SECTION II: APPLYING YOUR KNOWLEDGE

Activity D

CASE STUDY: Extracellular Fluid Volume Deficit

1. a drop in postural blood pressure
2. The nurse should obtain orthostatic vital signs to include blood pressure and pulse with the patient lying down, then sitting up, and then standing.
3. monitoring urinary output to assess kidney perfusion, positioning the patient flat in bed with legs elevated to maintain adequate circulating volume, teaching leg exercises to promote venous return and prevent postural hypotension when the patient stands

CASE STUDY: Congestive Heart Failure

1. a full pulse, edema, and neck vein distention.
2. rapid weight gain
3. auscultating for abnormal breath sounds, inspecting for leg edema, and weighing the patient daily.

CASE STUDY: Diabetes

1. metabolic acidosis
2. hypertension, lethargy, and hypokalemia
3. hyperkalemia
4. sodium bicarbonate

CASE STUDY: Intravenous Therapy

1. air embolism, febrile reaction, and circulatory overload.

2. subclavian or internal jugular
3. total volume divided by the total time equals the mL/hr

SECTION III: PRACTICING FOR NCLEX

Activity E

1. a	**2.** c	**3.** c	**4.** b	**5.** c
6. a	**7.** b	**8.** b, c, e	**9.** a, c, d	**10.** c
11. a, c, d	**12.** a	**13.** c	**14.** a	**15.** c
16. a	**17.** b	**18.** c	**19.** b	**20.** d
21. c				

CHAPTER 14

SECTION I: ASSESSING YOUR UNDERSTANDING

Activity A

1. inadequate tissue perfusion; poor oxygen and nutrient delivery, cellular starvation, cell death, organ dysfunction leading to organ failure, eventual death
2. glucose; adenosine triphosphate (ATP)
3. blood volume, cardiac pump, vasculature
4. stroke volume, heart rate; diameter of the arterioles
5. carotid sinus, aortic arch; aortic arch, carotid arteries
6. cellular, tissue
7. lactated Ringer's solution, 0.9% sodium chloride solution (normal saline solution)
8. B-type natriuretic peptide (BNP)

Activity B

1. *Mean arterial pressure (MAP)* is the average pressure at which blood flows through the vasculature. MAP must exceed 65 mm Hg.
2. limit additional myocardial damage, increase cardiac contractility, and decrease ventricular afterload
3. loss of sympathetic tone, release of biochemical mediators from cells
4. spinal cord injury, spinal anesthesia, the depressant action of medications and glucose deficiency

Activity C

1. c	**2.** a	**3.** a	**4.** e	**5.** f
6. d	**7.** c	**8.** b	**9.** b	**10.** e

SECTION II: APPLYING YOUR KNOWLEDGE

Activity D

CASE STUDY: Hypovolemic Shock

1. 700 to 1500 mL of blood
2. In the compensatory stage of shock, the BP remains within normal limits. Vasoconstriction, increased heart rate, and increased contractility of the heart contribute to maintaining adequate cardiac output.
3. output <30 mL/hr
4. colloids, Ringer's lactate, and normal saline

CASE STUDY: Septic Shock

1. severe clinical insult that causes an overwhelming inflammatory response

2. lactic acidosis, oliguria, altered level of consciousness, thrombocytopenia, and altered hepatic function
3. urine, blood, sputum, and wound drainage
4. cardiovascular overload and pulmonary edema

SECTION III: PRACTICING FOR NCLEX

Activity E

1. b, c, d	**2.** c	**3.** d	**4.** b	**5.** a, d, e
6. a, b, c	**7.** c	**8.** d	**9.** d	**10.** d
11. a	**12.** a, b, c	**13.** b	**14.** b	**15.** c
16. d	**17.** d	**18.** b	**19.** d	**20.** d

CHAPTER 15

SECTION I: ASSESSING YOUR UNDERSTANDING

Activity A

1. Men: lung, prostate, colorectal area; women: breast, lung, colorectal area.
2. Carcinoembryonic antigen (CEA), prostate-specific antigen (PSA)
3. lymph, blood
4. 75%
5. tobacco smoke
6. Cabbage, broccoli, cauliflower. Fats, alcohol, salt-cured and smoked meats (ham), nitrite/nitrate-containing foods (bacon and red and processed meats)
7. nausea, vomiting
8. leucopenia, neutropenia, anemia, thrombocytopenia; infection, bleeding
9. cisplatin, methotrexate, mitramycin

Activity B

1. Cancer begins when an abnormal cell, after being transformed by the genetic mutation of DNA, forms a clone and begins to proliferate abnormally, ignoring growth-regulating signals.
2. breast and ovarian cancer syndrome (*BRCA1* and *BRCA2*), and multiple endocrine neoplasia syndrome (*MEN1* and *MEN2*)
3. Answer should include four of the following: mouth, pharynx, larynx, esophagus, liver, colorectum, and breast.
4. antibodies produced by B-lymphocytes, lymphokines, macrophages, natural killer (NK) cells, and T-lymphocytes
5. Answer should include three from each of the following choices:
   a. Skin: alopecia, erythema, desquamation
   b. Oral mucosal membrane: xerostomia, stomatitis, decreased salivation, loss of taste
   c. Stomach or colon: anorexia, nausea, vomiting, diarrhea
   d. Bone marrow–producing sites: anemia, leukopenia, and thrombocytopenia

6. Answer should include five of the following: redness; pain; swelling; a mottled appearance; phlebitis; loss of blood return; resistance to flow; tissue necrosis; or damage to underlying tendons, nerves, and blood vessels.

Activity C

PART I

1. a **2.** b **3.** f **4.** e **5.** d
6. g **7.** h **8.** c

PART II

1. b **2.** a **3.** a **4.** b **5.** b

PART III

Refer to Table 15-7, Select Antineoplastic Agents, in the text.

1. a; bone marrow suppression
2. c; nausea, vomiting, and diarrhea
3. f; masculinization and feminization
4. a; bone marrow suppression
5. b; delayed and cumulative myelosuppression
6. d; bone marrow suppression
7. a; nausea, vomiting, and cystitis
8. c; proctitis, stomatitis, and renal toxicity
9. e; neuropathies
10. h; bone marrow suppression
11. g; hepatotoxicity

SECTION II: APPLYING YOUR KNOWLEDGE

Activity D

CASE STUDY: Cancer of the Breast

1. genetics
2. attitudes toward her body image, feelings of self-esteem, social and sexual values
3. denial
4. tissue manipulation during surgery, apprehension regarding the prognosis of her condition, anger stemming from her change in body image
5. Her lungs may possibly produce more mucus, the skin at the treatment area may become red and inflamed, she may tire more easily and require additional rest periods.
6. Handle the area gently, avoid irritation with soap and water, wear loose-fitting clothing.
7. bone marrow depression, altered nutrition, leukopenia

CASE STUDY: Cancer of the Lung

1. denial
2. Answer questions and concerns, identify resources and support persons, communicate and share concerns, help frame questions for the physician.
3. weight loss
4. elevated white blood cell count

SECTION III: PRACTICING FOR NCLEX

Activity E

1. a **2.** a, b, c **3.** c **4.** a **5.** c
6. b **7.** c **8.** b **9.** a **10.** d
11. b **12.** b **13.** a **14.** d **15.** a
16. a

CHAPTER 16

SECTION I: ASSESSING YOUR UNDERSTANDING

Activity A

1. Kübler-Ross, *On Death and Dying*
2. Assisted suicide
3. Physician-assisted suicide
4. neurodegenerative diseases (dementia and Parkinson's), cardiovascular diseases
5. bronchodilators, corticosteroids
6. Decadron (dexamethasone), Megace (megestrol acetate), Marinol (dronabinol)

Activity B

1. Structure and process, physical aspects, psychological and psychiatric, social, cultural, care of the imminently dying, ethical and legal, and spiritual/religious/existential.
2. *Palliative care* and *hospice care* involve coordinated programs of interdisciplinary services provided by professional caregivers and trained volunteers to patients with serious, progressive illnesses who are not responsive to curative treatments. However, palliative care does not focus primarily on preparation for death, as does hospice care.
3. Kübler-Ross's work revealed that, given open discussion, adequate time, and some help in working through the process, patients could reach a stage of acceptance in which they were neither angry nor depressed about their fate.
4. Durable power of attorney for health care—a legal document through which the signer appoints and authorizes another individual to make medical decisions on the signer's behalf when the signer is no longer able to speak for him/herself. This is also known as a health care power of attorney or a proxy directive. Living will—a type of advance directive in which the individual documents treatment preferences. It provides instructions for care in the event that the signer is terminally ill and not able to communicate his/her wishes directly and often is accompanied by a durable power of attorney for health care. This is also known as a medical directive or treatment directive.
5. The ANA acknowledges the complexity of the assisted-suicide debate but clearly states that nursing participation in assisted suicide is a violation of the Code for Nurses.

SECTION II: APPLYING YOUR KNOWLEDGE

Activity C

1. dexamethasone (Decadron), megestrol acetate (Megace), dronabinol (Marinol)
2. The medication should only be used as short-term therapy because it interferes with the synthesis of muscle protein.
3. The nurse can make a referral to hospice.

SECTION III: PRACTICING FOR NCLEX

Activity D

1. b	**2.** c	**3.** c	**4.** d	**5.** d
6. a	**7.** d	**8.** d	**9.** c	**10.** a, b, c

CHAPTER 17

SECTION I: ASSESSING YOUR UNDERSTANDING

Activity A

1. when the decision to do surgery is made, is transferred onto the operating room table
2. is transferred to the operating room table, the patient is admitted to the PACU
3. the number and severity of coexisting health problems, the nature and duration of the operative procedure
4. respiratory, cardiac
5. hypoglycemia, hyperglycemia, acidosis, glucosuria
6. 7 to 10 days; inhibiting platelet aggregation

Activity B

1. it is invasive, it requires sedation or anesthesia, it involves radiation, and/or it has more than a slight risk of potential harm
2. dehydration, hypovolemia, electrolyte imbalances
3. improve circulation, prevent venous stasis, promote optimal respiratory function
4. Refer to Chart 17-4, Risk Factors—Surgical Complications, in the text.

Activity C

Refer to Table 17-2, Nutrients Important for Wound Healing, in the text.

1. d	**2.** a	**3.** e	**4.** c	**5.** b

Activity D

Medication Administration

Refer to Table 17-3, Examples of Medications With the Potential to Affect the Surgical Experience, in the text.

Preoperative Nursing

A wide range of interventions are used to prepare the patient physically and psychologically and to maintain safety. Beginning with the nursing history and physical examination, listing of medications taken routinely, allergies, surgical and anesthetic histories, the patient's overall health status, and level of experience and understanding may be established. For more information, refer to chapter heading "Preoperative Nursing Interventions" in the text.

SECTION II: APPLYING YOUR KNOWLEDGE

Activity E

1. Instruct the patient about diaphragmatic breathing, coughing, leg exercises, turning to the side, and how to get out of the bed. For more information, see Chart 17-6, Patient Education—Preoperative Instructions to Prevent Postoperative Complications, in the text.
2. Ingesting even moderate amounts of alcohol prior to surgery can weaken a patient's immune system and increase the likelihood of developing postoperative infections. In addition, the use of illicit drugs and alcohol may impede the effectiveness of some medications. People who abuse drugs or alcohol frequently deny or attempt to hide it. In such situations, the nurse who is obtaining the patient's health history needs to ask frank questions with patience, care, and a nonjudgmental attitude. See Chapter 5 for an assessment of alcohol and drug use.
3. Patients who smoke are urged to stop 4 to 8 weeks before surgery to significantly reduce pulmonary and wound healing complications. Preoperative smoking cessation interventions can be effective in changing smoking behavior and reducing the incidence of postoperative complications. Patients who smoke are more likely to experience poor wound healing, a higher incidence of surgical site infection, and complications that include venous thromboembolism and pneumonia.

SECTION III: PRACTICING FOR NCLEX

Activity F

1. c	**2.** b	**3.** a	**4.** c	**5.** a
6. a	**7.** a	**8.** c	**9.** a	**10.** b
11. a	**12.** a, b, c	**13.** d	**14.** a	**15.** a
16. c, d, e	**17.** d	**18.** c	**19.** d	**20.** c

CHAPTER 18

SECTION I: ASSESSING YOUR UNDERSTANDING

Activity A

1. moderate sedation; Versed, Valium
2. thiopental sodium (Pentothal), respiratory depression
3. the subarachnoid space at the lumbar level (usually between L4 and L5)
4. epidural
5. 104°F or 42°C
6. Ultane
7. 3 hours

Activity B

1. *Restricted zone:* area in the operating room where scrub attire and surgical masks are required; includes operating room and sterile core areas. *Semirestricted zone:* area in the operating room where scrub attire is required; may include areas where surgical instruments are processed. *Unrestricted zone:* area in the operating room that interfaces with other departments; includes patient reception area and holding area.
2. Anesthesia is reduced with age because the percentage of fatty tissue increases as one gets older. Fatty tissue has an affinity for anesthetic agents.
3. Handling tissue, providing exposure at the operative field, suturing, maintaining hemostasis
4. Answer may include five of the following: exposure to blood and body fluids, hazards associated with laser beams, exposure to latex and adhesive substances, exposure to radiation and toxic agents, faulty equipment, improper use of equipment, surgical plume (smoke generated by electrosurgical cautery), cuts, needlestick injuries.
5. Complete return of sensation in the patient's toes, in response to a pinprick, indicates recovery.
6. nausea and vomiting, anaphylaxis, hypoxia, hypothermia, malignant hypothermia
7. Refer to chapter heading "Types of Anesthesia and Sedation" in the text.
8. Refer to Chart 18-2, Potential Adverse Effects of Surgery and Anesthesia, in the text.
9. The elderly have a variety of age-related cardiovascular and pulmonary changes as well as changes in the liver and kidneys. Refer to chapter heading "Gerontologic Considerations" in the text.
10. Refer to chapter heading "Health Hazards Associated With the Surgical Environment" in the text
11. *Anesthesia awareness* is a condition in which patients are partially awake while under general anesthesia. Cardiac, obstetric, and major trauma patients are most at risk.

Activity C

Inhalation Anesthetic Agents

Refer to Table 18-1, Inhalation Anesthetic Agents, in the text.

1. d   **2.** b   **3.** a   **4.** c   **5.** e

Common Intravenous Medications

Refer to Table 18-2, Commonly Used Intravenous Medications, in the text.

1. d   **2.** b   **3.** a   **4.** c   **5.** e

SECTION II: APPLYING YOUR KNOWLEDGE

Activity D

CASE STUDY: General Anesthesia

1. fast recovery, low incidence of respiratory depression, rapid induction and recovery, not explosive or flammable
2. It may produce hypoxia.
3. Respiratory depression, ECG abnormalities

CASE STUDY: Moderate Sedation

1. Moderate sedation involves the IV administration of sedatives or analgesic medications to reduce patient anxiety and control pain during diagnostic or therapeutic procedures.
2. The continual assessment of the patient's vital signs, level of consciousness, and cardiac and respiratory function is an essential component of moderate sedation. Pulse oximetry, ECG monitor, and frequent measurement of vital signs are used to monitor the patient.
3. The goal is to depress a patient's level of consciousness to a moderate level to enable surgical, diagnostic, or therapeutic procedures to be performed while ensuring the patient's comfort and cooperation during the procedure.

SECTION III: PRACTICING FOR NCLEX

Activity E

1. b	**2.** a	**3.** c	**4.** a, b, c	**5.** b
6. c	**7.** c	**8.** a	**9.** b, c, d	**10.** a, b, c
11. b	**12.** b	**13.** d	**14.** b	**15.** b
16. c	**17.** a	**18.** c	**19.** a	

CHAPTER 19

SECTION I: ASSESSING YOUR UNDERSTANDING

Activity A

1. respiratory function (ventilation); hypoxemia and hypercapnia
2. hypovolemic, cardiogenic, neurogenic, anaphylactic, septic
3. respiratory
4. paralytic ileus and intestinal obstruction
5. bowel sounds, the passage of flatus
6. the stress response; muscle tension and local vasoconstriction
7. sympathetic activity; myocardial demand, oxygen consumption
8. blood viscosity, platelet aggregation; phlebothrombosis, pulmonary embolism

Activity B

1. The answer should include five of the following: medical diagnosis; type of surgery performed; patient's general condition, including age, airway patency, vital signs; anesthetic and other medications used; any intraoperative problems that might influence postoperative care (shock, hemorrhage, cardiac arrest); any pathology encountered; fluid administered; patent IV site; blood loss and replacement; tubing, drains, catheters, or other supportive aids; and specific information about which surgeon or anesthesiologist wishes to be notified.
2. *Primary* hemorrhage occurs at the time of the operation. *Intermediary* hemorrhage occurs within the

first few hours after surgery when a return of blood pressure to its normal level dislodges insecure clots. *Secondary* hemorrhage occurs some time after the operation as a result of the slipping of a ligature, which may happen because of infection, insecure tying, or erosion of a vessel by a drainage tube.

3. Patient-controlled analgesia refers to self-administration of pain medication by way of intravenous or epidural routes within prescribed time/dosage limits.

4. Atelectasis and hypostatic pneumonia are reduced with early ambulation because ventilation is increased and the stasis of bronchial secretions in the lungs is reduced.

5. Wound *dehiscence* refers to the disruption of the wound or surgical incision. Wound *evisceration* refers to the protrusion of wound contents.

6. Pallor; cool, moist skin; tachypnea; cyanosis (lips, gums, tongue); rapid, weak, and thready pulse; narrowing pulse pressure; hypotension; and concentrated urine.

7. Refer to chapter heading "Managing Potential Complications" in the text.

8. Refer to Figure 19-3 and chapter heading "Determining Readiness for Postanesthesia Care Unit Discharge" in the text.

9. The respiratory depressive effects of opioids, decreased lung expansion secondary to pain, and decreased mobility are three conditions that put patients at risk for atelectasis, pneumonia, and hypoxemia.

10. See Table 19-3, Factors Affecting Wound Healing, and chapter heading "Caring for Wounds" in the text.

SECTION II: APPLYING YOUR KNOWLEDGE

Activity C
CASE STUDY: Hypopharyngeal Obstruction

1. The primary objective in the immediate postoperative period is to maintain ventilation and thus prevent hypoxemia and hypercapnia.

2. The signs of occlusion include: choking; noisy and irregular respirations; decreased oxygen saturation scores; and within minutes, a blue dusky color of the skin.

3. The treatment of hypopharyngeal obstruction involves tilting the head back and pushing forward on the angle of the lower jaw, as if to push the lower teeth in front of the upper teeth. This maneuver pulls the tongue forward and opens the air passages.

CASE STUDY: Wound Healing

1. Surgical wound healing occurs in three phases: first-intention, second-intention, and third-intention wound healing.

2. Ongoing assessment of the surgical site involves inspection for approximation of wound edges, integrity of sutures or staples, redness, discoloration, warmth, swelling, unusual tenderness, or

drainage. Inspect for a reaction to tape or trauma from tight bandages.

3. pain, redness, and warmth

4. encouraging coughing and deep breathing to enhance pulmonary and cardiovascular function

SECTION III: PRACTICING FOR NCLEX

Activity E
1. c	**2.** d	**3.** b	**4.** a	**5.** b, c, d
6. d	**7.** a	**8.** d	**9.** a	**10.** c
11. b	**12.** c	**13.** d	**14.** d	**15.** a
16. c	**17.** a, b, d	**18.** a	**19.** d	**20.** d

CHAPTER 20

SECTION I: ASSESSING YOUR UNDERSTANDING

Activity A

1. the *apneustic center* in the lower pons, the *pneumotaxic center* in the upper pons

2. 50

3. pleura

4. one less lobe

5. lobar bronchi, segmented bronchi, subsegmented bronchi, bronchioles

6. Type II cells

7. respiration

8. expiratory reserve volume

9. 1000

10. diffusion

11. high-pressure, high-resistance system

12. PaO_2

Activity B

1. *Ventilation* refers to the movement of air in and out of the airways, whereas *respiration* refers to gas exchange between atmospheric air and blood and between the blood and the cells of the body.

2. The epiglottis is a flap of cartilage that covers the opening of the larynx during swallowing.

3. Low or decreased compliance occurs with certain pathology. Answer should include four of the following: morbid obesity, atelectasis, pneumothorax, hemothorax, pulmonary fibrosis or edema, pleural effusion, ARDS.

4. *Partial pressure* is the pressure exerted by each type of gas (e.g., oxygen, carbon dioxide) in a mixture of gases.

5. Answer should include six of the following: dyspnea, cough, sputum production, chest pain, wheezing and hemoptysis, tachypnea, hypoxia.

6. asthma, COPD, cystic fibrosis, alpha-1 antitrypsin deficiency

7. Cheyne–Stokes respirations are characterized by alternating episodes of apnea (cessation of breathing) and periods of deep breathing. It is usually associated with heart failure and damage to the respiratory center.

8. Cilia move the mucus back to the larynx.
9. *Streptococcus pneumoniae, Haemophilus influenzae, Staphylococcus aureus,* and *Moraxella catarrhalis*
10. Diffusion is the exchange of oxygen and carbon dioxide at the air–blood interface. Pulmonary perfusion is the actual flow of blood through the pulmonary circulation.

SECTION II: APPLYING YOUR KNOWLEDGE

Activity C

CASE STUDY: Bronchoscopy

1. in the bronchus, larynx, or trachea
2. supplying information about the procedure, withholding food and fluids for at least 6 hours, ensuring that informed consent is obtained
3. aspiration, infection, pneumothorax
4. Monitor the patient's respiratory status and observe for hypoxia, hypotension, tachycardia, dysrhythmias, hemoptysis, and dyspnea.
5. Offer ice chips and eventually fluids after the gag and cough reflex return.

CASE STUDY: Thoracentesis

1. informing Mrs. Lomar about pressure sensations that will be experienced during the procedure, making sure that chest roentgenograms ordered in advance have been completed, seeing that the consent form has been explained and signed
2. sitting on the edge of the bed with the patient's feet supported and arms and head on a padded overbed table
3. second and third intercostal space
4. blood-tinged mucus, signs of hypoxemia, tachycardia.

SECTION III: PRACTICING FOR NCLEX

Activity D

1. a	**2.** c, d, e	**3.** c	**4.** d	**5.** c, d, e
6. d	**7.** a	**8.** a	**9.** c	**10.** c
11. b	**12.** b	**13.** a, c, d	**14.** c	**15.** a, b, c
16. b	**17.** a	**18.** c	**19.** b	**20.** d

CHAPTER 21

SECTION I: ASSESSING YOUR UNDERSTANDING

Activity A

1. cardiac output, arterial oxygen content, hemoglobin concentration, metabolic requirements
2. 50, >48 hours
3. hypoxia
4. vitamin E, vitamin C, beta-carotene
5. chronic obstructive pulmonary disease (COPD)
6. No Smoking sign
7. nasal cannula
8. Venturi
9. T-piece
10. 2

11. decreases venous return, decreases cardiac output
12. 1–3 and 1.5
13. 6
14. 15 and 20, 6–8
15. 10–15, 6, 7–9
16. histotoxic
17. pneumonectomy
18. 2.0

Activity B

1. Answer should include five of the following: substernal discomfort, paresthesias, dyspnea, restlessness, fatigue, malaise, progressive respiratory difficulty, refractory hypoxemia, alveolar atelectasis, and alveolar infiltrates on x-ray.
2. decreased blood oxygen rather than elevated carbon dioxide levels
3. nasal cannula, oropharyngeal catheter, simple mask, partial-rebreather, nonrebreather
4. dislodge mucus and remove bronchial secretions, improve ventilation, and increase the efficiency of the respiratory muscles
5. Bi-PAP ventilation offers independent control of inspiratory and expiratory pressures while providing pressure support ventilation. It delivers two levels of positive airway pressure provided via a nasal or oral mask, nasal pillow, or mouthpiece with a tight seal and portable ventilator.
6. Positive pressure ventilators inflate the lungs by exerting pressure on the airway, pushing air in, forcing the alveoli to expand during inspiration.
7. A patient "bucks the ventilator" when his or her breathing is out of phase with the machine. This occurs when the patient attempts to breathe out during the ventilator's mechanical inspiratory phase or when there is jerky and increased abdominal muscle effort.
8. Refer to chapter heading "The Patient Receiving Mechanical Ventilation" in the text.
9. Refer to Chart 21-19, Risk Factors—Surgery-Related Atelectasis and Pneumonia, in the text.

Activity C

1. d	**2.** c	**3.** e	**4.** f	**5.** b
6. a				

SECTION II: APPLYING YOUR KNOWLEDGE

Activity D

CASE STUDY: Pneumonectomy: Preoperative Concerns

1. breathing patterns, smoking history, cardiac status
2. the renal system
3. evaluate the arterial blood gases

CASE STUDY: Pneumonectomy: Postoperative Concerns

1. maintain a patent airway
2. hypovolemia
3. pulmonary edema
4. dyspnea and tachypnea

CASE STUDY: Patient with Mechanical Ventilation

1. breath sounds
2. bradycardia and bradypnea
3. Reposition the patient every 2 hours to diminish the pulmonary effects of immobility.
4. hypercarbia, hypoxia, inadequate minute volume

CASE STUDY: Weaning from the Ventilator

1. The patient should maintain an inspiratory pressure force of at least 20 cm H_2O pressure, have a PaO_2 greater than 60% and an FiO_2 lower than 40%, and be able to generate a minimum vital capacity of 10–15 mL/kg of body weight.
2. See Chart 21-17, Care of the Patient Being Weaned from Mechanical Ventilation.
3. 70–100 mm Hg

SECTION III: PRACTICING FOR NCLEX

Activity E

1. a	**2.** a	**3.** d	**4.** b	**5.** c
6. d	**7.** a, b, d	**8.** d	**9.** a	**10.** c, d, e
11. c	**12.** a	**13.** a, b, c	**14.** c	**15.** b
16. b	**17.** a	**18.** c	**19.** a	**20.** b

CHAPTER 22

SECTION I: ASSESSING YOUR UNDERSTANDING

Activity A

1. viral; hoarseness, aphonia, severe cough
2. symptom relief
3. Antihistamines
4. acute, subacute, chronic
5. Peritonsillar abscess
6. hemorrhage

Activity B

1. Rhinitis causes the nasal passages to become inflamed, congested, and edematous. The swollen conchae block the sinus openings and cause sinusitis.
2. *Streptococcus pneumoniae, Haemophilus influenzae, Staphylococcus aureus, Moraxella catarrhalis*
3. Answer should include four of the following: severe orbital cellulitis, subperiosteal abscess, cavernous sinus thrombosis, meningitis, encephalitis, and ischemic infarction.
4. Refer to chapter heading "The Patient With Upper Airway Infection" in the text.
5. Complications may include sepsis, a peritonsillar abscess, otitis media, sinusitis, and meningitis.
6. Obstructive sleep apnea is defined as frequent loud snoring and breathing cessation for 10 seconds or longer with five or more episodes per hour. This is followed by awakening abruptly with a loud snort when the blood oxygen level drops.
7. esophageal speech, an artificial larynx, tracheo-esophageal puncture

Activity C

1. b	**2.** e	**3.** c	**4.** a	**5.** d

SECTION II: APPLYING YOUR KNOWLEDGE

Activity D

CASE STUDY: Tonsillectomy and Adenoidectomy

1. bleeding from the surgical site
2. hemorrhage
3. In the immediate postoperative period, the most comfortable position is prone, with the patient's head turned to the side to allow drainage from the mouth and pharynx.
4. Offer her soft foods for several days to minimize local discomfort and supply her with necessary nutrients.

CASE STUDY: Epistaxis

1. Gilberta should sit upright with her head tilted forward to prevent swallowing and aspiration of blood. She should also pinch the soft outer portion of the nose against the midline spectrum for 5–10 continuous minutes.
2. Application of nasal decongestants (phenylephrine, one or two sprays) to act as vasoconstrictors may be necessary.
3. The packing may remain in place for 3–4 days if necessary to control bleeding.

CASE STUDY: Cancer of the Larynx

1. palpation of the neck for swelling
2. "You will most likely have radiation or surgery."
3. The nurse should inform Brenda that the highest risk for laryngeal cancer is within 2–3 years.

CASE STUDY: Laryngectomy

1. supraglottic laryngectomy
2. The nurse should inform him that there are ways he will be able to carry on a conversation without his voice, making sure that he knows he will require a permanent tracheal stoma, and reminding him that he will not be able to sing, whistle, or laugh.
3. 1 week
4. The nurse should inform him that the laryngectomy tube will be removed when the stoma is well healed.

SECTION III: PRACTICING FOR NCLEX

Activity E

1. b, c, d	**2.** a	**3.** a	**4.** c, d, e	**5.** a
6. a, b, c	**7.** a, b, d	**8.** c	**9.** a	**10.** b
11. c	**12.** d	**13.** d	**14.** b	**15.** a

CHAPTER 23

SECTION I: ASSESSING YOUR UNDERSTANDING

Activity A

1. impaired host defenses, an inoculum of organisms that reach the lower respiratory tract, the presence of a highly virulent organism
2. 60%; nonpulmonary multiple-system organ failure
3. 16%
4. Tachypnea, dyspnea, mild to moderate hypoxemia
5. silent aspiration
6. *Streptococcus pneumoniae, Haemophilus influenzae,* and *Staphylococcus aureus*
7. alcoholism, chronic obstructive pulmonary disease (COPD), acquired immunodeficiency syndrome (AIDS), diabetes, heart failure
8. hypotension, shock, respiratory failure
9. impaired central nervous system (CNS) function, neuromuscular, musculoskeletal, pulmonary dysfunction

Activity B

1. Refer to Figure 23-1 and chapter heading "Atelectasis" in the text.
2. dyspnea, cough, sputum production, tachycardia, tachypnea, pleural pain, and central cyanosis
3. frequent turning, early mobilization, deep breathing maneuvers, assistance with the use of spirometry, suctioning, postural drainage, aerosol nebulizer treatments, and chest percussion
4. *Superinfection* is suspected when a subsequent infection occurs with another bacterium during antibiotic therapy.
5. hypoxemia that does not respond to supplemental oxygen
6. enlargement of the right ventricle of the heart because of diseases affecting the structure or functions of the lung
7. Refer to Chart 23-8, Etiologic Factors Related to Acute Respiratory Distress Syndrome, in the text.

Activity C

1. d   2. c   3. f   4. b   5. a
6. e

SECTION II: APPLYING YOUR KNOWLEDGE

Activity D

CASE STUDY: Community-Acquired Pneumonia

1. Provide Theresa with fluids, at least 1 L/day.
2. fever, stabbing or pleuritic chest pain, tachypnea
3. Bronchospasm causes alveolar collapse, which decreases the surface area necessary for perfusion. Mucosal edema occludes the alveoli, thereby producing a drop in alveolar oxygen; venous blood is shunted from the right to the left side of the heart.
4. atelectasis, hypotension and shock, pleural effusion

CASE STUDY: Tuberculosis

1. he has been exposed to *M. tuberculosis* or has been vaccinated with BCG.
2. sputum culture
3. rifampin

CASE STUDY: Acute Respiratory Distress Syndrome

1. dysrhythmias and hypotension, contraction of the accessory muscles of respiration, tachypnea, and tachycardia.
2. drowsiness, irritability, confusion
3. 44%

CASE STUDY: Pulmonary Embolism

1. "Most of the time, the clots form from venous stasis due to immobility."
2. dyspnea
3. cardiac output

SECTION III: PRACTICING FOR NCLEX

Activity E

1. a, b, c	2. a	3. c	4. d	5. a
6. c	7. d	8. a	9. c	10. b
11. a	12. b	13. d	14. a	15. d
16. c	17. a, b, d, e	18. a	19. b	20. b

CHAPTER 24

SECTION I: ASSESSING YOUR UNDERSTANDING

Activity A

1. third
2. Passive smoking
3. respiratory insufficiency, chronic respiratory failure
4. Spirometry
5. bullectomy
6. cessation of smoking
7. tracheobronchial infection, air pollution
8. *Streptococcus pneumoniae, Haemophilus influenzae*
9. allergy; cough, wheezing, and dyspnea
10. status asthmaticus, respiratory failure, pneumonia, atelectasis
11. 37 years

Activity B

1. Chronic inflammation results in the following: increased goblet cells and enlarged submucosal glands (proximal airways), inflammation and airway narrowing (peripheral airways), and narrowing of the airway lumen.
2. *Emphysema* is an abnormal distention of the air spaces, beyond the terminal bronchioles, that results in destruction of the walls of the alveoli.
3. A genetic risk factor for COPD is a deficiency in alpha-antitrypsin, an enzyme inhibitor that protects the lungs.

4. chronic cough, sputum production, and dyspnea on exertion
5. Answer should include five of the following: history of cigarette smoking, passive smoking exposure, age, rate of decline of FEV_1, hypoxemia, weight loss, reversibility of airflow obstruction, pulmonary artery pressure, and resting heart rate.
6. alter smooth muscle tone, reduce airway obstruction, and improve alveolar ventilation

Activity C

1. f   **2.** c   **3.** e   **4.** d   **5.** b
6. a

SECTION II: APPLYING YOUR KNOWLEDGE

Activity D
CASE STUDY: Emphysema

1. "air trapping" in the lungs
2. dyspnea
3. respiratory acidosis
4. dysrhythmias, central nervous system excitement, tachycardia
5. decreased respiratory rate, increased alveolar ventilation, reduction of functional residual capacity
6. a Venturi mask that delivers a predictable oxygen flow at about 24%.

SECTION III: PRACTICING FOR NCLEX

Activity E

1. b   **2.** a   **3.** b   **4.** a, b, c   **5.** b
6. d   **7.** a   **8.** c   **9.** d   **10.** d
11. c   **12.** a, c, d   **13.** a   **14.** c   **15.** c

CHAPTER 25

SECTION I: ASSESSING YOUR UNDERSTANDING

Activity A

1. 20, 10
2. Cholesterol, triglycerides, lipoproteins
3. atherosclerosis
4. size, contour, position
5. 2 to 6
6. preload, afterload, contractility
7. hyperlipidemia, hypertension, diabetes
8. <70 mg/dL; <140/90 mm Hg; <110 mg/day; 18.5 to 24.9 kg/m²
9. creatine kinase (CK), isoenzyme CK-MB; troponin T and I, myoglobin

Activity B

1. hypertension, CAD, heart failure, stroke, congenital cardiovascular defects
2. The atrioventricular (AV) valves separate the atria from the ventricles. The tricuspid separates the right atrium and ventricle; the bicuspid separates the left atrium and ventricle. The AV valves permit blood to flow from the atria into the ventricles. The semilunar valves are situated between each ventricle and its corresponding artery. The pulmonic valve is between the right ventricle and the pulmonary artery; the aortic valve is between the left ventricle and the aorta. These valves permit blood to flow from the ventricles into the arteries.
3. Depolarization is said to have occurred when the electrical difference between the inside and the outside of the cell is reduced. The inside of the cell becomes less negative, membrane permeability to calcium is increased, and muscle contraction occurs.
4. Cardiac output (stroke volume × heart rate) would equal 5,320 mL.
5. Starling's law of the heart refers to the relationship between increased stroke volume and increased ventricular end-diastolic volume for a given intrinsic contractility.
6. Physiologic effects of the aging process may include: reduction in the size of the left ventricle, decreased elasticity and widening of the aorta, thickening and rigidity of cardiac valves, and increased connective tissue in the sinoatrial and atrioventricular nodes and bundle branches.
7. below the fifth intercostal space and lateral to the mid-clavicular line
8. Cardiac catheterization is used most frequently to assess the patency of the patient's coronary arteries and to determine readiness for coronary bypass surgery. It is also used to measure pressures in the various heart chambers and to determine oxygen saturation of the blood by sampling specimens.
9. Selective angiography refers to the technique of injecting a contrast medium into the vascular system to outline a particular heart chamber or blood vessel.
10. A lowered central venous pressure reading indicates that the patient is hypovolemic. Serial measurements are more reflective of a patient's condition and should be correlated with the patient's clinical status.
11. Answer should include any four of the following: infection, pulmonary artery rupture, pulmonary thromboembolism, pulmonary infarction, catheter kinking, dysrhythmias, and air embolism.

Activity C
PART I

1. c   **2.** e   **3.** a   **4.** d   **5.** b
6. f

PART II

1. d   **2.** g   **3.** a   **4.** f   **5.** i
6. k   **7.** b   **8.** j   **9.** c   **10.** h
11. e

Activity D

	Pericarditis	Musculoskeletal Disorders
Duration of pain	Intermittent	Hours to days
Precipitating events and aggravating factors	Sudden onset; pain increases with inspiration, coughing, and trunk rotation.	Most often follows respiratory tract infection with significant coughing, vigorous exercise, or posttrauma. Some cases are idiopathic. Exacerbated by deep inspiration, coughing, sneezing, and movement of upper torso or arms.
Alleviating factors	Sitting upright, analgesics, and anti-inflammatory agents	Rest, ice, or heat Analgesic or anti-inflammatory medications

SECTION III: APPLYING YOUR KNOWLEDGE

Activity E

CASE STUDY: Cardiac Assessment for Chest Pain

1. peripheral cyanosis
2. d
3. c
4. 45 degrees
5. 5th intercostal space

SECTION III: PRACTICING FOR NCLEX

Activity F

1. a	2. c	3. d	4. a	5. b
6. c	7. d	8. d	9. c	10. a
11. a	12. b	13. c	14. b	15. a, b, c

CHAPTER 26

SECTION I: ASSESSING YOUR UNDERSTANDING

Activity A

1. dysrhythmic
2. automaticity
3. conductivity
4. depolarization
5. diastole

6. Ablation
7. QT interval
8. 0.12 and .20 seconds
9. premature atrial complex
10. atrial flutter
11. 100 beats/min

Activity B

1. atria, atrioventricular node or junction, sinus node, and ventricles
2. Electrical conduction through the heart begins in the sinoatrial node (SA), travels across the atria to the atrioventricular node (AV), and then travels down the right and left bundle branches and Purkinje fibers to the ventricular muscle.
3. Answer should include five of the following: fever, hypovolemia, anemia, exercise, pain, congestive heart failure, anxiety, and sympathomimetic or parasympatholytic drugs.
4. Ventricular tachycardia occurs when there is more than three premature ventricular contractions (PVCs) in a row and the rate exceeds 100 beats per minute (bpm).
5. a thromboembolic event, heart failure, and cardiac arrest
6. The difference is in the timing of the electrical current. With cardioversion, the current is synchronized with the patient's electrical events; with defibrillation, the current is unsynchronized and immediate.
7. The standard procedure is to place one paddle to the right of the upper sternum below the right clavicle and the other paddle just to the left of the cardiac apex.
8. An on-demand pacemaker is set for a specific rate and stimulates the heart when normal ventricular depolarization does not occur; the fixed-rate pacemaker stimulates the ventricle at a preset constant rate, independently of the patient's rhythm.
9. Small incisions are made throughout the atria so that scar tissue forms and prevents reentry conduction of the electrical impulse.

Activity C

1. b	2. d	3. f	4. h	5. g
6. e	7. c	8. a		

SECTION II: APPLYING YOUR KNOWLEDGE

Activity D

Graph Analysis

1. a. T wave
   b. PR interval
   c. P wave
   d. QRS complex
   e. ST segment
2. a. Q wave is larger.
   b. ST segment is elevated.
   c. T wave is inverted.

Graphic Recordings

1. P waves come early in cycle and close to T wave of previous heartbeat.
2. QRS complex is bizarre. P waves are hidden in QRS complexes.
3. Three or more PVCs in a row, occurring at a rate of 100 bpm.

Activity E
CASE STUDY: Permanent Pacemaker

1. Yes. Heart rate can vary as much as 5 bpm faster or slower than the preset rate.
2. bleeding, hematoma formation, and infection
3. dislodgment of the pacing electrode
4. the pacemaker model, date and time of insertion, stimulation threshold, pacer rate, incision appearance, patient tolerance
5. Nursing interventions would include the education of the patient and sterile wound care. Expected outcomes are that Mr. Woo will be free from infection, adhere to a self-care program, maintain pacemaker function, understand signs and symptoms of infection and when to seek medical attention, assess pulse rate at regular intervals, and experience no abrupt changes in pulse rate or rhythm.

SECTION III: PRACTICING FOR NCLEX
Activity F

1. d	**2.** c	**3.** b	**4.** a	**5.** c
6. a	**7.** d	**8.** a	**9.** c	**10.** d
11. a, b, c	**12.** b	**13.** d	**14.** a	**15.** c

CHAPTER 27

SECTION I: ASSESSING YOUR UNDERSTANDING
Activity A

1. acute MI, sudden death
2. smoking
3. Oral contraceptive
4. 140/90
5. supplemental oxygen, aspirin, nitroglycerine, morphine
6. cardiovascular disease
7. atherosclerosis
8. chest pain referred to as *angina pectoris*
9. age—more than 50% are older than 65 years of age
10. less than 200 mg/dL; 3.5:1.0; less than 100 mg/dL; greater than 60 mg/dL; 150 mg/dL
11. 25% to 35%
12. an elevated ST segment in two contiguous leads
13. greater saphenous vein
14. the formation of a thrombus

Activity B

1. Answer should include four of the following: hyperlipidemia, cigarette smoking, obesity, hypertension, diabetes mellitus, metabolic syndrome, and physical activity.
2. insulin resistance, central obesity, dyslipidemia, hypertension (>130/85 mm Hg), increased levels of C-reactive protein (proinflammation), and elevated fibrinogen levels (prothrombotic)
3. Answer should include three of the following: acute coronary syndrome or MI, dysrhythmias, cardiac arrest, heart failure, and cardiogenic shock.
4. Answer should include four of the following: fever, pericardial pain, pleural pain, dyspnea, pericardial effusion, pericardial friction rub, and arthralgia.
5. An atheroma, also called plaque, is a fibrous cap of smooth muscle cells that form over lipid deposits within the arterial vessels, protrude and narrow the lumen, and then obstruct blood flow.
6. Because the duration of oxygen deprivation determines the number of myocardial cells that die, the time from the patient's arrival in the emergency department (ED) to the time PCI is performed should be less than 60 minutes. This is frequently referred to as *door-to-balloon time.*

Activity C

1. f	**2.** e	**3.** b	**4.** c	**5.** d
6. a				

SECTION II: APPLYING YOUR KNOWLEDGE
Activity D
CASE STUDY: Angina Pectoris

1. There is not enough blood flow in your coronary arteries to get adequate oxygen to the heart muscle."
2. It is relieved by rest and is predictable.
3. causing venous pooling throughout the body, dilating the coronary arteries to increase the oxygen supply, lowering systemic blood pressure.
4. Administer a third nitroglycerin and give her oxygen at 2 L/min via nasal cannula.

CASE STUDY: Decreased Myocardial Tissue Perfusion

1. the first hour after symptoms begin
2. enlarged T wave
3. elevations in troponin levels, CK-MB, myoglobin
4. cardiogenic shock

SECTION III: PREPARING FOR NCLEX
Activity E

1. a	**2.** c	**3.** a	**4.** c	**5.** b
6. a	**7.** b, c, d	**8.** b, c, d	**9.** b	**10.** c
11. c	**12.** a, b, c	**13.** c	**14.** a	**15.** a, b, c

CHAPTER 28

SECTION I: ASSESSING YOUR UNDERSTANDING

Activity A

1. systolic click
2. left ventricle, left atrium
3. stenosis
4. Commissurotomy
5. chordotomy
6. caffeine, alcohol, cigarettes
7. at the third and fourth intercostal spaces at the left sternal border, a blowing diastolic murmur
8. prophylactic antibiotics
9. penicillin therapy, rheumatic fever
10. streptococci, enterococci, pneumococci, staphylococci
11. digitalis, digitalis toxicity

Activity B

1. MVP is usually an inherited connective tissue disorder that causes enlargement of both mitral valve leaflets. Usually there are no symptoms. It can result in valve incompetency and regurgitation. As valve dysfunction progresses, symptoms of heart failure ensue.
2. Answer should include four of the following: congestive heart failure, ventricular dysrhythmias, atrial dysrhythmias, cardiac conduction defects, pulmonary or cerebral embolism, and valvular dysfunction.
3. cardiomyopathy, ischemic heart disease, valvular disease, rejection of previously transplanted hearts, and congenital heart disease
4. An inflamed endothelium causes a fibrin clot to form (vegetation), which converts to scar tissue that thickens, contracts, and causes deformities. The result is leakage or valvular regurgitation and stenosis.
5. Myocarditis is an inflammatory process that usually results from an infection. The infectious process can cause heart dilation, thrombi formation, infiltration of blood cells around the coronary vessels and between the muscle fibers, and eventual degeneration of the muscle fibers themselves.
6. Listen at the left sternal edge of the thorax in the fourth intercostal space where the pericardium comes in contact with the left chest wall.
7. Answer should include six of the following: idiopathic, infection, disorders of connective tissue, sarcoidosis, hypersensitivity states, disorders of adjacent structures, neoplastic disease, radiation therapy of chest and upper torso, trauma, kidney failure, and uremia.

Activity C

1. a   2. e   3. d   4. b   5. c

SECTION II: APPLYING YOUR KNOWLEDGE

Activity D

CASE STUDY: Infective Endocarditis

1. Roth's spots
2. The nurse should report headache; temporary or transient cerebral ischemia; and strokes, which may be caused by emboli to cerebral arteries. Embolization may be a presenting symptom; it may occur at any time and may involve other organ systems.
3. 5 days

CASE STUDY: Acute Pericarditis

1. Pain may be relieved with a forward-leaning or sitting position.
2. Determine the cause, administer therapy for treatment and symptom relief, and detect signs and symptoms of cardiac tamponade. When cardiac output is impaired, the patient should be placed on bed rest until fever, chest pain, and friction rub have subsided.
3. left sternal edge in the fourth intercostal space

SECTION III: PRACTICING FOR NCLEX

Activity E

1. a	2. a	3. c	4. b	5. d
6. b	7. c	8. c	9. b	10. a
11. a	12. b	13. b	14. a	15. b

CHAPTER 29

SECTION I: ASSESSING YOUR UNDERSTANDING

Activity A

1. venous return, ventricular compliance; the diameter/distensibility of the great vessels, the opening/competence of the semilunar valves
2. jugular venous distention, mean arterial blood pressure, a positive hepatojugular test
3. pulmonary embolism
4. 100; 30:2
5. coronary artery disease, cardiomyopathy, hypertension, valvular disorders
6. dilated, hypertrophic, restrictive; dilated
7. dyspnea, cough, pulmonary crackles, low oxygen saturation, extra heart sound (ventricular gallop)
8. dependent edema, hepatomegaly, ascites, anorexia, nausea, weakness, weight gain (fluid retention)
9. Angiotensin-converting enzyme (ACE) inhibitors, beta-blockers, diuretics, digitalis
10. hypoxia, acidosis, the accumulation of lactic acid

Activity B

1. Cardiac output equals the heart rate times the stroke volume (the amount of blood pumped out with each contraction).

2. Preload is the amount of myocardial stretch created by the volume of blood within the ventricle before systole. Afterload refers to the amount of resistance to the ejection of the blood from the ventricle.

3. Answer should include four of the following: symptomatic hypotension, hyperuricemia, ototoxicity, electrolyte imbalances, dizziness, and balance problems.

4. weak pulse, faint heart sounds, hypotension, muscle flabbiness, diminished deep tendon reflexes, and generalized weakness

5. end-stage heart failure, cardiac tamponade, pulmonary embolism, cardiomyopathy, myocardial ischemia, and dysrhythmias

Activity C

1. a	**2.** b	**3.** a	**4.** b	**5.** b
6. a	**7.** a	**8.** b	**9.** a	**10.** b

SECTION II: APPLYING YOUR KNOWLEDGE

Activity D

CASE STUDY: Pulmonary Edema

1. Rest decreases blood pressure, increases the heart reserve, and reduces the work of the heart.

2. The patient should maintain an upright position with the feet and legs dependent to reduce left ventricular workload.

3. Symptoms of toxicity include anorexia, bradycardia and tachycardia, nausea and vomiting. Mr. Wolman should call his doctor if any of these symptoms occur.

4. bananas, raisins, orange juice

SECTION III: PRACTICING FOR NCLEX

Activity E

1. b	**2.** d	**3.** b	**4.** c	**5.** c
6. c, d, e	**7.** a	**8.** a	**9.** c	**10.** d
11. d	**12.** b	**13.** a	**14.** a	**15.** b

CHAPTER 30

SECTION I: ASSESSING YOUR UNDERSTANDING

Activity A

1. resistance vessels
2. intermittent claudication
3. C-reactive protein
4. edema, altered pigmentation, pain, stasis dermatitis
5. the use of tobacco products

Activity B

1. pain, pallor, pulselessness, paresthesia, poikilothermia (coldness), and paralysis
2. venous stasis, vessel wall injury, and altered blood coagulation

3. The rate of blood flow through a vessel is determined by dividing the pressure difference (ΔP) (arterial and venous) by the resistance to flow (R).

4. The pain in intermittent claudication is caused by the inability of the arterial system to provide adequate blood flow to the tissues in the face of increased demands for oxygen and nutrients during exercise.

5. Refer to chapter headings "Thoracic Aortic Aneurysm" and "Abdominal Aortic Aneurysm."

6. Refer to Chart 30-5, Home Care Checklist—Foot and Leg Care in Peripheral Vascular Disease.

7. chronic venous occlusion, pulmonary emboli from dislodged thrombi, valvular destruction, venous obstruction

Activity C

1. a	**2.** b	**3.** a	**4.** a	**5.** b
6. b	**7.** a	**8.** a		

SECTION II: APPLYING YOUR KNOWLEDGE

Activity D

CASE STUDY: Peripheral Arterial Occlusive Disease

1. intermittent claudication
2. 0.50
3. a planned program involving systematic lowering of the extremity below heart level, Buerger-Allen exercises, graded extremity exercises
4. The examiner should use light touch and avoid using only the index finger for palpation because this finger has the strongest arterial pulsation of all the fingers. The thumb should not be used for the same reason.

SECTION III: PRACTICING FOR NCLEX

Activity E

1. d	**2.** a, c, d	**3.** b	**4.** a, b, c	**5.** a, b, c
6. a	**7.** b	**8.** c	**9.** d	**10.** a
11. d	**12.** d	**13.** a, b, d	**14.** d	**15.** c
16. b				

CHAPTER 31

SECTION I: ASSESSING YOUR UNDERSTANDING

Activity A

1. cardiac output; peripheral resistance
2. heart rate; stroke volume
3. 30%
4. cardiovascular damage
5. 130 mm Hg
6. 50%
7. rebound hypertension
8. Hypertensive emergency, hypertensive urgency

Activity B

1. Cigarette smoking does not cause high blood pressure; however, if a person with hypertension smokes, that person's risk of dying from heart disease or related disorders increases significantly.
2. noncompliance with recommended therapeutic regimen
3. hypertension that has been poorly controlled, undiagnosed hypertension, patients who have abruptly discontinued their medications
4. weight reduction, DASH diet, dietary sodium restriction, increasing physical activity, moderation of alcohol consumption
5. a diet rich in fruits, vegetables, and low-fat dairy products with a reduced content of saturated fats and total fat

Activity C

1. d	2. b	3. f	4. a	5. c
6. e				

SECTION II: APPLYING YOUR KNOWLEDGE

Activity D

CASE STUDY: Secondary Hypertension

1. releasing renin in response to decreased renal perfusion
2. An eye examination with an ophthalmoscope is particularly important because retinal blood vessel damage indicates similar damage elsewhere in the vascular system. The patient is questioned about blurred vision, spots in front of the eyes, and diminished visual acuity.
3. blocks reabsorption of sodium, chloride, and water in the kidneys
4. adhere to dietary regimens, become involved with a regular exercise program, and take her medication as prescribed

SECTION III: PRACTICING FOR NCLEX

Activity E

1. a	2. d	3. a, b	4. b	5. c
6. b	7. a	8. c	9. d	10. a, c, d
11. a	12 c	13. b	14. a	15. d

CHAPTER 32

SECTION I: ASSESSING YOUR UNDERSTANDING

Activity A

1. 5 to 6 L
2. bone marrow
3. ribs, vertebrae, pelvis, sternum
4. hemoglobin; transport oxygen between the lungs and the tissues
5. 15 g
6. 2 mg

7. C
8. albumin, globulins
9. the sternum, the iliac crest

Activity B

1. An intricate clotting mechanism is activated when necessary to seal any leak in the blood vessels. Excessive clotting is equally dangerous, because it can obstruct blood flow to vital tissues. To prevent this, the body has a fibrinolytic mechanism that eventually dissolves clots formed within blood vessels.
2. The stroma is important in an indirect manner, in that it produces the colony-stimulating factors needed for hematopoiesis.
3. Iron, vitamin B_{12}, folic acid, pyridoxine, protein, and other factors are required. A deficiency of these factors during erythropoiesis can result in decreased red cell production.
4. An increased number of band cells is sometimes call a left shift or shift to the left. A shift to the left indicates that more immature cells are present in the blood than normal.
5. NK cells accumulate in the lymphoid tissues (especially spleen, lymph nodes, and tonsils), where they mature. When activated, they serve as potent killers of virus-infected and cancer cells. They also secrete chemical messenger proteins, called cytokines, to mobilize the T and B cells into action.
6. Knowledge of correct administration techniques and possible complications is required. It is very important to be familiar with the agency's policies and procedures for transfusion therapy.

Activity C

1. e	2. j	3. g	4. o	5. a
6. p	7. f	8. b	9. q	10. h
11. k	12. c	13. r	14. g	15. n
16. d	17. m	18. i		

SECTION II: APPLYING YOUR KNOWLEDGE

Activity D

CASE STUDY: Blood Transfusion

1. Check for the abnormal presence of gas bubbles and cloudiness in the blood bag; check that the blood has been typed and cross-matched and that the recipient's blood numbers match the donor's blood numbers.
2. Determine any history of previous transfusions as well as previous reactions to transfusion. The history should include the type of reaction, its manifestations, the interventions required, and whether any preventive interventions were used in subsequent transfusions.
3. The nurse knows that reactions are usually mild and should respond to an antihistamine such as diphenhydramine (Benadryl).

SECTION III: PRACTICING FOR NCLEX

Activity E

1. d	**2.** b	**3.** a	**4.** a	**5.** a
6. c	**7.** d	**8.** d	**9.** b, c, d, e	**10.** b, c, d
11. a	**12.** c, d, e	**13.** a	**14.** b	**15.** a

CHAPTER 33

SECTION I: ASSESSING YOUR UNDERSTANDING

Activity A

1. Anemia
2. 50%
3. heart failure, paresthesias, delirium
4. 4% to 6%, 13% to 14%
5. neurologic
6. Antacids, dairy products
7. Aplastic anemia
8. Proton pump inhibitors (PPIs), metformin (Glucophage)
9. skin, mucous membranes, tongue
10. Sickle cell anemia
11. Heparin infusion

Activity B

1. Factors include the rapidity with which the anemia has developed, the duration of the anemia, the metabolic requirements of the patient, other concurrent disorders or disabilities, and complications or concomitant features of the condition that produced the anemia.
2. correcting or controlling the cause of the anemia
3. Answer may include decreased mobility, increased depression, increased risk for falling, and delirium. The heart rate and cardiac output do not increase as quickly; thus fatigue, dyspnea, and confusion may be seen more readily in the anemic older adult.
4. Dietary teaching sessions should be individualized, involve family members, and include cultural aspects related to food preferences and food preparation. Additional amounts of iron, up to 2 mg daily, must be absorbed by women of childbearing age to replace that lost during menstruation.
5. bleeding from ulcers, gastritis, inflammatory bowel disease (IBD), or gastrointestinal (GI) tumors
6. Chemical agents potentially responsible for bone marrow aplasia include benzene and benzene derivatives such as airplane glue, paint remover, and dry-cleaning solutions. Certain toxic materials—such as inorganic arsenic, glycol ethers, plutonium, and radon—have also been implicated as potential causes.
7. The patient with sickle cell trait usually has a normal hemoglobin level, a normal hematocrit, and a normal blood smear. In contrast, the patient with sickle cell anemia has a low hematocrit and sickled cells on the smear. The diagnosis is confirmed by hemoglobin electrophoresis.

8. Answer may include the following: in an acute exacerbation of anemia, in the prevention of severe complications from anesthesia and surgery, in improving the response to infection, in the case of acute chest syndrome and multi-organ failure, in thwarting the evolution of a stroke or an acute neurologic defect, and in diminishing episodes of sickle cell crisis in pregnant women.
9. sepsis, trauma, cancer, shock, abruption placentae, toxins, and allergic reactions

Activity C

1. c	**2.** a	**3.** b	**4.** a	**5.** c
6. b				

SECTION II: APPLYING YOUR KNOWLEDGE

Activity D

1. The patient is experiencing DIC.
2. If possible, the nurse should avoid administering medications that interfere with platelet function, such as aspirin, nonsteroidal anti-inflammatory drugs (NSAIDs), and beta-lactam antibiotics.
3. neurological checks, hemodynamics, abdominal girth, urine output, amount of external bleeding
4. heparin

SECTION III: PRACTICING FOR NCLEX

Activity E

1. b	**2.** a	**3.** c	**4.** c	**5.** c
6. a	**7.** d	**8.** c	**9.** d	**10.** b
11. a	**12.** b	**13.** a, b, c	**14.** c	**15.** a

CHAPTER 34

SECTION I: ASSESSING YOUR UNDERSTANDING

Activity A

1. assess, monitor, educate, intervene
2. cells
3. B lymphocyte
4. leukemias
5. lymphoid, myeloid
6. acute, chronic
7. 55, 67
8. bleeding, infection
9. stem cell
10. dysplasia

Activity B

1. The signs and symptoms result from insufficient production of normal blood cells.
2. The results will show an excess of immature blast cells, which is the hallmark of the diagnosis.
3. The goal of treatment is to obtain remission without excess toxicity and with a rapid hematologic recovery so that additional therapy can be administered if needed.
4. because the illness is unpredictable

5. See Chart 34-2: Potential Long-Term Complications of Therapy for Hodgkin Lymphoma.

Activity C
1. h	**2.** c	**3.** d	**4.** g	**5.** a
6. e	**7.** f	**8.** i	**9.** b	

SECTION II: APPLYING YOUR KNOWLEDGE

Activity D
CASE STUDY: Multiple Myeloma

1. The classic presenting symptom of multiple myeloma is bone pain, usually in the back or ribs. The bone pain usually increases with movement and decreases with rest; he may report less pain when awakening but more during the day.
2. As more and more malignant plasma cells are produced, the marrow has less space for erythrocyte production, and anemia may develop. It is also caused by a diminished production of erythropoietin by the kidney.
3. chemotherapy
4. NSAIDs can cause gastritis and renal dysfunction, so renal function must be carefully monitored and patients assessed for gastritis; many patients are unable to use NSAIDs due to concurrent renal insufficiency.

SECTION III: PRACTICING FOR NCLEX

Activity E
1. a	**2.** b	**3.** c	**4.** d	**5.** a
6. a	**7.** b	**8.** d	**9.** b	**10.** c
11. d	**12.** a, c, d	**13.** a, b, c	**14.** a	**15.** c

CHAPTER 35

SECTION I: ASSESSING YOUR UNDERSTANDING

Activity A
1. bone marrow, lymphoid tissue, white blood cells
2. bone marrow
3. thymus
4. lymphocytes
5. neutrophils
6. monocytes
7. phagocytic immune response
8. lymphocytes
9. protein
10. natural deficiency
11. proliferation

Activity B
1. activation of complement, arrival of killer T cells, and attraction of macrophages
2. by altering the antigen's cell membrane, causing cellular lysis, and producing lymphokines, which destroy invading organisms
3. Disorders arise from excesses or deficiencies of immunocompetent cells, alterations in cellular

functioning, immunologic attack on self-antigens, and inappropriate or exaggerated responses to specific antigens.
4. Natural immunity, which is nonspecific, is present at birth. Acquired immunity is more specific and develops throughout life. Active acquired immunity refers to defenses developed by the person's own body. Passive acquired immunity is a temporary immunity transmitted from another source that has developed immunity through previous disease or immunization.
5. Complement is a term used to describe circulating plasma proteins that are made in the liver and activated when an antibody couples with an antigen. Complement defends the body against bacterial infection, bridges natural and acquired immunity, and disposes of immune complexes and byproducts associated with inflammation.
6. BMRs suppress antibody production and cellular immunity.
7. See Table 35-4, Age-Related Changes in Immunologic Function.
8. See Table 35-5, Selected Medication and Effects on the Immune System.

Activity C
Immunoglobulins
1. d	**2.** e	**3.** c	**4.** d	**5.** a
6. b	**7.** a			

Medications
1. d	**2.** b	**3.** a	**4.** c	**5.** b
6. a	**7.** e			

SECTION II: APPLYING YOUR KNOWLEDGE

Activity D
1. The first line of defense, the *phagocytic immune response,* primarily involves the WBCs (granulocytes and macrophages), which have the ability to ingest foreign particles and destroy the invading agent; eosinophils are only weakly phagocytic. Phagocytes also remove the body's own dying or dead cells. Dying cells in necrotic tissue release substances that trigger an inflammatory response.
2. A second protective response, the *humoral immune response* (sometimes called the *antibody response*), begins with the B lymphocytes, which can transform themselves into plasma cells that manufacture antibodies. These antibodies are highly specific proteins that travel in the bloodstream and attempt to disable invaders.
3. The third mechanism of defense, the *cellular immune response,* also involves the T lymphocytes, which can turn into special cytotoxic (or killer) T cells that can attack the pathogens.

SECTION III: PRACTICING FOR NCLEX

Activity E

1. a   **2.** c   **3.** a, b, c   **4.** c   **5.** a, b, d
6. b, c, d   **7.** b   **8.** b   **9.** a   **10.** d
11. d   **12.** d   **13.** a, b, c, d   **14.** b   **15.** b

CHAPTER 36

SECTION I: ASSESSING YOUR UNDERSTANDING

Activity A

1. severe infections, autoimmunity, cancer
2. humoral immunity, T-cell defects, combined B- and T-cell defects, phagocytic disorders, complement production
3. mature B cells, plasma cells
4. pernicious anemia
5. severe malnutrition

Activity B

1. Immunodeficiency disorders may be caused by a defect in or a deficiency of phagocytic cells, B lymphocytes, T lymphocytes, or the complement system.
2. The cardinal symptoms of immunodeficiency include chronic or recurrent and severe infections, infections caused by unusual organisms or by organisms that are normal body flora, poor response to standard treatment for infections, and chronic diarrhea. In addition, the patient is susceptible to a variety of secondary disorders, including autoimmune disease and lymphoreticular malignancies.
3. Common primary immunodeficiencies include disorders of humoral immunity (affecting B-cell differentiation or antibody production), T-cell defects, combined B- and T-cell defects, phagocytic disorders, and complement deficiencies.
4. Patients with neutropenia are at increased risk for developing severe infections.
5. Infants with X-linked agammaglobulinemia usually become symptomatic after the natural loss of maternally transmitted immunoglobulins, which occurs at about 5 to 6 months of age. Symptoms of recurrent pyogenic infections usually occur by that time.

Activity C

1. d   **2.** c   **3.** b   **4.** a

SECTION II: APPLYING YOUR KNOWLEDGE

Activity D

1. The nurse should monitor for the following adverse effects: complaints of flank and back pain, shaking chills, flushing, dyspnea, and tightness in the chest; headache, fever, muscle cramps, nausea/vomiting, and local reaction at the infusion site; hypotension (possible with severe reactions); transfusion-related acute lung injury; elevated BUN/creatinine. Serious

conditions can include aseptic meningitis, kidney failure, thromboembolic events, Stevens-Johnson syndrome, and anaphylaxis. Anaphylactic reactions typically occur 30 to 60 minutes after the start of the infusion. The potential increases as the dose of IVIG increases.
2. See Chart 36-1, Pharmacology—Managing an Intravenous Immunoglobulin Infusion.
3. See Chart 36-1, Pharmacology—Managing an Intravenous Immunoglobulin Infusion.

SECTION III: PRACTICING FOR NCLEX

Activity E

1. d   **2.** a, c, d   **3.** b   **4.** b   **5.** d
6. d   **7.** b   **8.** a, b, c   **9.** a   **10.** a

CHAPTER 37

SECTION I: ASSESSING YOUR UNDERSTANDING

Activity A

1. 1.2 million
2. unprotected sex and the sharing of injection drug use equipment (refer to Chart 37-1, Risk Factors—Risks Associated With HIV Infection and AIDS, in the text)
3. blood, seminal fluid, vaginal secretions, amniotic fluid, and breast milk
4. retroviruses that carry their genetic material in the form of RNA rather than DNA
5. Ora Quick test
6. the ability of pathogens to withstand the effects of medications that are intended to produce toxicity
7. candidiasis
8. alpha-interferon
9. B-cell lymphomas

Activity B

1. Refer to Chart 37-2, Health Promotion—Protecting Against HIV Infection, in the text.
2. Refer to Chart 37-4, Recommendations for Standard Precautions, in the text.
3. Refer to Chart 37-5, Postexposure Prophylaxis for Health Care Providers, in the text.
4. *Primary infection* is that period from infection with HIV to the development of HIV-specific antibodies. It is the time during which the viral burden set point is achieved and includes the acute symptoms and early infection phases. During primary infection, a window period occurs in which the person is infected but tests negative on the HIV antibody blood test.
5. Adverse effects associated with all HIV treatment regimens include hepatotoxicity, nephrotoxicity, and osteopenia, along with increased risk of cardiovascular disease and myocardial infarction (see Table 37-3, Antiretroviral Agents, in the text). Many of the antiretroviral agents that prolong life may simultaneously cause fat redistribution syndrome

and metabolic alterations such as dyslipidemia and insulin resistance, which put the patient at risk for early-onset heart disease and diabetes. The fat redistribution syndrome (lipodystrophy) consists of lipoatrophy (localized subcutaneous fat loss in the face, arms, legs, and buttocks) and lipohypertrophy (central visceral fat [lipomata] accumulation in the abdomen, although possibly in the breasts, dorsocervical region [buffalo hump], and within the muscle and liver).

6. Refer to chapter heading "Immune Reconstitution Inflammatory Syndrome" in the text.
7. The lesions are usually brownish pink to deep purple. They may be flat or raised and surrounded by hemorrhagic patches and edema.
8. Refer to chapter heading "HIV Encephalopathy" in the text.
9. Refer to chapter heading "Treatment of Opportunistic Infections" in the text.

Activity C

1. c	2. b	3. c	4. a	5. c
6. b	7. a	8. c		

SECTION II: APPLYING YOUR KNOWLEDGE

Activity D

CASE STUDY: Acquired Immunodeficiency Syndrome

1. Wasting syndrome
2. poor skin turgor, dry mucous membranes
3. octreotide acetate (Sandostatin)
4. Encourage him to rest before eating, limit fluids 1 hour before meals, have 5 to 6 small meals a day.

SECTION III: PRACTICING FOR NCLEX

Activity E

1. c	2. b	3. b	4. a	5. b, d, e
6. d	7. a	8. c	9. b	10. d
11. c	12. b	13. a	14. a	15. a

CHAPTER 38

SECTION I: ASSESSING YOUR UNDERSTANDING

Activity A

1. neutralizing toxic antigens, precipitating the antigens out of solution, coating the surface of the antigens
2. IgE
3. immunoglobulins
4. the pain and fever seen with inflammatory responses
5. Answer should include two of the following: systemic lupus erythematosus, rheumatoid arthritis, serum sickness, certain types of nephritis, and some types of bacterial endocarditis.

6. contact dermatitis, latex allergy
7. penicillin
8. epinephrine, in a 1:1,000 dilution given subcutaneously
9. 4 to 10

Activity B

1. An allergic reaction occurs when the body is invaded by an *antigen,* usually a protein that the body recognizes as foreign. The body responds in an effort to destroy the invading antigen. *Antibodies* (protein substances) are produced. When an interaction between the antigen and antibody results in tissue injury, an allergic reaction occurs and chemical mediators are released into the body.
2. Refer to chapter heading "Histamine" in the text.
3. Refer to Figure 38-2 in the text.
4. The three types of allergy tests are skin testing (including prick skin tests, scratch tests, and intradermal skin testing), which entails the intradermal injection or superficial application (epicutaneous) of solutions at several sites; provocative testing, which involves the direct administration of the suspected allergen to the sensitive tissue, such as the conjunctiva, nasal or bronchial mucosa, or gastrointestinal tract (by ingestion of the allergen), with observation of target organ response; and radioallergosorbent testing (RAST), in which a sample of the patient's serum is exposed to a variety of suspected allergen particle complexes. Refer to the chapter headings "Skin Tests," "Provocative Testing," and "Radioallergosorbent Test" in the text for more information.
5. Refer to chapter heading "Allergic Disorders" in the text.
6. The systemic reactions of flushing, warmth, and itching rapidly progress to bronchospasm, laryngeal edema, severe dyspnea, cyanosis, and hypotension. Cardiac arrest and coma can occur. Onset can begin within 2 hours postexposure.
7. Refer to chapter heading "Anaphylaxis" and Chart 38-2, Nonallergenic Anaphylaxis (Anaphylactoid Reaction) in the text.
8. Refer to Table 38-4, Types, Testing, and Treatment of Contact Dermatitis in the text.

Activity C

1. c	2. b	3. d	4. a

SECTION II: APPLYING YOUR KNOWLEDGE

Activity D

CASE STUDY: Allergic Rhinitis

1. breathing difficulties, pruritus, and tingling sensations
2. hoarseness, a rash or hives, and wheezing
3. information about reducing exposure to allergens, desensitization procedures, and the correct use of medications

CASE STUDY: Latex Allergy

1. Irritant contact dermatitis, a nonimmunologic response, may be caused by mechanical skin irritation or an alkaline pH associated with latex gloves.
2. These symptoms can be eliminated by changing glove brands or by using powder-free gloves.
3. Use of hand lotion before donning latex gloves can worsen the symptoms, because lotions may leach latex proteins from the gloves, increasing skin exposure and the risk of developing true allergic reactions.
4. Sensitization is detected by skin testing, RAST, EIA, ELISA or level of Hevea latex-specific IgE antibody in the serum. Testing for the chemicals used in latex rubber production is performed using the patch test. Skin patch testing is the preferred method for patients with contact allergies.

SECTION III: PRACTICING FOR NCLEX

Activity E

1. a	**2.** b	**3.** d	**4.** a	**5.** a
6. a	**7.** b	**8.** d	**9.** a, b, c	**10.** c
11. b	**12.** c	**13.** d	**14.** c	**15.** a

CHAPTER 39

SECTION I: ASSESSING YOUR UNDERSTANDING

Activity A

1. pain
2. T lymphocytes
3. milky, cloudy, dark yellow
4. collagen
5. synovial tissue

Activity B

1. One theory of *degradation* is that genetic or hormonal influences, mechanical factors, and prior joint damage cause cartilage failure. Degradation of cartilage ensues, and increased mechanical stress on bone ends causes stiffening of bone tissue. Another theory is that bone stiffening occurs and results in increased mechanical stress on cartilage, which in turn initiates the processes of degradation. For more information, refer to chapter heading "Rheumatic Diseases" in the text.
2. *Exacerbation* is a period of time when the symptoms of a disorder occur or increase in intensity and frequency. *Remission* is a period of time when symptoms are reduced or absent.
3. In *inflammatory* rheumatic disease, the inflammation occurs as the result of an immune response. Newly formed synovial tissue is infiltrated with inflammatory cells (pannus formation), and joint degeneration occurs as a secondary process. In *degenerative* rheumatic disease, synovitis results from mechanical irritation. A secondary inflammation occurs.

4. Refer to Table 39-2, Management Goals and Strategies for Rheumatic Diseases, in the text.
5. Range-of-motion (ROM), isometric, dynamic, aerobic, and pool exercises are used to promote mobility for patients with rheumatic diseases. For more information, including the purpose of and precautions for each type of exercise, refer to Table 39-4, Exercise to Promote Mobility, in the text.
6. PMR is characterized by severe proximal muscle discomfort with mild joint swelling. Severe aching in the neck, shoulder, and pelvic muscles is common. Stiffness, noticeable most often in the morning and after periods of inactivity, can become so severe that patients struggle putting on a coat or combing their hair. Systemic features include low-grade fever, weight loss, malaise, anorexia, and depression. For more information, refer to chapter heading "Polymyalgia Rheumatica and Giant Cell Arteritis" in the text.
7. The primary clinical manifestations of OA are joint pain, stiffness, and functional impairment. For more information, refer to chapter heading "Osteoarthritis (Degenerative Joint Disease)" in the text.
8. Manifestations of gout include acute gouty arthritis (recurrent attacks of severe articular and periarticular inflammation), tophi (crystalline deposits accumulating in articular tissue, osseous tissue, soft tissue, and cartilage), gouty nephropathy (renal impairment), and uric acid urinary calculi. For more information, refer to chapter heading "Gout" in the text.
9. Nurses need to pay special attention to supporting patients with fibromyalgia and providing encouragement as they begin their program of therapy. Patient support groups may be helpful. Careful listening to patients' descriptions of their concerns and symptoms is essential to help them make the changes that are necessary to improve their quality of life. Refer to chapter heading "Fibromyalgia" in the text.

Activity C

1. c	**2.** d	**3.** e	**4.** a	**5.** f
6. b	**7.** h	**8.** g		

SECTION II: APPLYING YOUR KNOWLEDGE

Activity D

CASE STUDY: Diffuse Connective Tissue Disease

1. Symmetric joint pain, swelling, warmth, erythema, and lack of function are classic symptoms of RA.
2. Rheumatoid factor is present in about 80% of patients with RA, but its presence alone is not diagnostic of RA, and its absence does not rule out the diagnosis.
3. 2 to 6 weeks after treatment begins
4. Research suggests that methotrexate combined with low-dose prednisone improves patient outcome, compared to use of methotrexate alone for early RA.

CASE STUDY: Systemic Lupus Erythematosus (SLE)

1. Cardiovascular assessment includes auscultation for pericardial friction rub, possibly associated with myocarditis and accompanying pleural effusions.
2. The mainstay of SLE treatment is based on pain management and nonspecific immunosuppression. Therapy includes NSAIDs, corticosteroids, antimalarials, and cytotoxic agents. Each of these medications has potentially serious side effects, including organ damage.
3. One of the most important risk factors associated with corticosteroid usage in SLE is osteoporosis and fractures. Osteopenia is reported in 25% to 74% and osteoporosis in 1.4% to 68% of SLE patients.

SECTION III: PRACTICING FOR NCLEX

Activity E

1. a, b, d	**2.** d	**3.** b	**4.** d	**5.** b
6. c	**7.** d	**8.** a	**9.** a	**10.** d
11. b	**12.** a, b, c	**13.** b	**14.** a	**15.** c

CHAPTER 40

SECTION I: ASSESSING YOUR UNDERSTANDING

Activity A

1. arthritis
2. 98%
3. 206
4. 1,000 to 1,200
5. sternum, ilium, vertebrae, ribs
6. parathyroid hormone, calcitonin
7. Crepitus

Activity B

1. The musculoskeletal system provides protection for vital organs, including the brain, heart, and lungs; provides a sturdy framework to support body structures; and makes mobility possible.
2. *Osteoblasts* function in bone formation by secreting bone matrix. The matrix consists of collagen and ground substances (glycoproteins and proteoglycans) that provide a framework in which inorganic mineral salts are deposited. These minerals are primarily composed of calcium and phosphorus. *Osteocytes* are mature bone cells involved in bone maintenance; they are located in lacunae (bone matrix units). *Osteoclasts,* located in shallow Howship's lacunae (small pits in bones), are multinuclear cells involved in dissolving and resorbing bone.
3. Vitamin D increases calcium in the blood by promoting calcium absorption from the gastrointestinal tract and by accelerating the mobilization of calcium from the bone.
4. The sex hormones testosterone and estrogen have important effects on bone remodeling. Estrogen stimulates osteoblasts and inhibits osteoclasts; therefore, bone formation is enhanced and resorption is inhibited. Testosterone has both direct and indirect effects on bone growth and formation. It directly causes skeletal growth in adolescence and has continued effects on skeletal muscle growth throughout the lifespan.
5. Phase I, reactive phase; phase II, reparative phase; phase III, remodeling
6. During isometric contraction, almost all of the energy is released in the form of heat; during isotonic contraction, some of the energy is expended in mechanical work. In some situations (i.e., shivering), the need to generate heat is the primary stimulus for muscle contraction.
7. Refer to Table 40-1, Age-Related Changes of the Musculoskeletal System, in the text.
8. **kyphosis:** increase in the convex curvature of the thoracic spine, **lordosis:** increase in concave curvature of the lumbar spine, **scoliosis:** lateral curving of the spine.

Activity C

See Chart 40-2, Assessment—Assessing for Peripheral Nerve Function, in the book.

1. c	**2.** a	**3.** d	**4.** b	**5.** e

SECTION II: APPLYING YOUR KNOWLEDGE

Activity D

1. If joint motion is compromised or the joint is painful, the joint is examined for *effusion* (excessive fluid within the capsule), swelling, and increased temperature that may reflect active inflammation. An effusion is suspected if the joint is swollen and the normal bony landmarks are obscured. The most common site for joint effusion is the knee. If large amounts of fluid are present in the joint spaces beneath the patella, it may be identified by assessing for the balloon sign and for ballottement of the knee (see Fig. 40-5 in the text).
2. Jewelry, hair clips, hearing aids, credit cards with magnetic strips, and other metal-containing objects must be removed before the MRI is performed; otherwise, they can become dangerous projectile objects or cause burns. Credit cards with magnetic strips may be erased, and nonremovable cochlear devices can become inoperable. Also, transdermal patches (e.g., nicotine patch [NicoDerm], nitroglycerin transdermal [Transderm-Nitro], scopolamine transdermal [Transderm Scop], clonidine transdermal [Catapres-TTS]) that have a thin layer of aluminized backing must be removed before MRI because they can cause burns. The primary provider should be notified before the patches are removed.
3. arthrocentesis

SECTION III: PRACTICING FOR NCLEX

Activity E

1. a	**2.** b	**3.** c	**4.** b	**5.** c
6. d	**7.** a	**8.** d	**9.** c	**10.** b
11. a, b, c	**12.** d	**13.** a, c, d		

CHAPTER 41

SECTION I: ASSESSING YOUR UNDERSTANDING

Activity A

1. chlorhexidine solution
2. osteomyelitis
3. unilateral calf tenderness, warmth, redness, swelling (increased calf circumference)
4. burning, numbness, tingling
5. 25 pounds
6. an acetabular socket, a femoral shaft, a spherical ball
7. 4 months
8. 3 to 6 months
9. 3 months
10. necrosis, impaired tissue perfusion, pressure ulcer formation, possible paralysis

Activity B

1. reducing a fracture, correcting a deformity, applying uniform pressure to underlying soft tissue, providing support and stability for weak joints
2. A fiberglass cast is light in weight and water resistant. It is more durable than plaster and water resistant.
3. The toes or fingers should be pink, warm, and easily moved (wiggled). There should be minimal swelling and discomfort. The blanch test should be carried out to determine rapid capillary refill.
4. pain, pallor, pulselessness, paresthesia, and paralysis
5. Answer should include unrelieved pain, swelling, discoloration, tingling, numbness, inability to move fingers or toes, or any temperature changes.
6. compartment syndrome, pressure ulcers, and disuse syndrome
7. to minimize muscle spasms; to reduce, align, and immobilize fractures; to lessen deformities; and to increase space between opposing surfaces within a joint
8. pressure ulcers, atelectasis, pneumonia, constipation, anorexia, urinary stasis and infection, and venous thromboemboli with PE or DVT
9. Compartment syndrome occurs when the circulation and function of tissue within a confined area (casted area) is compromised. Treatment requires that the cast be bivalved; a fasciotomy may be necessary.
10. Volkmann's contracture is a serious complication of impaired circulation in the arm. Contracture of the fingers and wrist occurs as the result of

obstructed arterial blood flow to the forearm and the hand. The patient is unable to extend the fingers, describes abnormal sensation, and exhibits signs of diminished circulation to the hand. Permanent damage develops within a few hours if action is not taken.

11. Methods for preventing hip prosthesis dislocation include the following:
    - Keep the knees apart at all times.
    - Put a pillow between the legs when sleeping.
    - Never cross the legs when seated.
    - Avoid bending forward when seated in a chair.
    - Avoid bending forward to pick up an object on the floor.
    - Use a high-seated chair and a raised toilet seat.
    - Do not flex the hip to put on clothing such as pants, stockings, socks, or shoes.

Activity C

1. f	**2.** i	**3.** g	**4.** h	**5.** c
6. b	**7.** a	**8.** d	**9.** e	

SECTION II: APPLYING YOUR KNOWLEDGE

Activity D

CASE STUDY: External Fixator

1. Benefits of external fixation, as opposed to other modes of treatment, include immediate fracture stabilization, minimization of blood loss (as compared to use of internal fixation), increased patient comfort, improved wound care, and promotion of early mobilization and weight-bearing on the affected limb, and active exercise of adjacent uninvolved joints.
2. Patients must be prepared psychologically for application of the external fixator, as they may be at risk for an altered body image related to the overwhelming size and bulk of the apparatus. To promote acceptance of the device, patients should be given comprehensive information about the frame, reassurance that the discomfort associated with the device is minimal and that early mobility is anticipated. Clothing and other materials may need to be altered or used to cover the device.
3. every 2 to 4 hours
4. The nurse assesses each pin site at least every 8 to 12 hours for redness, swelling, pain around the pin sites, warmth, and purulent drainage, as these are the most common indicators of pin-site infections.

CASE STUDY: Total Hip Replacement

1. With joint replacement, patients may expect pain relief, return of joint motion, and improved functional status and quality of life.
2. The use of certain medications, such as selected hormones and NSAIDs, should be discontinued a week before surgery because they increase the risk of clotting.
3. Tom should be in a supine position with his head slightly elevated and the affected leg in a neutral position. The use of an abduction splint, a wedge pillow or two or three pillows placed between the

legs prevent adduction beyond the midline of the body. A cradle boot may be used to prevent leg rotation and to support the heel off the bed, preventing development of a pressure ulcer. When he is turned in bed to the unaffected side, it is important to keep the operative hip in abduction. He should not turn or be turned to the operative side, which could cause dislocation, unless specified by the surgeon.

4. Tom is informed of increased pain at the surgical site, swelling, and immobilization; acute groin pain in the affected hip or increased discomfort; shortening of the affected extremity; abnormal external or internal rotation of the affected extremity; restricted ability or inability to move the leg; and reported "popping" sensation in the hip.

SECTION III: PRACTICING FOR NCLEX

Activity E

1. a, c, d	**2.** b	**3.** a, b, c	**4.** d	**5.** a, b, c
6. b	**7.** b	**8.** b	**9.** a	**10.** a
11. a	**12.** c	**13.** a	**14.** b	**15.** c

CHAPTER 42

SECTION I: ASSESSING YOUR UNDERSTANDING

Activity A

1. bone fracture
2. 45 and 55, after menopause
3. a deficiency in activated vitamin D (calcitriol)
4. calcitonin, bisphosphonates, plicamycin
5. L4, L5, S1
6. ingrown toenail
7. diabetes, peripheral vascular disease
8. 1,000 to 1,500
9. calcium intake, muscular activity, weight bearing
10. osteochondroma

Activity B

1. Answer should include five of these conditions: acute lumbosacral strain, unstable lumbosacral ligaments, weak lumbosacral muscles, osteoarthritis of the spine, spinal stenosis, intervertebral disk problems, and unequal leg length.
2. Refer to chapter heading "Bursitis and Tendinitis" in the text.
3. Impingement syndrome is a general term that describes impaired movement of the rotator cuff of the shoulder. Impingement usually occurs from repetitive overhead movement of the arm or from acute trauma resulting in irritation and eventual inflammation of the rotator cuff tendons or the subacromial bursa as they grate against the coracoacromial arch.
4. Tinel's sign may be elicited in patients with carpal tunnel syndrome by percussing lightly over the median nerve, located on the inner aspect of the wrist. If the patient reports tingling, numbness, and pain, the test for Tinel's sign is considered positive.

5. Refer to Figure 42-7 in the text.
6. The patient with acute septic arthritis presents with a warm, painful, swollen joint with decreased range of motion (ROM). Systemic chills, fever, and leukocytosis are sometimes present. Although any joint may be infected, 50% of cases involve a knee.

Activity C

1. c	**2.** b	**3.** d	**4.** a	**5.** e
6. f				

SECTION II: APPLYING YOUR KNOWLEDGE

Activity D

CASE STUDY: Osteoporosis

1. Patient education focuses on factors influencing the development of osteoporosis, interventions to arrest or slow the process, and measures to relieve symptoms. The nurse emphasizes that people of any age need sufficient calcium, vitamin D, and weight-bearing exercise to slow the progression of osteoporosis. Patient education related to medication therapy as described previously is important. Patients must understand that having one fracture increases the probability of sustaining another.
2. Women have a lower peak bone mass than men, and estrogen loss affects the development of the disorder.
3. Refer to chapter heading "Risk Factors" under "Osteoporosis" in the text.
4. 1,000 to 1,500 mg

SECTION III: PRACTICING FOR NCLEX

Activity E

1. b	**2.** b	**3.** c	**4.** c	**5.** c
6. c	**7.** b	**8.** d	**9.** a, b, c	**10.** b
11. c, d, e	**12.** d	**13.** c	**14.** a	**15.** b

CHAPTER 43

SECTION I: ASSESSING YOUR UNDERSTANDING

Activity A

1. strain
2. neck
3. osteomyelitis, tetanus, gas gangrene
4. Colles' fracture
5. deep vein thrombosis
6. atelectasis, pneumonia
7. abduction, external rotation, flexion
8. flexion contracture of the hip
9. 10, 4
10. tibial shaft

Activity B

1. AVN is tissue death due to anoxia and diminished blood supply.
2. The sensation is caused by the rubbing of bone fragments against each other; the nurse would document it as crepitus.

3. Early: Answer should include three of the following: shock, fat embolism, compartment syndrome, deep vein thrombosis, thromboembolism, DIC, and infection. Delayed: Answer should include three of the following: delayed union and nonunion, avascular necrosis of bone, reaction to internal fixation devices, complex regional pain syndrome (CRPS), and heterotrophic ossification.

4. stabilizing the fracture to prevent further hemorrhage, restoring blood volume and circulation, relieving the patient's pain, providing proper immobilization, and protecting against further injury

5. deep vein thrombosis, thromboembolism, and pulmonary embolus

6. With an open fracture, the wound is covered with a sterile dressing to prevent contamination of deeper tissues. No attempt is made to reduce the fracture, even if one of the bone fragments is protruding through the wound. Splints are applied for immobilization.

7. Closed reduction is performed without a surgical incision and can be done when there is a dislocation of a fracture. Cast may be applied after the procedure. Open reduction is usually performed with plate and screws to provide mobilization of the bone, especially if there is displacement of the fracture.

8. See Chart 43-2, Factors That Affect or Inhibit Fracture Healing.

Activity C

PART I

1. c   **2.** a   **3.** b   **4.** e   **5.** d

PART II

1. c   **2.** b   **3.** a   **4.** d   **5.** e

SECTION II: APPLYING YOUR KNOWLEDGE

Activity D

CASE STUDY: Above-the-Knee Amputation

1. color and temperature, palpable responses, palpable pulses

2. the circulatory status of the affected limb, the type of prosthesis to be used, the ability to understand and use the prosthetic device

3. triceps brachii

4. Keep him as active as possible and encourage self-expression.

5. monitoring vital signs to detect any indication of bleeding, placing the residual limb in an extended position with brief periods of elevation, keeping a tourniquet nearby in case of hemorrhage

6. abduction deformities of the hip, flexion deformities, nonshrinkage of the residual limb

7. Begin vertical turns on the anterior surface of the residual limb.

SECTION III: PRACTICING FOR NCLEX

Activity E

1. b   **2.** d   **3.** b   **4.** c   **5.** a, b, c
6. a   **7.** b   **8.** d   **9.** a   **10.** d
11. b   **12.** a, b, c **13.** a **14.** a, b, e **15.** c

CHAPTER 44

SECTION I: ASSESSING YOUR UNDERSTANDING

Activity A

1. trypsin, amylase, lipase

2. mixed waves that move the intestinal contents back and forth in a churning motion; a movement that propels the contents of the small intestine toward the colon.

3. 4 hours; 12 hours

4. decreased motility and emptying, weakened gag reflex, decreased resting pressure of the lower sphincter

5. cardiac sphincter

6. ptyalin

7. 1.0

8. B_{12}

9. secretin

10. Bile

11. cardia, fundus, body, pylorus

12. glucose

Activity B

1. Both the sympathetic and parasympathetic portions of the autonomic nervous system innervate the GI tract. In general, sympathetic nerves exert an inhibitory effect on the GI tract, decreasing gastric secretion and motility and causing the sphincters and blood vessels to constrict. Parasympathetic nerve stimulation causes peristalsis and increases secretory activities. The sphincters relax under the influence of parasympathetic stimulation, except for the sphincter of the upper esophagus and the external anal sphincter, which are under voluntary control.

2. Obstruction of the GI tract increases the force of intestinal contraction. Distention occurs above the point of obstruction, causing pain and a sense of bloating.

3. 16 to 20 inches

4. Red meats, aspirin, nonsteroidal anti-inflammatory drugs, turnips, and horseradish should be avoided for 72 hours prior to the study, because they may cause a false-positive result. Also, ingestion of vitamin C from supplements or foods can cause a false-negative result.

5. MRI is contraindicated when the patient has any of the following: permanent pacemakers, artificial heart valves, and implanted insulin pumps.

6. Intrinsic factor, also secreted by the gastric mucosa, combines with dietary vitamin B_{12} so that the vitamin can be absorbed in the ileum. In the absence of

intrinsic factor, vitamin B_{12} cannot be absorbed, and pernicious anemia results.

Activity C

1. f   **2.** a   **3.** e   **4.** c   **5.** b
6. d

SECTION II: APPLYING YOUR KNOWLEDGE

Activity D

1. Adequate colon cleansing provides optimal visualization and decreases the time needed for the procedure.
2. Colonoscopy is performed while the patient is lying on the left side with the legs drawn up toward the chest. The patient's position may be changed during the test to facilitate advancement of the scope.
3. The patient's cardiac and respiratory function and oxygen saturation are monitored continuously, with supplemental oxygen used as necessary.
4. Complications during and after the procedure can include cardiac dysrhythmias and respiratory depression resulting from the medications administered, vasovagal reactions, and circulatory overload or hypotension resulting from overhydration or underhydration during bowel preparation.

SECTION III: PRACTICING FOR NCLEX

Activity E

1. c	**2.** b	**3.** a	**4.** a	**5.** c
6. d	**7.** c	**8.** c	**9.** a, b, c	**10.** b
11. c	**12.** a	**13.** d	**14.** d	**15.** b

CHAPTER 45

SECTION I: ASSESSING YOUR UNDERSTANDING

Activity A

1. 4
2. receive, process
3. peristaltic
4. pylorus, prokinetic agents
5. Nasoduodenal, nasojejunal
6. leakage of fluid
7. seepage of gastric acid, spillage of feeding

Activity B

1. The purpose of gastric intubation is to decompress the stomach and remove gas and fluid; lavage (flush with water or other fluids) the stomach and remove ingested toxins or other harmful materials; diagnose GI disorders; administer tube feedings, medications, and fluids; compress a bleeding site; and aspirate GI contents for aspirate.
2. Gastric aspirate is most frequently cloudy and green, tan, off-white, or brown and may be large volume. Intestinal aspirate is primarily clear and yellow to bile colored and typically smaller volume.

3. Possible causes for constipation include: concomitant use of opioids; administration of fiber-free tube feeding formulas; and inadequate water intake (tube feedings typically do not meet total fluid needs, so additional water must be administered).
4. control of bleeding esophageal varices
5. Caution is required when inserting feeding tubes with a stylet because there is a risk of tissue puncture or placement error.

Activity C

1. e	**2.** b	**3.** d	**4.** a	**5.** c

SECTION II: APPLYING YOUR KNOWLEDGE

Activity D

CASE STUDY: Dumping Syndrome

1. caloric density, tubing size, speed of infusion, temperature and volume of feeding, zinc deficiency, contaminated formula, malnutrition, and medication therapy
2. Return the solution through the tube and administer the next feeding.
3. Administer the feeding at room temperature.
4. dehydration, hypotension, tachycardia

CASE STUDY: Total Parenteral Nutrition

1. approximately 1,500 calories per day
2. 1,000 calories
3. chills, fever, and nausea

SECTION III: PRACTICING FOR NCLEX

Activity E

1. a	**2.** a	**3.** c	**4.** d	**5.** b
6. a, b, c	**7.** b	**8.** d	**9.** d	**10.** a
11. b	**12.** b	**13.** a	**14.** c	**15.** b

CHAPTER 46

SECTION I: ASSESSING YOUR UNDERSTANDING

Activity A

1. mouth
2. Fifteen
3. aphthous stomatitis
4. sugar
5. 5 years
6. parotid
7. 60%
8. mouth

Activity B

1. Tooth decay is an erosive process that begins with the action of bacteria on fermentable carbohydrates in the mouth, which produces acids that dissolve tooth enamel.
2. Measures used to prevent and control dental caries include practicing effective mouth care, reducing

the intake of starches and sugars (refined carbohydrates), applying fluoride to the teeth or drinking fluoridated water, refraining from smoking, controlling diabetes, and using pit and fissure sealants. Regular dental visits are an important method of preventive dental maintenance.

3. In the early stages of an infection, a dentist or oral surgeon may perform a needle aspiration or drill an opening into the pulp chamber to relieve pressure and pain, and to provide drainage.
4. Sialadenitis is an inflammation of the salivary gland; sialolithiasis are calculi in the submandibular gland.
5. hemorrhage, chyle fistula, nerve injury

Activity C

Refer to Table 46-1, Disorders of the Lips, Mouth, and Gums, in the text.

1. f	**2.** g	**3.** e	**4.** a	**5.** d
6. b	**7.** c	**8.** h		

SECTION II: APPLYING YOUR KNOWLEDGE

Activity D

CASE STUDY: Radical Neck Dissection

1. shoulder drop and poor cosmesis (visible neck depression)
2. altered respiratory status, wound infection, and hemorrhage
3. Fowler's position
4. stridor
5. hypoglossal nerve
6. Referral for a home health nurse to visit and educate the wife about the care of the patient.

CASE STUDY: Mandibular Fracture

1. on his side with his head slightly elevated to prevent aspiration
2. Nasogastric suctioning is needed to remove stomach contents, thereby reducing the danger of aspiration.
3. a wire cutter or scissors
4. clear liquids

CASE STUDY: Cancer of the Mouth

1. The typical lesion is a painless, indurated (hardened) ulcer with raised edges.
2. pain
3. a sore, roughened area that has not healed in 3 weeks; minor swelling in an area adjacent to the lesion; numbness in the affected area in the mouth

SECTION III: PRACTICING FOR NCLEX

Activity E

1. a	**2.** b	**3.** a, c, d	**4.** b	**5.** c
6. a	**7.** a	**8.** a	**9.** b, c, d	**10.** b
11. c	**12.** d	**13.** d	**14.** b	**15.** a

CHAPTER 47

SECTION I: ASSESSING YOUR UNDERSTANDING

Activity A

1. duodenum
2. 40, 60
3. Nexium
4. hemorrhage
5. 60%
6. *Helicobacter pylori*
7. Hemorrhage, perforation, penetration, pyloric obstruction
8. 30

Activity B

1. Dilute and neutralize the offending agent. To neutralize a corrosive acid, use common antacids such as milk and aluminum hydroxide. To neutralize an alkali, use diluted lemon juice or diluted vinegar.
2. Patients with gastritis due to a vitamin deficiency exhibit antibodies against intrinsic factor, which interferes with vitamin B_{12} absorption.
3. Hypersecretion of acid pepsin and a weakened gastric mucosal barrier predispose to peptic ulcer development.
4. hypersecretion of gastric juice, multiple duodenal ulcers, hypertrophied duodenal glands, and gastrinomas (islet cell tumors) in the pancreas
5. A stress ulcer refers to acute mucosal ulceration of the duodenal or gastric area that occurs after a stressful event.
6. Cushing's ulcers, which are common in patients with brain trauma, usually occur in the esophagus, stomach, or duodenum. Curling's ulcers occur most frequently after extensive burns and usually involve the antrum of the stomach and duodenum.
7. The objective of the ulcer diet is to avoid oversecretion and hypermotility in the gastrointestinal tract. Extremes of temperature should be avoided, as well as overstimulation by meat extractives, coffee (including decaffeinated), alcohol, and diets rich in milk and cream. Current therapy recommends three regular meals per day if an antacid or histamine blocker is taken.
8. When peptic ulcer perforation occurs, the patient experiences severe upper abdominal pain, vomiting, fainting, and an extremely tender abdomen that can be board-like in rigidity; signs of shock will be present (hypotension and tachycardia).
9. Bariatric surgery works by restricting a patient's ability to eat and by restricting ingested nutrient absorption.

Activity C

Pharmacologic Therapy for Peptic Ulcer Disease and Gastritis

1. b	**2.** a	**3.** d	**4.** e	**5.** c

SECTION II: APPLYING YOUR KNOWLEDGE

Activity D

CASE STUDY: Gastric Cancer

1. ascites and hepatomegaly
2. esophagogastroduodenoscopy and barium x-ray of the upper gastrointestinal tract; endoscopic ultrasound; computed tomography
3. wide resection of the middle and distal portions of the stomach (removal of about 75% of the stomach)
4. 5-fluorouracil (5-FU)

SECTION III: PRACTICING FOR NCLEX

Activity E

1. a, b, c	**2.** b	**3.** b	**4.** a, b, c	**5.** c
6. a	**7.** b, c, d	**8.** a	**9.** a	**10.** d
11. c	**12.** c	**13.** a	**14.** c	**15.** d

CHAPTER 48

SECTION I: ASSESSING YOUR UNDERSTANDING

Activity A

1. irritable bowel syndrome, diverticular disease
2. 25 to 30 g/day; three
3. *Clostridium difficile*
4. adhesions, hernias, neoplasms
5. adenocarcinoid tumors
6. Zollinger-Ellison syndrome
7. vitamin B$_{12}$
8. sigmoid
9. abdominal pain, diarrhea
10. 2 to 3

Activity B

1. peritonitis, abscess formation, fistulas, and bleeding
2. *Escherichia coli, Klebsiella, Proteus,* and *Pseudomonas*
3. Answer should include six of the following: increasing age; family history of colon cancer (Lynch syndrome) or polyps (familial adenomatous polyposis (FAP); previous colon cancer or adenomatous polyps; high consumption of alcohol; cigarette smoking; obesity; history of gastrectomy; history of IBD; high-fat, high-protein (with high intake of beef), low-fiber diet; genital cancer (e.g., endometrial cancer, ovarian cancer) or breast cancer (in women).
4. forcible exhalation against a closed glottis followed by a rise in intrathoracic pressure and subsequent possible dramatic rise in arterial pressure
5. These may include cholinergic agents (e.g., bethanechol [Urecholine]), cholinesterase inhibitors (e.g., neostigmine [Prostigmin]), or prokinetic agents (e.g., metoclopramide [Reglan]). Prokinetic agents including serotonin (5-HT4) receptor agonists like prucalopride (Resolor) and prostones like lubiprostone (Amitiza) stimulate chloride channels in the gut. Medical probiotics (i.e., ingested live organ-isms) may help some constipated individuals by creating improved bacterial balance.
6. Although no anatomic or biochemical abnormalities have been found that account for its common symptoms, various factors are associated with the syndrome: heredity, psychological stress or conditions such as depression and anxiety, a diet high in fat and stimulating or irritating foods, alcohol consumption, and smoking.
7. The hallmarks of malabsorption syndrome from any cause are diarrhea or frequent, loose, bulky, foul-smelling stools that have increased fat content and are often grayish (steatorrhea).

Activity C

PART 1: Key Terms

1. e	**2.** m	**3.** i	**4.** o	**5.** a
6. g	**7.** k	**8.** b	**9.** p	**10.** j
11. c	**12.** n	**13.** d	**14.** l	**15.** h
16. f				

PART 2: Laxative Classification and Action

1. b-5	**2.** d-3	**3.** e-6	**4.** a-1	**5.** c-2
6. f-4				

SECTION II: APPLYING YOUR KNOWLEDGE

Activity D

CASE STUDY: Appendicitis

1. Vague epigastric or periumbilical pain progresses to right lower quadrant pain and is usually accompanied by a low-grade fever and nausea, and sometimes by vomiting. Loss of appetite is common. In up to 50% of presenting cases, local tenderness is elicited at McBurney's point when pressure is applied. Rebound tenderness may be present.
2. A pregnancy test should be performed to rule out pregnancy prior to any x-rays or medications administered.
3. The appendix has ruptured.

SECTION III: PRACTICING FOR NCLEX

Activity E

1. b	**2.** c	**3.** c	**4.** b	**5.** a
6. d	**7.** b	**8.** c	**9.** c	**10.** a
11. b	**12.** b	**13.** a	**14.** c	**15.** b

CHAPTER 49

SECTION I: ASSESSING YOUR UNDERSTANDING

Activity A

1. 70%
2. bleeding, bile peritonitis
3. 10%
4. hepatitis C
5. chronic liver disease, hepatitis B, hepatitis C, cirrhosis

6. infection
7. portal vein
8. vitamin K
9. cholesterol
10. 90%
11. Hepatitis C
12. Ruptured esophageal varices

Activity B

1. Refer to Chart 49-1, Age-Related Changes of the Hepatobiliary System, in the text.
2. producing ketone bodies, synthesizing albumin, and participating in gluconeogenesis
3. *Hemolytic jaundice* is the result of an increased destruction of red blood cells that overload the plasma with bilirubin so quickly that the liver cannot excrete the bilirubin as fast as it is formed. *Hepatocellular jaundice* is caused by the inability of damaged liver cells to clear normal amounts of bilirubin from the blood. *Obstructive jaundice* is usually caused by occlusion of the bile duct by a gallstone, an inflammatory process, a tumor, or pressure from an enlarged organ.
4. fat emulsification in the intestines
5. accidental exposure to HbAg-positive blood, perinatal exposure, sexual contact with those who are positive for HbAg
6. chloroform, gold compounds, and phosphorus
7. esophagus, lower rectum, and stomach
8. ascites, jaundice, portal hypertension

Activity C

1. c   2. e   3. b   4. a   5. d
6. g   7. f

SECTION II: APPLYING YOUR KNOWLEDGE

Activity D

CASE STUDY: Liver Biopsy

1. making sure that informed consent has been obtained and the permit is signed, compatible donor blood is obtained, vital signs are obtained and recorded, and coagulation studies are reviewed
2. recumbent, with her right upper abdomen exposed
3. Instruct the patient to inhale and exhale deeply several times, finally to exhale, and to hold breath at the end of expiration.
4. the right side-lying position with a pillow placed under the right costal margin

CASE STUDY: Paracentesis

1. 3 L
2. upright, with her feet resting on a support so that the puncture site will be readily visible
3. hypotension, oliguria, pallor

CASE STUDY: Alcoholic or Nutritional Cirrhosis

1. a liver decreased in size and nodular
2. 3,500 calories
3. 2,000 to 2,500/24 hours

CASE STUDY: Liver Transplantation

1. bleeding
2. nephrotoxicity, septicemia, thrombocytopenia
3. For patients with liver cancer anticipating surgery, support, education, and encouragement are provided to help them prepare psychologically for the surgery.

SECTION III: PRACTICING FOR NCLEX

Activity E

1. b   2. c, d   3. b   4. d   5. a
6. d   7. a   8. b   9. c   10. a
11. c   12. d   13. a   14. d   15. b

CHAPTER 50

SECTION I: ASSESSING YOUR UNDERSTANDING

Activity A

1. 30 to 50
2. insulin, glucagon, somatostatin
3. amylase; trypsin; lipase
4. Calculous cholecystitis
5. bile duct injury
6. pancreatic necrosis
7. gallbladder
8. secretin
9. multiparous, obese, over 40

Activity B

1. If a gallstone obstructs the cystic duct, the gallbladder becomes distended, inflamed, and eventually infected (acute cholecystitis).
2. The bile, which is no longer carried to the duodenum, is absorbed by the blood and gives the skin and mucous membranes a yellow color.
3. Because of the short hospital stay with uncomplicated laparoscopic cholecystectomies, it is important to provide patient education about managing postoperative pain and reporting signs and symptoms of intra-abdominal complications, including loss of appetite, vomiting, pain, distention of the abdomen, and temperature elevation.
4. patients with sepsis or severe cardiac, renal, pulmonary, or liver failure
5. Refer to Chart 50-3, Criteria for Predicting Severity of Pancreatitis, in the text.

Activity C

1. b   2. c   3. e   4. d   5. a

SECTION II: APPLYING YOUR KNOWLEDGE

Activity D

CASE STUDY: Cholecystectomy: Preoperative Situation

1. analgesics and antibiotics, intravenous fluids, nasogastric suctioning

2. Brenda should avoid foods high in fat, as well as eggs, cream, pork, fried foods, cheese, rich dressings, gas-forming vegetables, and alcohol.

3. Chenodeoxycholic acid may not be effective if taken with dietary cholesterol, estrogens, or oral contraceptives.

CASE STUDY: Cholecystectomy: Postoperative Situation

1. If the common bile duct is thought to be obstructed by a gallstone, an ERCP with sphincterotomy may be performed to explore the duct before laparoscopy.

2. indicators of infection, leakage of bile into the peritoneal cavity, obstruction of bile drainage

3. 4–6 weeks

SECTION III: PRACTICING FOR NCLEX

Activity E

1. c	**2.** b, c, d	**3.** d	**4.** d	**5.** a
6. a	**7.** b	**8.** a, c, d	**9.** a, b, c	**10.** a
11. c	**12.** d	**13.** a	**14.** c	**15.** b

CHAPTER 51

SECTION I: ASSESSING YOUR UNDERSTANDING

Activity A

1. 25.8

2. nontraumatic amputation, blindness, end-stage kidney disease

3. type I diabetes, type II diabetes, gestational

4. glycogenolysis, gluconeogenesis

5. osmotic diuresis

6. decreased

7. hyperglycemic hyperosmolar syndrome

8. 18%

9. 105 mg/dL, 130 mg/dL

10. polyuria, polydipsia, polyphagia

11. elevated blood glucose levels

12. seventh, 20%

13. 24 to 28 weeks

14. Ketoacidosis

15. Hyperglycemia, ketosis, metabolic acidosis

Activity B

1. because of increasing health care costs and an aging population

2. Hyperglycemia develops during pregnancy because of the secretion of placental hormones, which causes insulin resistance.

3. insulin resistance and impaired insulin secretion

4. One risk involved in suddenly increasing fiber intake is that it may require adjusting the dosage of insulin or oral agents to prevent hypoglycemia. Other problems may include abdominal fullness, nausea, diarrhea, increased flatulence, and constipation if fluid intake is inadequate.

5. Insulin regulates the production and storage of glucose. In diabetes, either the pancreas stops producing insulin or the cells stop responding to insulin. Hyperglycemia results and can lead to acute metabolic complications such as diabetic ketoacidosis and hyperglycemic hyperosmolar nonketotic syndrome. Long-term complications can contribute to macrovascular or microvascular complications.

6. Answer should include the following: hypotension, profound dehydration, tachycardia, and variable neurologic signs (seizures, hemiparesis, alteration of sensorium).

7. Sulfonylureas act by directly stimulating the beta cells of the pancreas to secrete insulin (cannot be used in patients with type 1 diabetes).

Activity C

1. c	**2.** a	**3.** b	**4.** e	**5.** d

SECTION II: APPLYING YOUR KNOWLEDGE

Activity D

CASE STUDY: Type 1 Diabetes

Refer to Table 51-3, Categories of Insulin, in the text.

1. between 11:30 AM and 7:30 PM

2. 16 to 20 hours

3. signs of hypoglycemia earlier than expected

CASE STUDY: Hypoglycemia

1. stress due to the breakup, lack of dietary intake

2. symptoms of rebound hypoglycemia

3. emotional changes, slurred speech and double vision, staggering gait, weakness, diaphoresis, and lack of coordination

4. eating regularly scheduled meals, eating snacks to cover the peak time of insulin, increasing food intake when engaging in increased levels of physical exercise

CASE STUDY: Diabetic Ketoacidosis

1. monitoring urinary output by means of an indwelling catheter, evaluating serum electrolytes, testing for glucosuria and acetonuria, blood glucose testing, and vital signs

2. 0.9% sodium chloride

3. hyperkalemia

4. When hanging the insulin drip, the nurse must flush the insulin solution through the entire IV infusion set and discard the first 50 mL of fluid. Insulin molecules adhere to the inner surface of plastic IV infusion sets; therefore, the initial fluid may contain a decreased concentration of insulin.

5. hypokalemia

SECTION III: PRACTICING FOR NCLEX

Activity E

1. a, b, d	**2.** a	**3.** a	**4.** a	**5.** c
6. a	**7.** a	**8.** a, b, c	**9.** a	**10.** c
11. b	**12.** c	**13.** d	**14.** a, b, c	**15.** d
16. b				

CHAPTER 52

SECTION I: ASSESSING YOUR UNDERSTANDING

Activity A

1. negative feedback
2. hypothalamus
3. vasopressin, the excretion of water by the kidneys; oxytocin, milk ejection during lactation
4. acromegaly, gigantism
5. diabetes insipidus; excessive thirst (polydipsia), large volumes of dilute urine
6. thyroxine, triiodothyronine, and calcitonin
7. autoimmune thyroiditis (Hashimoto's disease)
8. women; men
9. Graves' disease
10. methimazole (Tapazole) and propylthiouracil (PTU)
11. Trousseau's, Chvostek's
12. glucocorticoids, mineralocorticoids, androgens
13. kidney stones
14. Toxic nodular goiter

Activity B

1. adrenocorticotropic hormone (ACTH), follicle-stimulating hormone (FSH), thyroid-stimulating hormone (TSH)
2. Answer should include four of the following: steroids, proteins or peptides, polypeptides and glycoproteins, amines and amino acids, and fatty acid derivatives.
3. The objectives in the management of hypothyroidism are to restore a normal metabolic state by replacing the missing hormone, and prevention of disease progression and complications.
4. Several routes are available for administering radiation to the thyroid or tissues of the neck, including oral administration of radioactive iodine and external administration of radiation therapy.

Activity C

1. h	2. g	3. i	4. d	5. a
6. c	7. f	8. e	9. j	10. b

SECTION II: APPLYING YOUR KNOWLEDGE

Activity D

CASE STUDY: Primary Hypothyroidism

1. serum TSH, T_3 resin uptake test, immunoassay for antithyroid antibodies, radioactive iodine uptake, thyroid scan, radioscan, or scintiscan
2. Extreme fatigue, hair loss, brittle nails, dry skin, and numbness and tingling of the fingers may occur. Hoarseness, menstrual disturbances, weight gain are other potential clinical manifestations.
3. encouraging frequent periods of rest throughout the day, offering her additional blankets to help prevent chilling, using a cleansing lotion instead of soap for her skin

4. Connie must be instructed that many over-the-counter and prescription medications interact with Synthroid and caution must be maintained when taking anything. There is a decrease in thyroid hormone absorption when patients are also taking magnesium-containing antacids. See section heading "Prevention of Medication Interaction" in the text.

CASE STUDY: Hyperparathyroidism

1. exophthalmos
2. increased sensitivity to catecholamines or to changes in neurotransmitter turnover
3. The nurse instructs Emily to take the medication in the morning on an empty stomach 30 minutes before eating to avoid decrease in absorption associated with some foods such as walnuts, soybean flour, cottonseed meal, and dietary fiber. Emily is also informed that it may take several weeks until relief of symptoms occurs.

CASE STUDY: Subtotal Thyroidectomy

1. semi-Fowler's position, with his head supported by pillows
2. voice change
3. IV calcium gluconate

SECTION III: PRACTICING FOR NCLEX

Activity E

1. a	2. b	3. b, c, d	4. d	5. a, b, c
6. b	7. d	8. a	9. d	10. a, c, d
11. c	12. c	13. b	14. a	15. b
16. a, b, c				

CHAPTER 53

SECTION I: ASSESSING YOUR UNDERSTANDING

Activity A

1. nephron; cortex
2. 400 to 500
3. 300 mOsm/kg
4. aldosterone
5. increased
6. antidiuretic hormone (ADH)
7. 7.35 to 7.45; 4.5
8. urea; 20 to 30
9. creatinine clearance

Activity B

1. If the total number of functioning nephrons is less than 20% of normal, renal replacement therapy needs to be considered.
2. There are three narrowed areas of each ureter: the ureteropelvic junction, ureteral segment near the sacroiliac junction, and ureterovesical junction.

Study Guide for Brunner & Suddarth's Textbook of Medical-Surgical Nursing, 13th Edition.

3. Amino acids and glucose are usually filtered at the level of the glomerulus and reabsorbed so that neither is excreted in the urine.
4. It is secreted by the posterior portion of the pituitary gland in response to changes in osmolality of the blood.
5. The regulation of sodium volume excreted depends on aldosterone, a hormone synthesized and released from the adrenal cortex.

Activity C

1. b   **2.** d   **3.** a   **4.** c   **5.** e

SECTION II: APPLYING YOUR KNOWLEDGE

Activity D

1. Before the biopsy is carried out, coagulation studies are conducted to identify any risk of postbiopsy bleeding.
2. The sedated patient is placed in a prone position with a sandbag under the abdomen.
3. IV fluids may be administered to help clear the kidneys and prevent clot formation.

SECTION III: PRACTICING FOR NCLEX

Activity E

1. a   **2.** b   **3.** c   **4.** a, b, c   **5.** a
6. a   **7.** b   **8.** a, b, c   **9.** a   **10.** b

CHAPTER 54

SECTION I: ASSESSING YOUR UNDERSTANDING

Activity A

1. diabetes
2. prolonged hypertension, diabetes
3. creatinine, BUN
4. Arteriosclerotic cardiovascular disease
5. peritonitis
6. abdominal distention, paralytic ileus
7. weight
8. edema
9. 85%
10. initiation, oliguria, diuresis, recovery
11. Nephrotic syndrome

Activity B

1. Cardiomegaly, a gallop rhythm, distended neck veins, and other signs and symptoms of heart failure may be present. Crackles can be heard in the bases of the lungs.
2. Clinical findings include a marked increase in protein (particularly albumin) in the urine (proteinuria), a decrease in albumin in the blood (hypoalbuminemia), diffuse edema, high serum cholesterol, and low-density lipoproteins (hyperlipidemia).

3. *Autosomal dominant PKD* is the most common inherited form. Symptoms usually develop between the ages of 30 and 40, but they can begin earlier, even in childhood. About 90% of all PKD cases are autosomal dominant PKD. *Autosomal recessive PKD* is a rare inherited form. Symptoms of autosomal recessive PKD begin in the earliest months of life or in utero.
4. The nurse assists the patient to prepare physically and psychologically for these procedures and monitors carefully for signs and symptoms of dehydration and exhaustion.
5. Factors that influence mortality include increased age, comorbid conditions, and preexisting kidney and vascular diseases and respiratory failure.

Activity C

1. a   **2.** b   **3.** c   **4.** e   **5.** d
6. j   **7.** h   **8.** f   **9.** g   **10.** i

SECTION II: APPLYING YOUR KNOWLEDGE

Activity D

CASE STUDY: Continuous Ambulatory Peritoneal Dialysis (CAPD)

1. The procedure allows the patient reasonable freedom and control of daily activities but requires a serious commitment to be successful.
2. approximately 4 to 5 times per day with no night exchanges
3. 10 to 15 minutes
4. Edward should adopt a diet that is high in protein.

CASE STUDY: Acute Kidney Failure

1. reduced glomerular filtration, renal ischemia, tubular damage
2. 70 g/24 h
3. a high-protein diet
4. 6 to 12 months

SECTION III: PRACTICING FOR NCLEX

Activity E

1. d   **2.** a   **3.** a, c, d   **4.** c   **5.** b
6. a   **7.** b   **8.** a   **9.** b   **10.** b
11. c   **12.** d   **13.** a   **14.** d   **15.** c

CHAPTER 55

SECTION I: ASSESSING YOUR UNDERSTANDING

Activity A

1. glycosaminoglycan (GAG); urinary immunoglobulin (IgA); normal bacterial flora of the vagina and urethral area
2. *Escherichia coli, Pseudomonas, Enterococcus*
3. chronic bacterial prostatitis
4. bladder
5. stress incontinence

6. 1.5 mL
7. infection
8. kidney failure
9. 3 inches
10. pain

Activity B

1. See Chart 55-2, Risk Factors—Urinary Tract Infection, in the text.
2. Answer may include the following: high incidence of multiple chronic medical conditions, frequent use of antimicrobial agents, presence of infected pressure ulcers, immunocompromise, cognitive impairment, immobility, and incomplete bladder emptying.
3. Answer may include the following: pregnancy, menopause, GI surgery, pelvic muscle weakness, incompetent urethra, immobility, high-impact exercise, diabetes, stroke, age-related changes, morbid obesity, cognitive disturbance, medications (diuretics, sedatives, etc.), and caregiver or toilet unavailable.
4. Answer may include the following: delirium/confusion, UTI, atrophic vaginitis, urethritis, prostatitis, medications, psychological factors, excessive urine production, limited or restricted activity, stool impaction/constipation.
5. See Chart 55-10, Preventing Infection in the Patient With an Indwelling Urinary Catheter, in the text.
6. Answer includes the following: cigarette smoking, exposure to environmental carcinogens, recurrent or chronic bacterial infections of the urinary tract, bladder stones, high urine pH, high cholesterol intake, pelvic radiation, other cancers related to the urinary tract.

Activity C

1. d	2. f	3. e	4. c	5. a
6. b				

SECTION II: APPLYING YOUR KNOWLEDGE

Activity D

CASE STUDY: Acute Pyelonephritis

1. urine for culture and sensitivity
2. Physical examination reveals pain and tenderness in the area of the costovertebral angle.
3. an ultrasound or CT scan

SECTION III: PRACTICING FOR NCLEX

Activity E

1. c	2. b	3. c	4. a	5. b, c, d
6. a	7. b	8. c	9. d	10. d
11. b, c, e	12. a	13. c	14. d	15. c

CHAPTER 56

SECTION I: ASSESSING YOUR UNDERSTANDING

Activity A

1. 11 to 13 years; 10 years
2. follicle-stimulating; luteinizing
3. 45 to 52; 51; 35
4. the luteinizing hormone
5. 95% to 99%
6. 1 in 5
7. endometrial biopsy
8. Metrorrhagia
9. estrogens, progesterones
10. diaphragm

Activity B

1. In women, chronic pelvic pain is often associated with physical violence, emotional neglect, and sexual abuse in childhood.
2. to prevent cervical cancer
3. A patient who has received anesthesia for a surgical cone biopsy is advised to rest for 24 hours after the procedure and to leave any vaginal packing in place until it is removed (usually the next day). The patient is instructed to report any excessive bleeding.
4. Hysteroscopy allows direct visualization of all parts of the uterine cavity by means of a lighted optical instrument.
5. Premenstrual syndrome (PMS) is a cluster of physical, emotional, and behavioral symptoms that are usually related to the luteal phase of the menstrual cycle.
6. The tube can be resected (salpingostomy) or removed (salpingectomy) along with an ovary (salpingo-oophorectomy); methotrexate may be used to "dissolve" the ectopic pregnancy. The conservative approach may include "milking the tube."
7. Possible causes are salpingitis, peritubal adhesions, structural abnormalities of the fallopian tube, previous ectopic pregnancy or tubal surgery, the presence of an IUD, and multiple previous abortions.

Activity C

1. f	2. d	3. h	4. a	5. e
6. g	7. c	8. b		

SECTION II: APPLYING YOUR KNOWLEDGE

Activity D

1. The hot or warm flashes and night sweats reported by some women are thought to be caused by hormonal changes and denote vasomotor instability.
2. Hormone therapy (HT) or menopausal hormonal therapy (previously referred to as hormone replacement therapy [HRT]) has been found to increase some health disorders and to be less effective in preventing others than previously believed. Although HT decreases hot flashes and reduces the risk of

osteoporotic fractures as well as colorectal cancer, studies have shown that it increases the risk of breast cancer, heart attack, stroke, and blood clots. Thus, the benefits of HT are inadequate given the increased risk of these other disorders.

3. Problematic hot flashes have been treated with low-dose venlafaxine (Effexor) and other medications. Similarly, vitamin B_6 and vitamin E may be effective. Some women have expressed interest in other alternative treatments (e.g., natural estrogens and progestins, black cohosh, ginseng, dong quai, soy products, and several other herbal preparations); however, few data exist about their safety or effectiveness.

SECTION III: PRACTICING FOR NCLEX

Activity E

1. a	**2.** c	**3.** c	**4.** a	**5.** a
6. a	**7.** b	**8.** c	**9.** a, b, d	**10.** a
11. b	**12.** a	**13.** d	**14.** b	

CHAPTER 57

SECTION I: ASSESSING YOUR UNDERSTANDING

Activity A

1. *Lactobacillus acidophilus*
2. estrogen
3. fish-like
4. premature labor, premature rupture of membranes, endometritis
5. skin, cervix, vagina, anus, penis, oral cavity
6. 100
7. condylomata
8. dysplasia
9. 50 million
10. nine
11. Family history

Activity B

1. Refer to Chart 57-1, Risk Factors—Vulvovaginal Infections, in the text.
2. Estrogen breaks down glycogen into lactic acid, which is responsible for producing a low vaginal pH. A pH level of 3.5 to 4.5 suppresses bacterial growth.
3. Treatments include antifungal agents such as miconazole (Monistat), nystatin (Mycostatin), clotrimazole (Gyne-Lotrimin), and terconazole (Terazol) cream.
4. PID is a condition of the pelvic cavity that may involve the uterus, fallopian tubes, ovaries, pelvic peritoneum, or pelvic vascular system.
5. Vulvovaginal candidiasis occurs more commonly in pregnancy or with a systemic condition such as diabetes or human immunodeficiency virus (HIV) infection, or when patients are taking medications such as corticosteroids or oral contraceptives.

Activity C

1. f	**2.** d	**3.** p	**4.** e	**5.** h
6. c	**7.** n	**8.** o	**9.** i	**10.** a
11. j	**12.** m	**13.** k	**14.** b	**15.** l
16. g				

SECTION II: APPLYING YOUR KNOWLEDGE

Activity D

CASE STUDY: Bacterial Vaginosis

1. Risk factors include douching after menses, smoking, multiple sex partners, and other sexually transmitted infections (STIs) (also referred to as sexually transmitted diseases [STDs]).
2. a vaginal pH of over 4.7
3. Patients are strongly advised to abstain from alcohol during treatment and for 24 hours after taking metronidazole.

CASE STUDY: Pelvic Inflammatory Disease

1. Pelvic or generalized peritonitis, abscesses, strictures, and fallopian tube obstruction may develop. There is also the potential for bacteremia with septic shock; chronic pelvic and abdominal pain; and recurring PID.
2. Broad-spectrum antibiotic therapy is prescribed, usually a combination of ceftriaxone (Ceftin), azithromycin, and doxycycline.
3. gonorrhea and chlamydia

SECTION III: PRACTICING FOR NCLEX

Activity E

1. d	**2.** d	**3.** a, b, c	**4.** a	**5.** b
6. d	**7.** d	**8.** b	**9.** c	**10.** d
11. a, b, c	**12.** c	**13.** a	**14.** a	**15.** a

CHAPTER 58

SECTION I: ASSESSING YOUR UNDERSTANDING

Activity A

1. second, sixth
2. Cooper's ligament
3. 10
4. Gynecomastia
5. breastfeeding

Activity B

1. Refer to Chart 58-3, Patient Education—Breast Self-Examination, in the text.
2. The nurse plays a critical role in BSE education, a modality used for the early detection of breast cancer. BSE can be taught in a variety of settings—either on a one-to-one basis or in a group. It can also be initiated by a health care provider during a patient's routine physical examination. Current practice is shifting from teaching BSE to promoting

breast self-awareness, a woman's attentiveness to the normal appearance and feel of her breasts.

3. Variations in breast tissue occur during the menstrual cycle, pregnancy, and the onset of menopause.

4. Nipple discharge in a woman who is not lactating may be related to many causes, such as carcinoma, papilloma, pituitary adenoma, cystic breasts, and various medications. Oral contraceptives, pregnancy, hormone therapy (HT), chlorpromazine (Thorazine)-type medications, and frequent breast stimulation may be contributing factors. In some athletic women, nipple discharge may occur during running or aerobic exercises.

5. Research suggests that racial disparities in cancer mortality are driven in large part by differences in socioeconomic status.

Activity C

1. e	2. g	3. a	4. c	5. b
6. d	7. f			

SECTION II: APPLYING YOUR KNOWLEDGE

Activity D

CASE STUDY: Total Mastectomy (i.e., simple mastectomy)

1. upper outer quadrant

2. Common sensations include tenderness, soreness, numbness, tightness, pulling, and twinges. These sensations may occur along the chest wall, in the axilla, and along the inside aspect of the upper arm. After mastectomy, some patients experience phantom sensations and report a feeling that the breast or nipple is still present.

3. The nurse first assesses the patient's readiness and provides gentle encouragement. It is important to maintain the patient's privacy while assisting her as she views the incision; this allows her to express feelings safely to the nurse. Asking the patient what she perceives, acknowledging her feelings, and allowing her to express her emotions are important nursing actions. Reassuring the patient that her feelings are a normal response to breast cancer surgery may be comforting.

SECTION III: PRACTICING FOR NCLEX

Activity E

1. b	2. a	3. c	4. a	5. b
6. b	7. a	8. c	9. a	10. a, b, c
11. c	12. a	13. c	14. b	15. d

CHAPTER 59

SECTION I: ASSESSING YOUR UNDERSTANDING

Activity A

1. prostate-specific antigen (PSA), digital rectal examination (DRE)

2. *Escherichia coli*

3. androgen deprivation therapy (ADT); Lupron, Zoladex, Eulexin, Casodex and Nilandron

4. hemorrhage, infection, DVT, catheter obstruction, sexual dysfunction

5. human chorionic gonadotropin, alpha-fetoprotein

6. spermatogenesis, testosterone

7. Libido, potency

8. kidney, bladder, prostate, penis

9. prostate-specific antigen (PSA)

10. Retrograde ejaculation

11. Urinary incontinence

12. Phosphodiesterase-5 (PDE-5) inhibitors

Activity B

1. Answer may include the following: fever, perineal prostatic pain, dysuria, urinary tract symptoms (frequency, urgency, hesitancy, and nocturia).

2. Answer may include the following: frequency of urination, nocturia, urgency and a sensation that the bladder has not emptied completely, hesitancy in starting urination, abdominal straining, a decrease in the volume and force of the urinary stream, recurring urinary tract infections, interruption of the urinary stream, and dribbling.

3. Factors to consider in choosing a penile prosthesis are the patient's activities of daily living, social activities, and the expectations of the patient and his partner. Ongoing counseling for the patient and his partner is usually necessary to help them adapt to the prosthesis.

Activity C

1. c	2. f	3. e	4. a	5. d
6. h	7. g	8. b		

SECTION II: APPLYING YOUR KNOWLEDGE

Activity D

CASE STUDY: Prostatectomy

1. Depending on the type of surgery, the patient may experience sexual dysfunction related to erectile dysfunction, decreased libido, and fatigue. These issues may become a concern to the patient soon after surgery or in the weeks to months of rehabilitation. With nerve-sparing radical prostatectomy, the likelihood of recovering the ability to have erections is better for men who are younger and men in whom both neurovascular bundles are spared. A decrease in libido is usually related to the impact of the surgery on the body. Reassurance that the usual level of libido will return after recuperation from surgery is often helpful for the patient and his partner. The patient should be aware that he may experience fatigue during rehabilitation from surgery. This fatigue may also decrease his libido and alter his enjoyment of usual activities.

2. Patients experiencing bladder spasms may report an urgency to void, a feeling of pressure or fullness in the bladder, and bleeding from the urethra around the catheter.

3. Medications that relax the smooth muscles can help ease the spasms, which can be intermittent and severe; these medications include flavoxate (Urispas) and oxybutynin (Ditropan). Warm compresses to the pubis or sitz baths may also relieve the spasms.

SECTION III: PRACTICING FOR NCLEX

Activity E

1. a	**2.** b	**3.** a	**4.** a	**5.** a, b, c
6. b	**7.** c	**8.** d	**9.** a	**10.** c
11. b	**12.** c	**13.** c	**14.** a	**15.** b

CHAPTER 60

SECTION I: ASSESSING YOUR UNDERSTANDING

Activity A

1. epidermis, dermis, subcutaneous tissue
2. keratinocytes, Merkel cells, Langerhans cells
3. 2 to 3 weeks
4. adipose; temperature
5. alopecia
6. sebaceous, sweat
7. vitamin D
8. sclera, mucous membrane
9. hypoxia
10. Radiation, conduction, convection

Activity B

1. Melanin is controlled by a hormone secreted from the hypothalamus of the brain called *melanocyte-stimulating hormone.*
2. The hair of the skin provides thermal insulation in mammals with hair or fur. This function is enhanced during cold or fright by piloerection, caused by contraction of the tiny erector muscles attached to the hair follicle.
3. The receptor endings of nerves in the skin allow the body to constantly monitor the conditions of the immediate environment. They sense temperature, pain, light touch, and pressure.
4. Answer may include dryness, wrinkling, uneven pigmentation, and various proliferative lesions. Cellular changes associated with aging include a thinning at the junction of the dermis and epidermis.

Activity C

1. h	**2.** i	**3.** j	**4.** g	**5.** d
6. f	**7.** c	**8.** a	**9.** e	**10.** b

SECTION II: APPLYING YOUR KNOWLEDGE

Activity D

1. the color of the lesions; redness, heat, pain, or swelling; size and location of the involved area; pattern of eruption; and distribution of the lesion
2. diabetic dermopathy

3. Because of changes in peripheral nerves, patients with diabetes do not always sense minor injuries to the lower legs and feet. Infections can begin and, if left untreated, may lead to ulcerations. Ulcerations are often not noticed and become quite large before being treated.

SECTION III: PRACTICING FOR NCLEX

Activity E

1. b	**2.** a	**3.** a	**4.** a	**5.** b
6. c	**7.** c	**8.** d	**9.** d	**10.** b
11. a	**12.** d	**13.** b	**14.** b	**15.** d

CHAPTER 61

SECTION I: ASSESSING YOUR UNDERSTANDING

Activity A

1. acne
2. passive, interactive, active
3. debridement
4. anti-inflammatory, antipruritic, vasoconstrictive
5. sweat glands
6. *Sarcoptes scabiei*
7. *Staphylococcus aureus*
8. autoimmune
9. Gentle removal of the scales
10. topical, phototherapy, systemic
11. Infection

Activity B

1. Answer should include the following: prevent additional damage, prevent secondary infection, revise the inflammatory process, and relieve symptoms.
2. Moisture retentive dressings have a high moisture vapor transmission rate. Some dressings even have reservoirs to hold excessive exudate.
3. Cytokines are proteins with mitogenic activity that release increased amounts of growth factors into a wound. This process stimulates cell growth and granulation of skin.
4. Foam dressings are nonadherent, thus the nurse must apply a secondary dressing to keep them in place.
5. Keratoconjunctivitis, sepsis, and multiple organ dysfunction syndrome (MODS) are potential complications of TEN and SJS.
6. Risk factors for malignant melanoma include: Caucasian skin color (particularly fairer-skinned or freckled, blue-eyed, blond or red-haired people of Celtic or Scandinavian origin); history of sunburns, particularly in childhood; previous history of melanoma (multiple primary melanomas are not uncommon); family history of melanoma (10% of patients diagnosed with melanoma have a positive family history of melanoma); personal or family history of multiple atypical nevi (formerly called dysplastic nevi); family history of astrocytoma or pancreatic cancer.

Activity C

1. e	**2.** f	**3.** g	**4.** d	**5.** i
6. j	**7.** l	**8.** k	**9.** b	**10.** h
11. m	**12.** n	**13.** o	**14.** c	**15.** a

SECTION II: APPLYING YOUR KNOWLEDGE

Activity D

CASE STUDY: Acne Vulgaris

1. Diet is not believed to play a major role in therapy. However, the elimination of a specific food or food product associated with a flare-up of acne, such as chocolate, cola, fried foods, or milk products, should be promoted.
2. tetracycline
3. Major nursing activities include patient education, particularly in proper skin care techniques, and managing potential problems related to the skin disorder or therapy. Providing positive reassurance, listening attentively, and being sensitive to the feelings of the patient with acne are essential for the patient's psychological well-being and understanding of the disease and treatment plan.

CASE STUDY: Malignant Melanoma

1. a superficial spreading melanoma
2. excisional biopsy
3. Metastasis is probable. The physician will include education about biopsy and treatment options.

SECTION III: PRACTICING FOR NCLEX

Activity E

1. d	**2.** c	**3.** b	**4.** a, b, c	**5.** a
6. a	**7.** a	**8.** c	**9.** c	**10.** a
11. d	**12.** b	**13.** b	**14.** c	**15.** b, c, d

CHAPTER 62

SECTION I: ASSESSING YOUR UNDERSTANDING

Activity A

1. young children, older adults
2. one-third
3. Hypovolemia
4. the depth of the injury, the extent of injured body surface area
5. acute respiratory failure. acute respiratory distress syndrome (ARDS)
6. sepsis
7. 0.5 to 1.0 mL/kg/h
8. *Pseudomonas,* methicillin-resistant *Staphylococcus, Acinetobacter*
9. silver sulfadiazine (Silvadene), silver nitrate, mafenide acetate (Sulfamylon)
10. increased temperature, tachycardia, widened pulse pressure, flushed, dry skin in nonburned areas

Activity B

1. Advances in burn care over the past 80 years have contributed to significant improvements in morbidity and mortality of patients with burns. These advances include the introduction of systemic antibiotics and topical antimicrobials, advances in fluid resuscitation, aggressive nutrition, early excision and wound closure, the introduction of engineered tissue therapies, advances in critical care therapies, and the advent of specialized burn centers.
2. The central area of the wound is termed the *zone of coagulation* due to the characteristic coagulation necrosis of cells that occurs. The surrounding zone, the *zone of stasis,* describes an area of injured cells that may remain viable but, with persistent decreased blood flow, will undergo necrosis within 24 to 48 hours. The *zone of hyperemia,* the outermost zone, sustains minimal injury and may fully recover over time.
3. The first is a thermal effect, which results in cutaneous burn injuries. The second effect is damage to the cellular DNA, which may be localized or affect the whole body.
4. Carbon monoxide, a byproduct of the combustion of organic materials, combines with hemoglobin to form carboxyhemoglobin. Carboxyhemoglobin competes with oxygen for available hemoglobin-binding sites.
5. primary survey, prevention of shock, prevention of respiratory distress, detection and treatment of concomitant injuries, wound assessment, and initial care
6. The depth of the injury depends on the temperature of the burning agent and the duration of contact with the agent.
7. Inhalation injury below the vocal cords results from inhaling the products of incomplete combustion or noxious gases, and is often the source of death at the scene of a fire.
8. The secondary survey focuses on obtaining a history, the completion of the total body system assessment, initial fluid resuscitation, and provision of psychosocial support of the conscious patient.
9. Preventive treatment modalities are used to prevent scar contractures and excess hypertrophic tissue. Compression is introduced early in burn wound treatment. Elastic bandage wraps are used initially to help promote adequate circulation, but they can also be used as the first form of compression for scar management, followed by elasticized tubular bandage until the patient can be measured for a customized garment.
10. Fluid overload may occur when fluid is mobilized from the interstitial compartment back into the intravascular compartment. If the cardiac system cannot compensate for the excess volume, congestive heart failure may result.

Activity C

1. b   **2.** f   **3.** c   **4.** e   **5.** d
6. a   **7.** g

SECTION II: APPLYING YOUR KNOWLEDGE

Activity D

1. Indicators of possible inhalation injury include the following: injury occurring in an enclosed space; burns of the face or neck; singed nasal hair; hoarseness, high-pitched voice change, stridor; soot in sputum; dyspnea or tachypnea and other signs of reduced oxygen levels (hypoxemia); and erythema and blistering of the oral or pharyngeal mucosa.
2. intubation and mechanical intubation, possible escharotomy to allow adequate chest expansion
3. 1,944 mL: 2 mL lactated ringers × patient's weight in kilograms (72) × %TBSA (13.5), second-, third-, and fourth-degree burns

SECTION III: PRACTICING FOR NCLEX

Activity E

1. b   **2.** c   **3.** d   **4.** c   **5.** a
6. a   **7.** b   **8.** a, b, d   **9.** d   **10.** b
11. a, b, d   **12.** c   **13.** c   **14.** a   **15.** c
16. b   **17.** c

CHAPTER 63

SECTION I: ASSESSING YOUR UNDERSTANDING

Activity A

1. 10–21 mm Hg
2. glaucoma
3. pallor (lack of blood supply), cupping of the optic nerve disc
4. laser trabeculoplasty, laser iridotomy
5. cataracts
6. irrigation with normal saline
7. *Streptococcus pneumoniae, Haemophilus influenzae, Staphylococcus aureus*
8. "pink eye," or dilation of the conjunctival blood vessels
9. diabetic retinopathy
10. cytomegalovirus (CMV)
11. lipoid, aqueous, mucoid
12. drooping of the eyelid

Activity B

1. Visual acuity is tested for both near (14 inches away) and distance (20 feet away) vision and performed on each eye separately with a standardized Snellen chart for distance and a Rosenbaum pocket screener for near vision.
2. Patients are cautioned to avoid squeezing the eyelids, holding the breath, or performing a Valsalva maneuver, as these may result in abnormally increased IOP.

3. The Amsler grid is a test often used for patients with macular problems, such as macular degeneration.

Activity C

PART I

1. b   **2.** c   **3.** f   **4.** j   **5.** a
6. e   **7.** g   **8.** d   **9.** h   **10.** i

PART II

1. g   **2.** n   **3.** e   **4.** l   **5.** o
6. a   **7.** b   **8.** j   **9.** c   **10.** k
11. d   **12.** m   **13.** f   **14.** i   **15.** h

SECTION II: APPLYING YOUR KNOWLEDGE

Activity D

CASE STUDY: Cataract Surgery

1. smoking, diabetes, alcohol abuse, and inadequate intake of antioxidant vitamins over time
2. painless blurring of vision, sensitivity to glare, and functional impairment due to reduced visual acuity
3. She cannot lie on the affected side for 2 nights.

SECTION III: PRACTICING FOR NCLEX

Activity E

1. a, b, c   **2.** c   **3.** d   **4.** d   **5.** d
6. c   **7.** a, b, c   **8.** c   **9.** a, b, c   **10.** a
11. c   **12.** c   **13.** c   **14.** a   **15.** b

CHAPTER 64

SECTION I: ASSESSING YOUR UNDERSTANDING

Activity A

1. cochlea
2. organ of Corti
3. eighth
4. 30
5. 70 to 90
6. functional
7. 85 to 90
8. 50%
9. seventh
10. eighth

Activity B

1. Hearing is conducted over two pathways: air and bone. Sounds transmitted by air conduction travel over the air-filled external and middle ear through vibration of the tympanic membrane and ossicles. Sounds transmitted by bone conduction travel directly through bone to the inner ear, bypassing the tympanic membrane and ossicles.
2. Rhine, Weber, and Whisper tests
3. inspection of the external, middle, and inner ear
4. frequency, pitch, and intensity

5. A tympanogram, or impedance audiometry, measures middle ear muscle reflex to sound stimulation and compliance of the tympanic membrane by changing the air pressure in a sealed ear canal.

Activity C

1. h	**2.** a	**3.** i	**4.** g	**5.** c
6. j	**7.** f	**8.** b	**9.** d	**10.** e

SECTION II: APPLYING YOUR KNOWLEDGE

Activity D

CASE STUDY: Mastoid Surgery: Postoperative Care

1. The patient's mastoid pressure dressing can be removed 24 to 48 hours after surgery.

2. Although infrequently injured, the facial nerve, which runs through the middle ear and mastoid, is at some risk for injury during mastoid surgery. As the patient awakens from anesthesia, any evidence of facial paresis should be reported to the physician.

3. Constant, throbbing pain accompanied by fever may indicate infection and should be reported to the primary provider.

CASE STUDY: Ménière's Disease

1. Answer may include vertigo, tinnitus, fluctuating and progressive sensorineural hearing loss, a feeling of pressure or fullness in the ear, episodic and incapacitating vertigo accompanied by nausea and vomiting.

2. Limit foods high in salt or sugar. Be aware of foods with hidden salts and sugars. Limit alcohol and caffeine. Avoid foods with monosodium glutamate (MSG).

3. aspirin or aspirin products

SECTION III: PRACTICING FOR NCLEX

Activity E

1. a	**2.** c	**3.** b	**4.** a	**5.** c
6. c	**7.** a	**8.** b	**9.** a, c, d	**10.** b
11. d	**12.** a	**13.** b	**14.** d	**15.** a

CHAPTER 65

SECTION I: ASSESSING YOUR UNDERSTANDING

Activity A

1. Serotonin
2. dopamine
3. frontal
4. temporal
5. frontal
6. hypothalamus
7. pituitary
8. thalamus
9. 150
10. C8 to L3

11. acetylcholine
12. cerebellum

Activity B

1. This barrier is formed by the endothelial cells of the brain's capillaries, which form continuous tight junctions, creating a barrier to macromolecules and many compounds.

2. The *autonomic nervous system* regulates the activities of internal organs such as the heart, lungs, blood vessels, digestive organs, and glands (see Fig. 65-10). Maintenance and restoration of internal homeostasis is largely the responsibility of the autonomic nervous system.

3. flaccid paralysis and atrophy of the affected muscles

4. Destruction or dysfunction of the basal ganglia leads not to paralysis but to muscle rigidity, disturbances of posture, and difficulty initiating or changing movement.

Activity C

Neurotransmitters and Nervous System Response

1. e	**2.** f	**3.** d	**4.** c	**5.** a
6. b				

Cranial Nerves

Nerve No.	Column I	Column II
I	Olfactory	Smell
II	Optic	Vision
III	Oculomotor	Eye movement
IV	Trochlear	Eye movement
V	Trigeminal	Facial sensation
VI	Abducens	Eye movement
VII	Facial	Taste and expression
VIII	Vestibulocochlear	Hearing and equilibrium
IX	Glossopharyngeal	Taste
X	Vagus	Swallowing, gastric motility, and secretion
XI	Spinal accessory	Trapezius and sternomastoid muscles
XII	Hypoglossal	Tongue movement

SECTION II: APPLYING YOUR KNOWLEDGE

Activity D

CASE STUDY: Mental Status

1. fall prevention measures

2. Procedures and preparations needed for diagnostic tests are explained, taking into account the possibility of impaired hearing and slowed responses in the older adult. Providing instruction at an unrushed pace and using reinforcement enhance learning and retention. Material should be short, concise, and concrete. Vocabulary is matched to the patient's ability, and terms are clearly defined. The older adult patient requires adequate time to receive and respond to stimuli, learn, and react. These measures allow comprehension, memory, and formation of association and concepts.

3. Delirium (transient mental confusion, usually with delusions and hallucinations) is seen in older adult patients who have underlying central nervous system damage or are experiencing an acute condition such as infection, adverse medication reaction, or dehydration. Drug toxicity and depression may produce impairment of attention and memory, and should be evaluated as a possible cause of mental status change. Delirium must be differentiated from dementia, which is a chronic and irreversible deterioration of cognitive status.

SECTION III: PRACTICING FOR NCLEX

Activity E

1. a	**2.** c	**3.** c	**4.** b, c, d	**5.** b
6. a	**7.** b	**8.** d	**9.** a	**10.** d
11. b	**12.** b	**13.** b	**14.** c	**15.** c

CHAPTER 66

SECTION I: ASSESSING YOUR UNDERSTANDING

Activity A

1. locked-in syndrome
2. pneumonia, aspiration, respiratory failure
3. a change in the level of consciousness (LOC)
4. brain stem herniation, diabetes insipidus, syndrome of inappropriate antidiuretic hormone (SIADH)
5. brain herniation resulting in death
6. cerebral edema, pain, seizures, increased ICP and neurologic status
7. cerebrovascular disease
8. status epilepticus

Activity B

1. An altered level of consciousness (LOC) is present when the patient is not oriented, does not follow commands, or needs persistent stimuli to achieve a state of alertness. LOC is gauged on a continuum, with a normal state of alertness and full cognition on one end and coma on the other end.
2. Answer should include five of the following: respiratory distress, pneumonia, aspiration, pressure ulcer, deep vein thrombosis, and contractures.
3. A neurologic examination should include evaluation of mental status, cranial nerve function, cerebellar function, reflexes, and motor and sensory function, as well as the score of the Glasgow Coma Scale.

4. Before and after suctioning, the patient is adequately ventilated to prevent hypoxia.
5. Alertness is measured by the patient's ability to open the eyes spontaneously or in response to a vocal or noxious stimulus (pressure or pain).

Activity C

1. a and f	**2.** c and e	**3.** b	**4.** a	**5.** c

SECTION II: APPLYING YOUR KNOWLEDGE

Activity D

CASE STUDY: Optimizing Cerebral Perfusion Pressure

1. Proper positioning helps reduce ICP. The patient's head is kept in a neutral (midline) position, maintained with the use of a cervical collar if necessary, to promote venous drainage. Elevation of the head is maintained at 30 to 45 degrees unless contraindicated. Extreme rotation of the neck and flexion of the neck are avoided, because compression or distortion of the jugular veins increases ICP. Extreme hip flexion is also avoided, because this position causes an increase in intra-abdominal and intrathoracic pressures, which can produce an increase in ICP.
2. Stool softeners may be prescribed. When Alex is awake and alert, a high-fiber diet may be indicated. Abdominal distention, which increases intraabdominal and intrathoracic pressure and ICP, should be noted. Enemas and cathartics are avoided if possible. When moving or being turned in bed, ask Alex to exhale (which opens the glottis) to avoid the Valsalva maneuver.
3. Space activities to avoid stress and strain. Maintain a calm atmosphere and decrease environmental stimuli.

SECTION III: PRACTICING FOR NCLEX

Activity E

1. d	**2.** a	**3.** c	**4.** b	**5.** c
6. a, b, c	**7.** d	**8.** c	**9.** d	**10.** c
11. a, c, d	**12.** c	**13.** a	**14.** d	**15.** c

CHAPTER 67

SECTION I: ASSESSING YOUR UNDERSTANDING

Activity A

1. stroke; brain attack
2. 4.5 hours
3. fourth
4. carotid enterectomy
5. Arteriosclerosis
6. hemiplegia
7. brain tissue, the ventricles, the subarachnoid space
8. rebleeding or hematoma expansion, cerebral vasospasm, acute hydrocephalus, seizures

9. hypertension
10. ischemic and hemorrhagic

Activity B

1. atrial fibrillation
2. Small, penetrating artery thrombotic strokes affect one or more vessels, and are the most common type of ischemic stroke.
3. The DASH diet is high in fruits and vegetables, moderate in low-fat dairy products, and low in animal protein (has a substantial amount of plant protein from legumes and nuts).
4. by dissolving the blood clot that is blocking blood flow to the brain

Activity C

1. d	**2.** h	**3.** e	**4.** a	**5.** b
6. g	**7.** c	**8.** f		

SECTION II: APPLYING YOUR KNOWLEDGE

Activity D

1. Before receiving t-PA, the patient is assessed using the National Institutes of Health Stroke Scale (NIHSS), a standardized assessment tool that helps evaluate stroke severity.
2. The nurse will administer 6.48 mg. (The dosage for t-PA is 0.9 mg/kg, with a maximum dose of 90 mg. Ten percent of the calculated dose is administered as an IV bolus over 1 minute.)
3. Bleeding is the most common side effect of t-PA administration, thus the patient is closely monitored for any bleeding (IV insertion sites, urinary catheter site, endotracheal tube, nasogastric tube, urine, stool, emesis, other secretions).

SECTION III: PRACTICING FOR NCLEX

Activity E

1. a	**2.** a	**3.** c	**4.** a	**5.** c
6. d	**7.** a, b, d	**8.** b	**9.** a	**10.** c
11. d	**12.** b	**13.** c	**14.** a, b, c	**15.** a

CHAPTER 68

SECTION I: ASSESSING YOUR UNDERSTANDING

Activity A

1. brain, blood, cerebrospinal fluid
2. Monro-Kellie doctrine
3. linear, comminuted, depressed; frontal, temporal, and basilar.
4. CT scan
5. hematoma (either epidural, subdural, or intracerebral)
6. coma, hypertension, bradycardia, bradypnea
7. coma, absence of brain stem reflexes, apnea
8. concussion
9. eye opening, verbal responses, motor responses to verbal commands or painful stimuli

10. systemic infections, neurosurgical infections, heterotrophic ossification
11. 5th cervical, 6th cervical, 7th cervical, 12th thoracic, 1st lumbar

Activity B

1. In Brown-Séquard syndrome, ipsilateral paralysis or paresis is noted, together with ipsilateral loss of touch, pressure, and vibration, and contralateral loss of sensation of pain and temperature.
2. The most common causes of TBI are falls (35.2%), motor vehicle crashes (17.3%), being struck by objects (16.5%), and assaults (10%).
3. *Primary injury* is the initial damage to the brain that results from the traumatic event. This may include contusions, lacerations, and torn blood vessels due to impact, acceleration/deceleration, or foreign object penetration. *Secondary injury* evolves over the ensuing hours and days after the initial injury and results from inadequate delivery of nutrients and oxygen to the cells. These processes include intracranial hemorrhage, cerebral edema, increased intracranial pressure, hypoxic brain damage, and infection.
4. A grade 1 concussion has symptoms of transient confusion, no loss of consciousness, and duration of mental status abnormalities on examination that resolve in less than 15 minutes.
5. Monitoring includes observing the patient for a decrease in LOC, worsening headache, dizziness, seizures, abnormal pupil response, vomiting, irritability, slurred speech, and numbness or weakness in the arms or legs.

Activity C

1. c	**2.** f	**3.** h	**4.** e	**5.** i
6. b	**7.** g	**8.** j	**9.** d	**10.** a

SECTION II: APPLYING YOUR KNOWLEDGE

Activity D

CASE STUDY: Spinal Cord Injury

1. independent in transfers and wheelchair
2. A major aspect of nursing care is educating the patient and family about complications and strategies to minimize risks. UTIs, contractures, infected pressure ulcers, and sepsis may necessitate hospitalization. Other late complications that may occur include lower extremity edema, joint contractures, respiratory dysfunction, and pain. To avoid these and other complications, the patient and a family member are educated about skin care, catheter care, range-of-motion exercises, breathing exercises, and other care techniques.
3. The diet for the patient with tetraplegia or paraplegia should be high in protein, vitamins, and calories to ensure minimal wasting of muscle and the maintenance of healthy skin, and high in fluids to maintain well-functioning kidneys. Excessive weight gain and obesity should be avoided, because they further limit mobility.

SECTION III: PRACTICING FOR NCLEX

Activity E

1. c	**2.** a	**3.** d	**4.** c	**5.** b
6. a	**7.** c	**8.** d	**9.** a, b, c, d	**10.** a, b, d
11. b	**12.** b	**13.** a	**14.** c	**15.** d

CHAPTER 69

SECTION I: ASSESSING YOUR UNDERSTANDING

Activity A

1. meningitis, brain abscesses, various types of encephalitis, Creutzfeldt-Jakob disease (CJD), variant CJD.
2. areflexia, ascending weakness
3. herpes simplex virus (HSV); acyclovir (Zovirax), ganciclovir (Cytovene)
4. immunologic assessment, electroencephalogram (EEG), magnetic resonance imaging (MRI)
5. myelin sheath
6. immunomodulating, immunosuppressive
7. acetylcholine receptors
8. double vision, ptosis
9. *Streptococcus pneumoniae, Neisseria meningitides*
10. Syndrome of inappropriate antidiuretic hormone (SIADH) with hyponatremia

Activity B

1. Risks for an unfavorable outcome include older age, a heart rate of greater than 120 bpm, decreased score on the Glasgow Coma Scale, cranial nerve palsies, and a positive Gram stain 1 hour after presentation to the hospital.
2. *Demyelination* refers to the destruction of myelin, the fatty and protein material that surrounds nerve fibers in the brain and spinal cord. This destruction results in impaired transmission of nerve impulses.
3. Avoiding hot temperatures, effective treatment of depression and anemia, and occupational and physical therapies may help control fatigue. Additional strategies include a balance of rest and activities, good nutrition to avoid being overweight and obese, and a healthy lifestyle, including avoidance of alcohol and cigarette smoking.

Activity C

1. b	**2.** b	**3.** e	**4.** d	**5.** f
6. f	**7.** g	**8.** h	**9.** h	**10.** d

SECTION II: APPLYING YOUR KNOWLEDGE

Activity D

CASE STUDY: Multiple Sclerosis

1. Exacerbations and remissions are characteristic of MS. During exacerbations, new symptoms appear and existing ones worsen; during remissions, symptoms decrease or disappear. Relapses may be associated with emotional and physical stress, which Toni is experiencing related to her clinical and classroom schedule.
2. Side effects include mood swings, weight gain, and electrolyte imbalances.
3. Nursing assessment should include neurologic deficits, secondary complications, and the impact of the disease on the patient and family. The patient's mobility and balance are observed to determine whether there is risk of falling. Assessment of function is carried out both when the patient is well rested and when fatigued. The patient is assessed for weakness, spasticity, visual impairment, incontinence, and disorders of swallowing and speech. Additional areas of assessment include how MS has affected the patient's lifestyle, how the patient is coping, adherence to the prescribed medication regimen, and what the patient would like to improve.

SECTION III: PRACTICING FOR NCLEX

Activity E

1. a, b, c	**2.** a	**3.** b	**4.** a	**5.** c
6. d	**7.** c	**8.** b, c, d	**9.** a	**10.** c
11. a	**12.** b	**13.** b	**14.** c	**15.** a

CHAPTER 70

SECTION I: ASSESSING YOUR UNDERSTANDING

Activity A

1. lung, breast, lower gastrointestinal tract, pancreas, kidney, skin
2. headache, nausea and vomiting, papilledema (70% to 75% occurrence)
3. hemiparesis, seizures, mental status changes
4. intramedullary
5. Answer may include five of the following seven: Parkinson's disease, Huntington's disease, Alzheimer's disease, amyotrophic lateral sclerosis, muscular dystrophies, degenerative disk disease, and postpolio syndrome.
6. tremor, rigidity, bradykinesia, postural instability
7. fatigue, progressive muscle weakness, cramps, fasciculations (twitching), incoordination
8. progressive muscle wasting and weakness, abnormal elevation in blood muscle enzymes
9. C5 to C6 or C6 to C7
10. hematoma at the surgical site, causing cord compression; and neurologic deficit and recurrent or persistent pain after surgery

Activity B

1. A variety of physiologic changes can occur, such as increased ICP and cerebral edema, seizure activity and focal neurologic signs, hydrocephalus, and altered pituitary function.
2. Brain tumors are classified according to origin: those arising from the covering of the brain, those developing in or on the cranial nerves, those

originating within brain tissue, and metastatic lesions originating elsewhere in the body.

3. Primary brain tumors originate from cells within the brain. Secondary, or metastatic, brain tumors develop from structures outside the brain and are twice as common as primary brain tumors.

4. Computer-assisted stereotactic (three-dimensional) biopsy is used to diagnose deep-seated brain tumors and to provide a basis for treatment and prognosis. Stereotactic approaches involve the use of a three-dimensional frame that allows very precise localization of the tumor; a stereotactic frame and multiple imaging studies (x-rays, CT scans, or MRIs) are used to localize the tumor and verify its position. Brain-mapping technology helps determine how close diseased areas of the brain are to structures essential for normal brain function.

5. Although symptoms are variable, a slow, unilateral resting tremor is present in the majority of patients at the time of diagnosis.

Activity C

1. d   **2.** c   **3.** g   **4.** a   **5.** h
6. f   **7.** b   **8.** e

SECTION II: APPLYING YOUR KNOWLEDGE

Activity D

CASE STUDY: Parkinson's Disease

1. A progressive program of daily exercise will increase muscle strength, improve coordination and dexterity, reduce muscular rigidity, and prevent contractures that occur when muscles are not used. Walking, riding a stationary bicycle, swimming, and gardening are all exercises that help maintain joint mobility. Stretching (stretch–hold–relax) and range-of-motion exercises promote joint flexibility. Postural exercises are important to counter the tendency of the head and neck to be drawn forward and down. A physical therapist may be helpful in developing an individualized exercise program and can provide instruction to the patient and caregiver on exercising safely. Faithful adherence to an exercise and walking program helps delay the progress of the disease. Warm baths and massage, in addition to passive and active exercises, help relax muscles and relieve painful muscle spasms that accompany rigidity.

2. Carbidopa is often added to levodopa to avoid metabolism of levodopa before it can reach the brain.

3. The goals for the patient may include improving functional mobility, maintaining independence in activities of daily living, achieving adequate bowel elimination, attaining and maintaining acceptable nutritional status, achieving effective communication, and developing positive coping mechanisms.

CASE STUDY: Huntington's Disease

1. The most prominent clinical features of the disease that this patient is experiencing are chorea (rapid, jerky involuntary movements) and impaired voluntary movement. Other prominent features include intellectual decline, and, often, personality changes.

2. The Huntington's Disease Society of America helps patients and families by providing information, referrals, family and public education, and support for research.

3. Selective serotonin reuptake inhibitors and tricyclics have been recommended for control of psychiatric symptoms. The threat of suicide is present particularly early in the course of the disease. Psychotic symptoms usually respond to antipsychotic medications. Psychotherapy aimed at allaying anxiety and reducing stress may be beneficial.

SECTION III: PRACTICING FOR NCLEX

Activity E

1. a, b, c   **2.** c   **3.** d   **4.** b   **5.** b
6. a   **7.** d   **8.** b   **9.** d   **10.** c
11. c   **12.** a   **13.** a   **14.** c   **15.** b

CHAPTER 71

SECTION I: ASSESSING YOUR UNDERSTANDING

Activity A

1. 50
2. measles, mumps, rubella, pertussis, tetanus, hepatitis B, varicella.
3. 100 mL/kg of oral rehydration solution (ORS)
4. The World Health Organization (WHO), Centers for Disease Control and Prevention (CDC)
5. coagulase-negative staphylococci, diphtheroids; *Staphylococcus aureus, Pseudomonas aeruginosa*
6. *Clostridium difficile,* methicillin-resistant *Staphylococcus aureus* (MRSA), vancomycin-resistant *Enterococcus* (VRE)
7. pneumococcus, meningococcus
8. skin; urethra, cervix, vagina, rectum, oropharynx.

Activity B

1. These essentials are a causative organism, a reservoir of available organisms, a portal or mode of exit from the reservoir, a mode of transmission from reservoir to host, a susceptible host, and a mode of entry to the host.
2. *Infectious disease* is the state in which the infected host displays a decline in wellness due to the infection.
3. spread of microorganisms by the hands of health care workers
4. avoidance of percutaneous injury
5. When hospitalized, a patient with tuberculosis should be in an airborne infection isolation room (AIIR), engineered to provide negative air pressure, rapid turnover of air, and air either highly filtered or exhausted directly to the outside. Health care providers should wear an N-95 respirator (i.e., protective mask) at all times while in the patient's

room. The nurse should be able to validate negative pressure when it is in place by reading a pressure manometer placed outside the room and/or by witnessing that a tissue held at the gap between the door and the floor will be pulled toward the room.

Activity C

1. a	**2.** d	**3.** b	**4.** e	**5.** f
6. c	**7.** g	**8.** h		

SECTION II: APPLYING YOUR KNOWLEDGE

Activity D

1. chlamydia
2. In women, pelvic inflammatory disease (PID), ectopic pregnancy, endometritis, and infertility are possible complications of either *N. gonorrhoeae* or *C. trachomatis* infection.
3. Diagnostic methods used in *N. gonorrhoeae* infection include Gram stain (appropriate only for male urethral samples), culture, and nucleic acid amplification tests (NAATs).
4. Along with reinforcing the importance of abstinence, when appropriate, education should address limiting the number of sexual partners and using condoms for barrier protection. Young women and pregnant women should also be instructed about the importance of routine screening for chlamydia.

SECTION III: PRACTICING FOR NCLEX

Activity E

1. b	**2.** c	**3.** a	**4.** c	**5.** a, c, d
6. b	**7.** d	**8.** a	**9.** b	**10.** a
11. c	**12.** c	**13.** d	**14.** a	**15.** c

CHAPTER 72

SECTION I: ASSESSING YOUR UNDERSTANDING

Activity A

1. primary
2. Emergency Medical Treatment and Active Labor Act (EMTALA)
3. speak, breathe, cough; 3 to 5 minutes
4. self-protection
5. muscle cramps; profound diaphoresis, profound thirst
6. drowning
7. 1, 9
8. 4, 12
9. 500, 1,000, normal saline solution

Activity B

1. Endotracheal intubation is indicated to establish an airway for a patient who cannot be adequately ventilated with an oropharyngeal airway, bypass an upper airway obstruction, prevent aspiration, permit connection of the patient to a resuscitation bag or mechanical ventilator, or facilitate the removal of tracheobronchial secretions.
2. Lactated Ringer's solution is initially useful because it approximates plasma electrolyte composition and osmolality, allows time for blood typing and screening, restores circulation, and serves as an adjunct to blood component therapy.
3. For older adult patients, especially those in extended-care facilities, sedatives and hypnotic medications, diseases affecting motor coordination (e.g., Parkinson's disease), and mental dysfunction (e.g., dementia, mental retardation) are risk factors for asphyxiation by food.
4. A quick neurologic assessment may be performed using the AVPU mnemonic:
   - *A* – *a*lert; is the patient alert and responsive?
   - *V* – *v*erbal; does the patient respond to verbal stimuli?
   - *P* – *p*ain; does the patient respond only to painful stimuli?
   - *U* – *u*nresponsive; is the patient unresponsive to all stimuli, including pain?
5. A basic and widely used triage system that has been in use for many years utilized three categories: emergent, urgent, and nonurgent. In this system, emergent patients have the highest priority, urgent patients are those with serious health problems but not immediately life-threatening ones, and nonurgent patients are those with episodic illnesses.

Activity C

1. g	**2.** h	**3.** b	**4.** f	**5.** d
6. a	**7.** c	**8.** e		

SECTION II: APPLYING YOUR KNOWLEDGE

Activity D

CASE STUDY: Heat Stroke

1. Clinical manifestations of heat stroke may include profound central nervous system (CNS) dysfunction (manifested by confusion, delirium, bizarre behavior, coma, seizures); elevated body temperature (40.6°C [105°F] or higher); hot, dry skin; and usually anhidrosis (absence of sweating), tachypnea, hypotension, and tachycardia.
2. The main goal is to reduce the high body temperature as quickly as possible, because mortality in heat stroke or morbid progression to heat stroke with less serious forms of heat-induced illnesses is directly related to the duration of hyperthermia. For the patient with heat stroke, simultaneous treatment focuses on stabilizing oxygenation using the CABs (*c*irculation, *a*irway, and *b*reathing) (formerly called the ABCs) of basic life support. This includes establishing intravenous (IV) access for fluid administration.
3. Urine output is measured frequently because acute tubular necrosis may occur as a complication of heat stroke from rhabdomyolysis (myoglobin in the urine).

SECTION III: PRACTICING FOR NCLEX

Activity E

1. b   **2.** d   **3.** b   **4.** b   **5.** b
6. a, b, c   **7.** c   **8.** a, b, d   **9.** c   **10.** b, c, d
11. a   **12.** a   **13.** c   **14.** c   **15.** c

CHAPTER 73

SECTION I: ASSESSING YOUR UNDERSTANDING

Activity A

1. anthrax; chlorine
2. Department of Health and Human Services, Department of Justice, Department of Defense, Department of Homeland Security
3. California, Colorado, North Carolina
4. Communication
5. anthrax, smallpox
6. ciprofloxacin, doxycycline; 100%
7. 13 years

Activity B

1. The Incident Command System is a management tool for organizing personnel, facilities, equipment, and communication for any emergency. Its activation during emergencies is mandated by the federal government.
2. Factors that influence a person's response to disaster include the degree and nature of the exposure to the disaster, loss of friends and loved ones, existing coping strategies, available resources and support, and the personal meaning attached to the event.
3. A critically ill individual with a high mortality rate would be assigned a low triage priority because it would be unethical to use limited resources on those with a low chance of survival. Others who are seriously ill and have a greater chance of survival should be treated.
4. Some cultural considerations include language differences, a variety of religious preferences (hygiene, diet, medical treatment), rituals of prayer, traditions for burying the dead, and the timing of funeral services.
5. A blast wave has four effects. These include spalling, which refers to the pressure wave itself; implosion, which refers to rupture of organs from entrapped gases; shearing, which refers to the blast response of different body tissues, dependent on their density; and irreversible work, which refers to the presence of forces that exceed the tensile strength of an organ or tissue.

Activity C

Triage Categories During a Mass Casualty Incident (MCI)

1. Green
2. Black
3. Red
4. Red
5. Black
6. Green
7. Green
8. Yellow
9. Red
10. Red
11. Black
12. Black
13. Yellow
14. Yellow

SECTION II: APPLYING YOUR KNOWLEDGE

Activity D

1. Disaster tags, which are numbered and include triage priority, name, address, age, location and description of injuries, and treatments or medications given, are used to communicate patient information.
2. In a disaster situation when health care providers are faced with a large number of casualties, the fundamental principle guiding resource allocation is to do the greatest good for the greatest number of people.
3. Traffic control within the facility is one of the most important components of managing the disaster and resources.

SECTION III: PRACTICING FOR NCLEX

Activity E

1. c   **2.** b   **3.** c   **4.** b   **5.** b
6. d   **7.** a   **8.** a   **9.** b   **10.** c
11. c   **12.** d   **13.** a   **14.** c   **15.** a